Erythropoietin

N

With love

Gidi

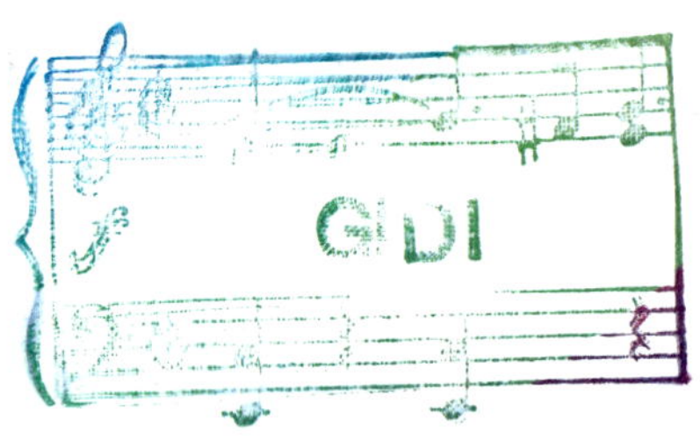

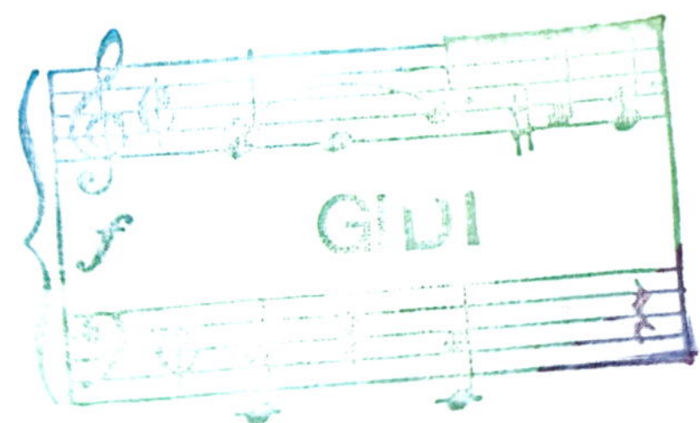

Erythropoietin

Molecular Physiology and Clinical Applications

edited by

C. Bauer
Institute of Physiology
University of Zürich-Irchel
Zürich, Switzerland

K. M. Koch
Zentrum Innere Medizin
Hannover, Germany

P. Scigalla
L. Wieczorek
Boehringer Mannheim GmbH
Mannheim, Germany

Marcel Dekker, Inc. New York • Basel • Hong Kong

Library of Congress Cataloging-in-Publication Data

Erythropoietin : molecular physiology and clinical applications /
  edited by C. Bauer ... [et al.].
      p. cm.
    Includes bibliographical references and index.
    ISBN 0-8247-9139-8 (alk. paper)
    1. Recombinant erythropoietin--Therapeutic use--Congresses.
  2. Erythropoietin--Physiological effect--Congresses. I. Bauer, C.
  (Christian).
    [DNLM: 1. Erythropoietin--metabolism--congresses.
  2. Erythropoietin--therapeutic use--congresses. 3. Anemia--drug
  therapy--congresses. 4. Neoplasms--drug therapy--congresses. WH
  150 E7397 1994]
  RM666.E834E78 1994
  612.1'11--dc20
  DNLM/DLC
  for Library of Congress   93-30025
                                                                        CIP

Great care has been taken to maintain the accuracy of the information contained in this volume. However, neither Marcel Dekker, Inc., nor the editors can be held responsible for errors or for any consequences arising from the use of the information contained herein.

The publisher offers discounts on this book when ordered in bulk quantities. For more information, write to Special Sales/Professional Marketing at the address below.

This book is printed on acid-free paper.

Marcel Dekker, Inc.
270 Madison Avenue, New York, New York 10016

Current printing (last digit):
10 9 8 7 6 5 4 3 2 1

PRINTED IN THE UNITED STATES OF AMERICA

Contents

Physiological Functions Under rhEPO Therapy

Panel Discussion

Mechanism of Erythropoietin Action/Immunogenicity of rhEPO

rhEPO Therapy in Neoplastic Disease

Panel Discussion

Application of rhEPO in Premature Infants and During/After Pregnancy

Use of rhEPO in Elective Surgery (Facilitation of Autologous Blood Donation, Transfusion Avoidance)

Panel Discussion

Preface

"My hands are of your colour, but I shame to wear a heart so white," whispers Lady Macbeth to her husband. A white heart is a bloodless heart, which, like a bloodless liver, indicates a lack of spirit and enthusiasm. These deficiencies were certainly not characteristic of the participants of a workshop held in Lucerne, Switzerland, that dealt with a hormone that stimulates the formation of red blood cells: erythropoietin (EPO). The Lucerne workshop, which took place in October 1992, was the fourth in a series of similar symposia that were held successively in Wolfenbüttel, Germany (1987), Cologne, Germany (1989), and Telfs, Austria (1990).

In recent years, many new basic findings have been made regarding the regulation of the EPO gene, the way in which the hormone acts on its target cells, and the postnatal shift of the production site from liver to kidney. Likewise, new and extensive data have been collected on the physiological and psychological effects of recombinant human EPO (rhEPO) in patients who suffer from renal anemia. And last but not least, new applications for rhEPO have opened further clinical and theoretical fields, such as its role in autologous blood donation programs, the treatment of anemia in the general framework of obstetrics, and the treatment of patients with the anemia of chronic inflammatory disease. About 200 basic scientists and clinicians from all over the world were present in Lucerne and, in lectures and discussions, contributed to a more thorough understanding of the molecular physiology and clinical application of this fascinating hormone.

Cell and molecular biologists have vividly tackled the question of how the lack of oxygen can activate the EPO gene. They found that the EPO gene contains a relative short stretch of DNA (cis-acting element) to which one or more nuclear proteins (trans-acting elements) can bind. This DNA stretch may constitute one member of a family of cis-acting elements that control the activity of the EPO gene but in itself is necessary and sufficient to convey oxygen control to the EPO gene. Interestingly, the intracellular machinery that activates this particular enhancer does not seem to be restricted to the cells that make EPO but is also found in a large variety of other cells. Erythroid precursor cells are critically dependent on EPO in order to survive and to enter the terminal differentiation program. The intracellular events that initiate and sustain this differentiation program are very complex, because nothing is known about the relative role of a given reaction in the entirety of the decision-making hierarchy within the cell. Nonetheless, it is now firmly established that EPO initiates phosphorylation–dephosphorylation reactions in its target cells, which in turn control the activity of defined proto-oncogenes. These findings set the stage for further efforts aimed at a better understanding of erythroid differentiation.

Quantitatively, one of the major products of erythroid differentiation is hemoglobin, whose synthesis requires iron. Only recently has it been appreciated that many patients who suffer from renal anemia or the anemia of chronic disease have a disturbed iron metabolism due either to an inhibition of iron transfer within the body or to iron losses. From these observations it follows that iron status must be carefully monitored under rhEPO therapy, and iron supplemented whenever deemed necessary. In point of fact, adequate iron therapy can even reduce the amount of rhEPO necessary to reach a given target hematocrit. These practical aspects have led to an impressive amount of studies that document an increase in the quality of life after the correction of anemia. Many factors can be considered in evaluating quality of life, including ability to perform analytical and sensory discrimination tasks and levels of physical fitness, fatigue, and resistance to psychosocial stress. All these variables significantly improve in patients with renal anemia during therapy with rhEPO. Noteworthy in this connection is the fact that the frequency of hypertension during rhEPO therapy in dialysis patients is only around 15% if care is taken to correct the anemia not too abruptly.

These and various other important clinical aspects of rhEPO were summarized and updated during a round-table discussion at the end of the workshop. Invited discussants and specialists from the audience formulated their points of view on three major subjects: 1) current questions and future aspects in the treatment of renal anemia with rhEPO, 2) the use of rhEPO in elective surgery, and 3) rhEPO in the therapy of neoplastic diseases. The entirety of the statements presented at this discussion represents the current state of the art in new and rapidly developing fields of application for rhEPO.

The rapid publication of the proceedings of this workshop, including the discussions after the lectures and the "round-table," should give this book a high degree of both immediacy and permanence. The editors are very grateful to Ms. Kerry Doyle of Marcel Dekker, Inc., for her most efficient help in resolving all the problems that seem to be ever-present in such an undertaking. My sincere thanks go to the Boehringer Mannheim Company for their support, without which this workshop could not have taken place. There are two individuals from the staff of Boehringer Mannheim to whom I owe a particularly large debt of gratitude: Mr. Edgar Rühl and Dr. Rudi Scherhag. Edgar Rühl was responsible for the technical organization of the workshop—and he did his job so well that nobody really noticed that there was an organization at all. Rudi Scherhag was exceedingly instrumental in helping to prepare the scientific part of the workshop and take care of many manuscripts which, of course, is essential for the publication of a book like the one you have in front of you. I hope you will enjoy reading it. Finally, I want to acknowledge that the Lucerne workshop was held under the auspices of the Federation of European Physiological Societies.

Christian Bauer

Mammalian Transcription Factors and Their Interaction with Enhancers and Promoters

Katja Seipel, Oleg Georgiev, David N. Arnosti, Walter Schaffner

Institute of Molecular Biology II, University of Zürich, Zürich, Switzerland

Summary

Regulatory regions of mammalian genes include promoter sequences close to the transcription initiation site and enhancer sequences located farther away. Both promoters and enhancers have modular structures and contain a variety of short DNA sequence motifs, which represent binding sites for sequence-specific transcription factors.

We reported previously that the lymphocyte-derived octamer transcription factor 2A (Oct-2A or OTF-2A) could activate promoters with an "octamer" sequence motif (ATGCAAAT) but was unable by itself to stimulate transcription from a remote enhancer position. We have addressed the question of proximal versus remote activation with respect to a larger set of transcription factors by fusing individual activation domains to the heterologous DNA-binding domain of GAL4 factor. According to their activity in transfected HeLa cells, we have identified at least two groups of qualitatively different activation domains. "General" activation domains, derived from factors VP16, GAL4, p65(NFκB), TFE3, ITF-1, and ITF-2, can activate transcription from remote as well as proximal positions. These domains contain many acidic amino acids and/or other features such as clusters of serine and threonine. "Proximal" activation domains, exemplified by glutamine-rich domains of Oct-1, Oct-2, and Sp1, stimulate transcription only from a position close to the TATA box, usually in response to a remote enhancer.

We have also tested in more detail the role of one of the above-mentioned transcription factors, Oct-2, in the process of transcription initiation in vitro using both nuclear extracts and purified basal transcription factors (in collaboration with Drs. A. Merino and D. Reinberg). Oct-2 specifically stimulates transcription from octamer sequence–containing promoters in both systems.

Thus, Oct-2 is a "true activator," rather than merely an "antirepressor" counteracting the effect of histones. In order-of-addition experiments, Oct-2 is required early, together with TFIID, to allow formation of a preinitiation complex. Oct-2 cannot functionally interact with cloned TATA-binding protein (TBP) but rather requires "coactivators" found in the TFIID fraction. In agreement with our studies in vivo, the N-terminal glutamine-rich activation domain of Oct-2 is required for full activity in vitro, indicating that this domain directly interacts with general transcription factors.

Introduction

Cis-acting transcriptional regulatory sequences include promoter sequences located around the initiation site (to about − 100 bp) and enhancer sequences located farther away (Fig. 1A). A promoter often consists of an initiation site, a TATA box, and one or more "upstream" sequence motifs, where sequence-specific transcription factors bind (Fig. 1B). Transcription initiation by RNA polymerase II involves the assembly of a multifactor complex at the promoter (Fig. 2). While the promoter is the regulatory center for the establishment of the preinitiation complex, enhancers confer additional regulatory information (e.g., cell-type specificity) to the promoter. Enhancers also have a modular structure and are composed of multiple binding sites for transcription factors. Eukaryotic transcriptional regulatory proteins belong to two major groups: the general transcription factors, which bind to common motifs (TATA box, initiator motif) [1], and the sequence-specific transcription factors, which bind to upstream promoter or enhancer elements [2]. Sequence-specific transcription factors are thought to influence the rate of transcription initiation by interacting with the general transcription factors, RNA polymerase II, and/or chromatin components [3]. The main components of a sequence-specific transcription factor are the DNA-binding domain, the nuclear localization signal, and the transactivation domain. These domains have been characterized in recent years.

Transcriptional activation domains have been characterized by a number of criteria: general amino acid content [4], requirement for coactivators [5, 6], activity in histone antirepression assays [7–10], and in vivo interference or "squelching" [11]. Our study provides a new classification of activation domains according to their ability to stimulate transcription from remote and/or proximal positions (Table 1).

We made a series of fusion protein constructions, all based on the yeast GAL4 DNA-binding domain (amino acid residues 1–93) fused to activation

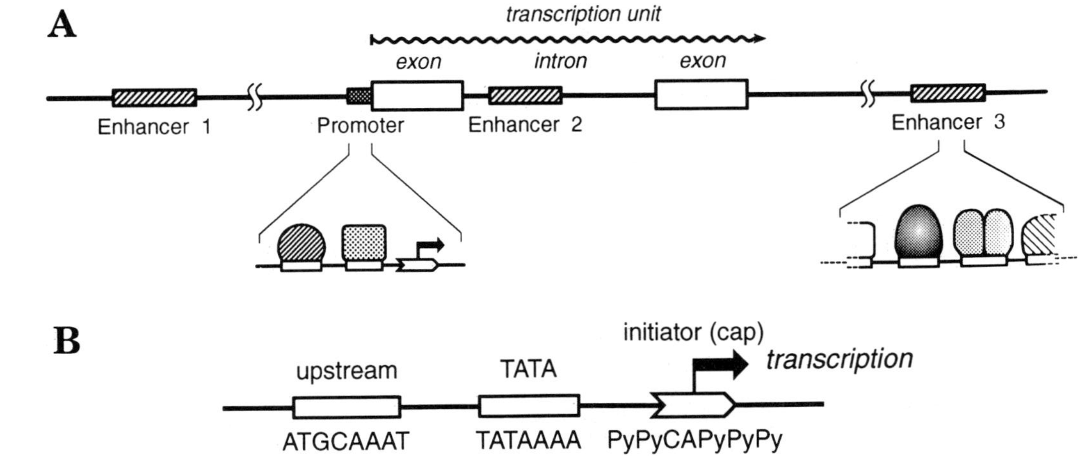

Fig. 1. (A) Schematic structure of a typical mammalian gene. Genes are divided into transcribed and nontranscribed (regulatory) regions. In higher eukaryotes, the primary transcript (wavy line above the gene structure) includes exon regions, which will be translated (open boxes) and untranslated regions. Splicing of the primary transcript in the nucleus yields the mRNA, which is transported to the cytoplasm. Introns are untranslated regions that will be spliced out before translation (region between the exons). The regulatory sequences include the promoter sequences located around the initiation site (dark stippled box) and enhancer sequences (striped boxes) located farther away, either upstream of the promoter (enhancer 1), within an intron (enhancer 2), or downstream of the transcribed region (enhancer 3). A magnification of the promoter and enhancer sequences is shown below. The promoter often consists of the initiation site (white arrow), where transcription starts (black arrow), the TATA box, where the TATA box–binding protein (TBP, stippled rectangle) and other general transcription factors assemble into the preinitiation complex, and one or more ''upstream'' sequences, where gene-specific regulatory factors can bind (striped circle). The enhancer also has a modular structure. It consists of recognition sites for gene-specific regulatory factors (indicated by various shapes). (B) Magnified scheme of a typical promoter sequence. The initiation site (white arrow) has the consensus sequence PyPy CAPyPyPy, the TATA box has the consensus sequence TATAAAA, the ''upstream'' sequences are recognition sites for transcription factors (the sequence motif ATGCAAAT, for example, binds Oct factors). While the sequences of the single elements can be inverted, the relative order upstream box/TATA box has to be maintained because it determines the direction of transcription [45].

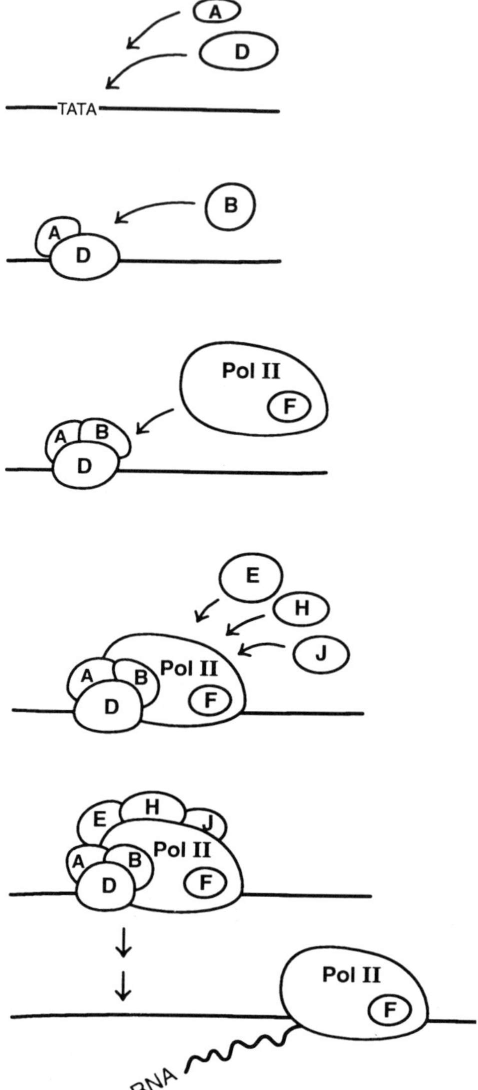

Fig. 2. Schematic drawing of the preinitiation complex assembly on a minimal promoter. The sequential assembly of the general transcription factors D, A, B on the TATA box is followed by the recruitment of RNA polymerase II and factor F to the DAB complex. The addition of factors E, H, and J to the DAB, Pol II, F complex completes the preinitiation complex assembly. This is a prerequisite for the initiation of transcription, which includes the release of the active RNA polymerase II from the preinitiation complex. Not shown is the binding of ''upstream'' factors (see Fig. 1). The binding of ''true activator'' factors (see Fig. 7) in proximity to the TATA box (usually about 20 bp upstream) facilitates the initiation complex formation possibly at every step. [Adapted from Ref. 1.]

Table 1.   Summary of transactivation results

GAL4 fusion constructs		Prevalent amino acids	Net charge	Activation proximal[a,c]	Activation remote[b,c]
GAL4(1-93)				$(+/-)$	$-$
GAL4(1-93)-Oct-1	(175-269)	Q	$+1$	$++$	$-$
GAL4(1-93)-Oct-2	(99-161)	Q	$+2$	$++$	$-$
GAL4(1-93)-Oct-2	$(143\text{-}160)_1$	Q	0	$+$	$-$
GAL4(1-93)-Oct-2	$(143\text{-}160)_2$	Q	0	$++$	$-$
GAL4(1-93)-Sp1	(132-243)	Q	0	$++$	$-$
GAL4(1-93)-Sp1	(340-485)	Q	$+1$	$++$	$-$
GAL4(1-93)-$[Q]_{43}$		Q	0	$(+/-)$	$-$
GAL4(1-93)-AP2	(31-76)	P>S+T	0	$+$	$(+/-)$
GAL4(1-93)-CTF	(399-499)	P>S+T	$+3$	$+$	$(+/-)$
GAL4(1-93)-$[P]_{43}$		P	0	$-$	$-$
GAL4(1-93)-GAL4	(753-881)	S+T>D+E	-8	$++$	$++$
GAL4(1-93)-VP16	(413-490)	D+E	-18	$++$	$++$
GAL4(1-93)-VP16(n)	(413-454)	D+E	-11	$++$	$++$
GAL4(1-93)-VP16(c)	(454-490)	D+E	-7	$+$	$+$
GAL4(1-93)-VP16	$(437\text{-}447)_1$	D+E	-5	$+$	$(+/-)$
GAL4(1-93)-VP16	$(437\text{-}447)_2$	D+E	-10	$++$	$++$
GAL4(1-93)-p65	(286-518)	P>S+T>D+E	0	$++$	$++$
GAL4(1-93)-p65	(520-550)	S>D+E	-5	$++$	$++$
GAL4(1-93)-ITF1	(1-427)	S+T>P	$+8$	$++$	$+$
GAL4(1-93)-ITF2	(2-451)	S+T>P	$+16$	$++$	$++$
GAL4(1-93)-TFE3	(2-216)	S+T>D+E	-6	$++$	$++$
GAL4(1-93)-Nuc	(170-277)	D+E	-57	$-$	$-$
GAL4(1-93)-cb12	(352-469)	D+E	-14	$-$	$-$
GAL4(1-93)-$[D]_{120}$		D	-120	$-$	$-$
GAL4(1-93)-$[E]_{120}$		E	-120	$-$	$-$

[a]Transcriptional activation on the reporter genes 1GAL/SV40, 2GAL/8MRE, 2GAL/SV40.
[b]Transcriptional activation on the reporter genes β-globin/5GAL, 1SP1/5GAL, 2SP1/5GAL, 1GAL/5GAL.
[c]$++$ indicates strong, $+$ weak, $(+/-)$ very weak, $-$ indicates no transcriptional activation by the corresponding activation domain.

domains from well-characterized mammalian transcription factors, with the assumption that these activation domains are independent functional units [12]. We tested glutamine-rich domains from Oct-1, Oct-2, and Sp1, proline-rich domains from CTF/NF1 and AP-2, negatively charged domains of VP16, GAL4, p65 (NFκB), and TFE-3, and serine-/threonine-rich domains of ITF-1 and ITF-2. All of these chimeric activators stimulated transcription when allowed to bind next to the TATA box. By contrast, only some of them were able to stimulate transcription from a remote position. The typical domains for promoter activation were found to be glutamine-rich, indicating that they are functionally distinct from the remote activation domains, which include domains with negatively charged residues. Therefore, our studies introduce evidence for differential function of promoters and enhancers.

According to the terminology of Croston et al. [7], activation can be classified as "antirepression," i.e., counteracting the negative effects of chromatin or other components, or "true activation," i.e., direct interaction with elements of the basal transcription apparatus (see Fig. 7). Several activators have been found to interact with TFIID, the multifactor complex that binds the TATA box. Transcription factor ATF and chimeric GAL4 derivatives have been found to alter TFIID footprinting patterns, while the pseudorabies immediate early protein and the EBV Zta protein have been found to facilitate TFIID-DNA interaction [13–17]. TFIIB also appears to be a target of activators. A GAL4/VP16 chimeric activator bound TFIIB directly and promoted stable association of TFIIB with the preinitiation complex [18, 19], while LSF, a factor that stimulates transcription from the SV40 major late promoter, increased the rate of TFIIB binding to the preinitiation complex [20].

The role of an activator after formation of the preinitiation complex remains to be elucidated. Experiments with the ATF activator suggested that once a transcription complex has been established, ATF can be removed without impairing transcription [21], implying that once activated, a target promoter would remain "on." In contrast, experiments with GAL4/VP16 suggested that antibody inhibition of the VP16 moiety shuts down transcription [22], although in this case, the promoter-bound antibody molecules may themselves be inhibitory. Recently, we have obtained good evidence that Oct-2 is continuously required at the promoter for multiple rounds of transcription [42]. This result argues against a "hit-and-run" mechanism whereby the activator becomes dispensable after organizing a TFIID-promoter complex.

In order to make functional comparisons between different transcription factors, we have initiated mechanistic studies to understand how Oct-2 activates transcription in vitro and to identify the targets of this factor. We found that Oct-2 acts together with TFIID to form preinitiation complexes. Glutamine-rich activation domains similar to those of Oct-2 are found in other transcription factors [4], thus these factors may all operate by a common mechanism.

Oct-2 is expressed specifically in nuclei of B lymphocytes where it is required for efficient transcription of immunoglobulin genes. This is an example of a simple regulation of gene expression induced by de novo protein synthesis of Oct-2. Other genes have a more sophisticated regulation with very fast induction and repression of transcription. This cannot be achieved by de novo protein synthesis, but by posttranslational modifications of the involved protein components. Phosphorylation is the best studied modification system [23]. Phosphorylation of a transcription factor can influence its nuclear translocation, DNA binding, and transactivation. Furthermore, any domain of a transcription factor can be masked either by intramolecular conformational changes or by a second protein (inhibitor), thereby preventing nuclear transport, DNA binding, or transactivation (Fig. 3).

Gene expression is also dependent on the phosphorylation status of the general transcription factors and the polymerases [23]. Phosphorylation and acetylation influence chromatin components [24], thereby changing the accessibility of regulatory regions on the DNA. In addition, methylation of DNA can indirectly repress transcription [25].

Results

The Activation Domains from Several Known Transcription Factors Can Be Divided into at Least Two Functional Groups

In order to study individual protein domains for transcriptional activation, we created a series of fusion constructions based on the DNA-binding domain of the yeast factor GAL4 fused to different activation domains from known transcription factors (Fig. 4A, Table 1): the glutamine-rich regions of Oct-1, Oct-2, and Sp1, the proline-rich regions of AP-2, CTF/NF1, and p65 (NFκB), the serine- and threonine-rich domains of ITF-1 and ITF-2, and the negatively charged regions from VP16, GAL4, p65 (NFκB), and TFE3. We also tested fusion proteins representing protein domains from nontranscription factors, namely the highly acidic regions of the oncogene cbl-2 and of nucleolin. The reporter genes were of two types (Fig. 4A). The "proximal GAL4" reporter genes contained one or two GAL4-binding sites next to the TATA box and either no enhancer, an SV40 enhancer, or eight metal-regulatory elements downstream of the reporter gene. The "remote GAL4" reporter genes contained five GAL4-binding sites downstream of the reporter gene and, as promoter, the β-globin TATA box in combination with one of the following proximal upstream elements: the rabbit β-globin upstream region (about 2 kb) [26], one of two Sp1 sites, one or two GAL4 sites, or an octamer site. With the exception of the

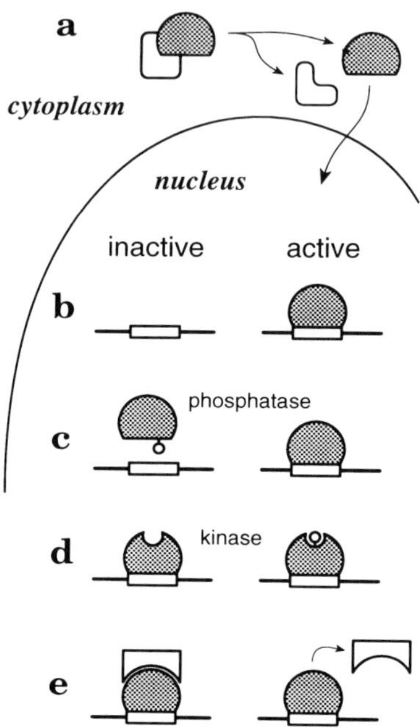

Fig. 3.   Regulation of gene expression by regulation of transcription factors. In a simple system, gene expression could be regulated merely by the presence or absence of a sequence-specific transcription factor. This might apply to the regulation of tissue-specific genes, e.g., activation of immunoglobulin gene expression in B lymphocytes by synthesis of Oct-2 (b). In most cases, however, regulation of gene expression is more complex and rapidly changing from activation to inactivation. Fast changes cannot be achieved by de novo protein synthesis but by posttranslational events. The transport of a transcription factor from the cytoplasm to the nucleus can be regulated (a). Transcription factors can be retained in the cytoplasm by the binding of inhibitors. A well-known example is NFκB [46]. Nuclear transport, DNA binding, and transactivation can be impaired by modifications. The best studied modification system is phosphorylation. Transcription factors inactive in the unphosphorylated state can be activated by protein kinases (d). This appears to be the case for CREB, SRF, c-Jun, and others. Likewise, transcription factors inactive in the phosphorylated state can be activated by the action of a phosphatase (c). This appears to be the case for c-Myb, c-Jun, and others [23, 47]. For c-Jun, both DNA binding and transcriptional activation are regulated by phosphorylation. Alternatively, transcription factors might bind to the DNA in complex with a repressor protein and only be activated by the release of this component as in the GAL4/GAL80 complex (e) [2, 48]. However, recent evidence suggests that GAL80 is not released from GAL4 upon activation and that phosphorylation plays a role in the activation by GAL4 [49], demonstrating that a combination of various regulatory events can influence a single transcription factor.

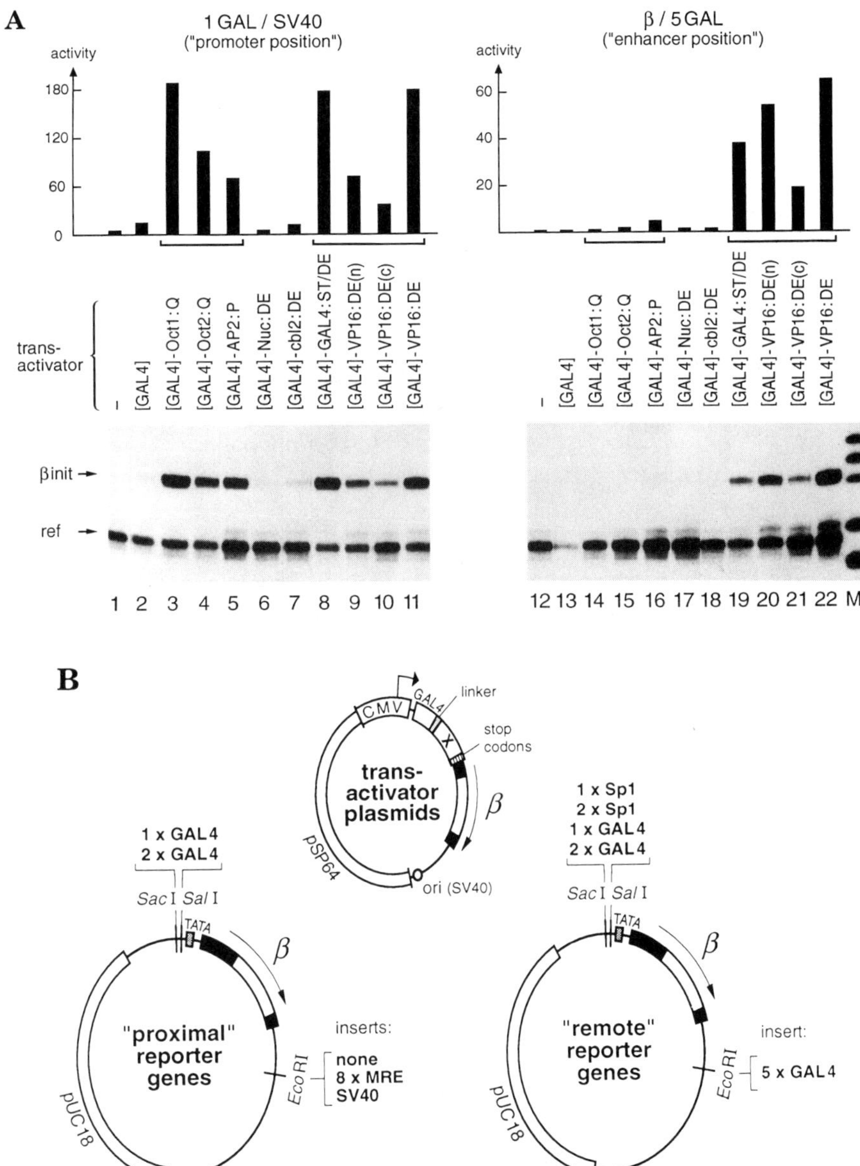

Fig. 4. The glutamine-rich activation domains from several known transcription factors fail to activate transcription from remote positions. (A) RNase protection analysis of a HeLa cell transfection with the reporter genes 1 GAL/SV40 and β-globin/5 GAL and the indicated GAL4-fusions as transactivators. Quantitation of the signals is shown above the autoradiographs. The ''activity'' numbers are arbitrary units of the signals from the reporter genes (βinit) relative to the signal from the reference gene (ref). (B) Schematic drawing of the transactivator and the reporter plasmids, described in detail in Seipel et al. [44].

glutamine-rich activation domains, all activation domains were able to activate transcription from proximal and remote positions, although to different extents (Fig. 4, summarized in Table 1). The glutamine-rich domains activate transcription only from a proximal position. The acidic clusters of the oncogene cbl-2 and of nucleolin and most of the homopolymers failed to activate the GAL4 reporter genes. The effects were not specific for a given promoter or enhancer, since different reporter gene constructions responded similarly (Table 1). All the fusion proteins were able to bind to the GAL4 DNA-binding site and were expressed at similar levels, as judged by gel retardation analysis with nuclear extracts from COS cells transfected with the same quantity of plasmid DNA as in the HeLa cell transfections (data not shown). From these experiments, we conclude that there exist at least two classes of transcriptional activating domains (Table 1): one exemplified by the glutamine-rich activation domains of Oct-1, Oct-2, and Sp1, the second exemplified by the negatively charged domains of VP16, GAL4, p65 (NFκB), and TFE-3, and the serine/threonine-rich domains of ITF-1 and ITF-2 (which would also be negatively charged in case of phosphorylation). The proline-rich domains of AP-2 and CTF/NF1 may belong to a third class, since they have considerable activity from proximal positions and also weak, but significant, activity from remote positions.

Activation of In Vitro Transcription by Oct-2

To study activation by the Oct-2 factor, test templates were transcribed in vitro using nuclear extracts derived from BJA-B (B lymphocyte) or HeLa cells. A κ light-chain promoter (Fig. 5A) and a composite promoter consisting of a single octamer site adjacent to the rabbit β-globin TATA box (Fig. 5B) were activated up to 10-fold by addition of recombinant Oct-2 produced in *E. coli*. Oct-2 stimulated transcription to similar maximal levels in both B-lymphocyte and nonlymphocyte systems (Fig. 5B), indicating that no B-cell–specific factors are required for Oct-2 activity, in accord with other in vitro studies [27–29] and with in vivo results obtained from transfections [30, 31]. Basal transcription from octamer promoters was higher with BJA-B extracts than with HeLa extracts (Fig. 5B), most likely because of endogenous Oct-2 in the BJA-B extract. A reference promoter lacking octamer binding sites was not activated by Oct-2 (Fig. 5B), indicating that the activation was specific.

It has been proposed that B-cell specific factors further enhance Oct factor activation on some promoters; Oct factors from B-cell nuclear extracts drive transcription in vitro from an immunoglobulin heavy-chain promoter and an MHC II DRA promoter more efficiently than the octamer factor(s) from HeLa

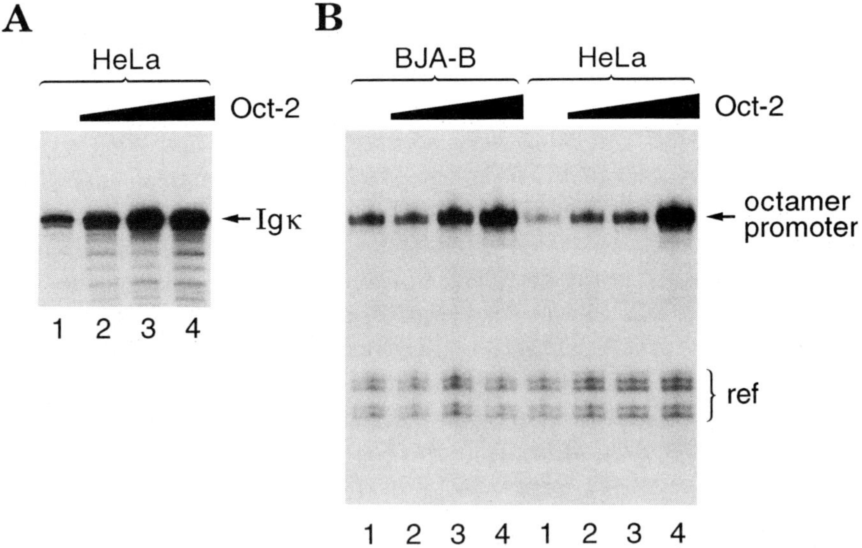

Fig. 5. (A) Oct-2 activation of an immunoglobulin κ light-chain promoter. Plasmid pκβ+21 (200 ng) bearing a −400 to +21 fragment of the MOPC-41 κ light chain promoter was transcribed with HeLa nuclear extract in the presence of 0, 1.7, 3.3, or 6.7 pmoles (Oct-2) (lanes 1–4), and transcripts were mapped by RNase protection. (B) Oct-2 activation of a composite octamer promoter in BJA-B and HeLa nuclear extracts. Plasmid p70Zhep⁻oct⁺ (400 ng) containing a single octamer-binding site upstream of the rabbit β-globin TATA box and the OVEC-ref plasmid (400 ng) driven by an SV40 enhancer sequence were transcribed in HeLa or BJA-B nuclear extracts in the presence of 0, 0.7, 1.6, or 6.7 pmoles Oct-2 (lanes 1–4), and transcripts were mapped by S1 nuclease analysis.

extracts [29, 32]. This and other studies show, however, that Oct-2 has an intrinsic ability to stimulate transcription. In fact, the Oct-2 glutamine-rich activation domain can by itself stimulate transcription when fused to a heterologous DNA binding domain (Fig. 4).

Oct-2 Functions as a "True Activator"

Stimulation of preinitiation complex formation might be the result of direct interaction of Oct-2 with the basal transcription machinery ("true activation") [7], or Oct-2 might counteract repressive effects of some component of the nuclear extracts (''antirepression''). While complete histone assembly is unlikely in a nuclear extract [33], the presence of histone H1 has been documented in Drosophila nuclear extracts [7]. We therefore tested the activity of Oct-2 in a fractionated system utilizing recombinant proteins (TFIIB, TFIIE) and purified fractions (TFIIA, TFIID, TFIIF/H, and RNA polymerase). Activation was observed with both a κ light-chain promoter and a composite promoter (Fig. 6), indicating that Oct-2 can interact with purified component(s) of the basal transcriptional machinery. While it is possible that trace amounts of a general repressor such as H1 are present in the purified fractions, we consider it unlikely that such a protein is involved in Oct-2 activation because, as noted below, Oct-2 functionally acts together with TFIID. Similar activation with Oct-2 is obtained using TFIID purified by three different methods, as well as crude extracts (data not shown). It is possible, however, that Oct-2 may counteract some transcriptional repressors thought to interact directly with TBP [34, 35].

Significant activation with Oct-2 is only observed when transcription is driven by TFIID, a fraction that contains both the TATA-binding protein (TBP) and TBP-associated proteins (TAFs) [36], but not with recombinant TBP alone (Fig. 6B). Thus, as has been observed for other transcriptional activators [37], Oct-2 requires ''coactivators'' present in the TFIID fraction for activity. We

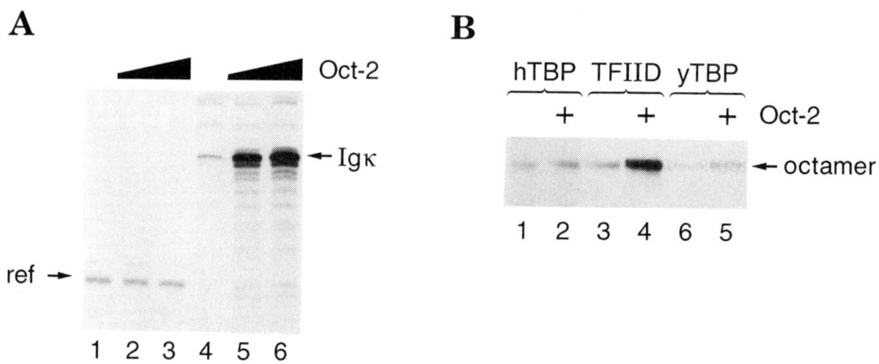

Fig. 6. Activation of promoters by Oct-2 in a fractionated system. (A) κ light chain promoter plasmid pκβ + 21 or REFΔ plasmid [30] driven by an SV40 enhancer element (90 ng) were transcribed in the presence of 0 (lanes 1 and 4), 0.17 (lanes 2 and 5), or 0.34 (lanes 3 and 6) pmoles Oct-2, and transcripts were analyzed by RNase protection. (B) Transcription with human TATA-binding protein (TBP), TFIID, or yeast TBP. Octamer promoter plasmid p70Zhep⁻oct⁺ (400 ng) was transcribed in presence of saturating amounts of TBP or with TFIID as indicated; 17 pmole Oct-2 was added to even-numbered lanes. RNA was analyzed by S1 analysis.

have not yet tested Oct-2 for antirepression activity on templates with reconstituted nucleosomes, but most transcription factors tested so far have this activity, including Sp1 [8], which has a glutamine-rich activation domain, as do Oct-1 and Oct-2. To date, it has not been reported whether antirepression also occurs in transcription reactions driven by TBP, where true activation is absent. If this is the case, then the requirement for TBP-associated factors (TAFs) may be a hallmark of true activation.

Discussion

Different Activation Domains Stimulate Transcription from Remote ("Enhancer") and Proximal ("Promoter") Positions

Transcriptional activation domains have been characterized by a number of criteria: general amino acid content [4], requirement for coactivators [5, 6], activity in histone antirepression assays [7–10], and in vivo interference or "squelching" [11]. This study introduces evidence for differential function of promoters and enhancers. Activation domains are classified according to their ability to stimulate transcription from remote and/or proximal positions (Table 1). The tested domains fall into at least two groups: one group, represented by the glutamine-rich domains, can activate only from a position close to the TATA box ("proximal" activation), usually in response to a remote enhancer, whereas another group, which includes the acidic domains, can activate from remote positions as well as from proximal positions ("general" activation). These two functional classes reflect qualitative differences rather than merely quantitative ones, i.e., "strong" versus "weak" activation. For example, the small acidic VP16 fragments, which are less effective than the glutamine-rich domains in a proximal position, nevertheless function well from a distance, unlike the glutamine-rich domains (Fig. 4). That the glutamine-rich domains qualify as bona fide activators is supported by our findings that they activate transcription in cell-free systems without the need for additional enhancer components. We have tested, in collaboration with Danny Reinberg and colleagues (University of Medicine and Dentistry of New Jersey, USA), the effect of Oct-2 factor in an in vitro transcription system with individually purified components. Oct-2 clearly stimulates transcription in the absence of nucleosomes (Fig. 5). A simple explanation would be that proximally active domains interact directly with the basal transcription machinery, while a major function of domains with long-range potential is to reorganize the chromatin for efficient transcription in vivo.

It is also possible that the two classes of activation domains interact with distinct proteins in the basal transcription complex. Furthermore, the target proteins the basal complex might be differentially accessible: while the target for proximal activation domains would be accessible only from positions close to the TATA box, the target for the general activation domains would be accessible from any position, presumably by looping out of the intervening DNA. If general and proximal activators have distinct pathways of activation, then one would expect to see synergistic activation when both elements are combined. Such a synergism is found with glutamine-rich domains of Oct-1, Oct-2, and Sp1. These "proximal" activation domains in vivo are weak activators in the absence of an enhancer but respond strongly to a remote enhancer. In contrast, acidic activation domains can be very active in vivo by themselves, with no need for an extra enhancer (our unpublished data). Thus the glutamine-rich activation domains, which have not been found in yeast so far, may be of particular importance in higher eukaryotes, where one gene can be independently controlled by several remote enhancers. We propose that the "proximal" activation domains have evolved to allow for efficient channeling of an enhancer effect to the responsive promoter.

Transcriptional Activation by Oct-2

Studies with the adenovirus 2 major late promoter (AdMLP) have pointed to a sequential process in which basal transcription factors associate with the promoter: first TFIID binds the TATA box, assisted by TFIIA, then TFIIB binds this DA complex, and the DAB complex is recognized by Pol II/TFIIF. Factors TFIIE, TFIIJ, and TFIIH associate and conformational changes occur prior to initiation (Fig. 2) [38]. Basal factors TFIIG and an initiator box binding factor have also been identified [39–41]. Although our understanding is far from complete, studies on natural and chimeric transcriptional activators have suggested that these factors can act either indirectly, by relieving histone repression [7–10], or directly, by facilitating association of general factors such as TFIID and TFIIB with the nascent preinitiation complex [13–16, 18, 20, 21]. Using an in vitro system, we determined that Oct-2 stimulated transcription from octamer promoters (Fig. 5) by facilitating formation of preinitiation complexes (Fig. 2). Oct-2 also stimulated transcription in a fractionated system (Fig. 6), showing that it interacts directly with components of the basal transcription machinery and is thus a "true activator" (Fig. 7). Activation was dependent upon "coactivators," components of the TFIID fraction distinct from TBP (Fig. 6B). We also examined the effect on transcription of removing Oct-2 from the promoter by addition of excess competitor oligonucleotide is single and multiple round transcriptions and found that Oct-2 is required continuously at the promoter for reinitiation

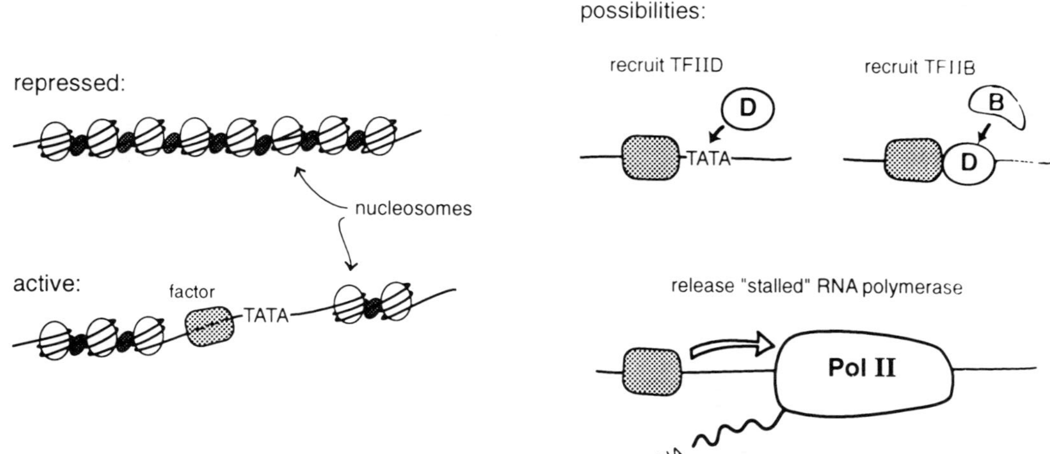

Fig. 7. Proposed models for the function of sequence-specific transcription factors (terminology of Croston et al. [7]). Activation can be classified as "antirepression," i.e., counteracting the negative effects of chromatin components (left side), or "true activation," i.e., direct interaction with elements of the basal transcription machinery (right side). Interactions of transcription factors have been found with the general factors TFIID and TFIIB, leading to a recruitment of these general factors to the preinitiation complex [13–20]. Direct interactions of transcription factors with the basal machinery are also implicated in the release of RNA polymerase II from the preinitiation complex [50].

(data shown in [42]). Furthermore, we tested the effect of Oct-2 deletion mutants on transcription. In accord with results obtained in vivo [43], the deletion of a glutamine-rich activation domain in the N terminus led to a severe loss of activity in vitro (data shown in [42]).

Our studies indicate that Oct-2 activates transcription by direct interaction with the basal machinery (''true activation'') and that the glutamine-rich domain activation previously found to be important for activity in vivo is required for assembly of preinitiation promoter complexes.

Materials and Methods

For a detailed description of the in vivo experiments (Fig. 4, Table 1) including the construction of plasmids, transfection and RNA analysis, preparation of nuclear extracts and bandshift experiments, see Seipel et al. [44]. For a detailed description of the in vitro experiments (Fig. 5, 6) containing the preparation of nuclear extracts, purification of basal transcription factors, overexpression and purification of Oct-2 and derivatives, expression vectors, and transcription assays, see Arnosti et al. [42].

Acknowledgments

We thank Dr. W. Herr for the human Oct-1 cDNA clone, Dr. M. Ptashne for the plasmids pG and pSGVP, Dr. A. Courey for the Sp1 plasmids, Dr. P. J. Mitchell for the human AP2 cDNA, Dr. N. Mermod for the plasmid pGAL-CTF1 (399-499), Dr. P. Bäuerle for the NFκB plasmids, Dr. T. Kadesch for the plasmids containing activation domains of ITF-1, ITF-2, and TFE3, Dr. W. Y. Langdon for the cDNA clone of the human cbl-2 gene, and Andreas Seiler for the cDNA clone ASA4 of the human nucleolin gene. We also are indebted to Dr. K. Harshman for the construction of the bacterial Oct-2 expression vectors, Dr. P. J. Mitchell for the critical reading of the manuscript, and F. Ochsenbein for excellent art work.

References

1   Weinmann R: The basic RNA polymerase II transcriptional machinery. Gene expression 1992;2:81–91.
2   Johnson PF, McKnight SL: Eukaryotic transcriptional regulatory proteins. Annu Rev Biochem 1989;58:799–839.
3   Felsenfeld G: Chromatin as an essential part of the transcriptional mechanism. Nature 1992;355:219–224.

4 Mitchell PJ, Tjian R: Transcriptional regulation in mammalian cells by sequence-specific DNA binding proteins. Science 1989;245:371–378.

5 Tanese N, Pugh BF, Tjian R: Coactivators for a proline-rich activator purified from the multisubunit human TFIID complex. Genes Dev 1992;5:2212–2224.

6 Berger SL, Pina B, Silverman N, Marcus GA, Agapite J, Regier JL, Triezenberg SJ, Guarente L: Genetic isolation of ada2: A potential transcriptional adaptor required for function of certain acidic activation domains. Cell 1992;70:251–265.

7 Croston GE, Kerrigan LA, Lira LM, Marshak DR, Kadonaga JT: Sequence-specific antidepression of histone H1-mediated inhibition of basal RNA polymerase II transcription. Science 1991;251:643–649.

8 Laybourn PJ, Kadonaga JT: Role of nucleosomal cores and histone H1 in regulation of transcription by RNA polymerase II. Science 1991;254:238–245.

9 Laybourn PJ, Kadonaga JT: Threshold phenomena and long-distance activation of transcription by RNA polymerase II. Science 1992;257:1682–1685.

10 Workman JL, Taylor IC, Kingston RE: Activation domains of stably bound GAL4 derivatives alleviate repression of promoters by nucleosomes. Cell 1991;64:533–544.

11 Tasset D, Tora L, Fromental C, Scheer E, Chambon P: Distinct classes of transcriptional activating domains function by different mechanisms. Cell 1990;62:1177–1187.

12 Brent R, Ptashne M: A eukaryotic transcriptional activator bearing the DNA specificity of a prokaryotic repressor. Cell 1985;43:729–736.

13 Abmayr SM, Workman JL, Roeder RG: The pseudorabies immediate early protein stimulates in vitro transcription by factilitating TFIID: promoter interactions. Genes Dev 1988;2:542–553.

14 Horikoshi M, Hai T, Lin YS, Green MR, Roeder RG: Transcription factor AFT interacts with the TATA factor to factilitate establishment of a preinitiation complex. Cell 1988;54:1033–1042.

15 Horikoshi M, Carey MF, Kakidani H, Roeder RG: Mechanism of action of a yeast activator: Direct effect of GAL4 derivatives on mammalian TFIID-promoter interactions. Cell 1988;54:665–669.

16 Stringer KF, Ingles CJ, Greenblatt J: Direct and selective binding of an acidic transcriptional activation domain to the TATA-box factor TFIID. Nature 1990;345:783–786.

17 Lieberman PM, Berk, AJ: The Zta trans-activator protein stabilizes TFIID association with promoter DNA by direct protein-protein interaction. Genes Dev 1991;5:2441–2454.

18 Lin YS, Green M: Mechanism of action of an acidic transcriptional activator in vitro. Cell 1991;64:971–981.

19 Lin YS, Ha I, Maldonado E, Reinberg D, Green MR: Binding of general transcription factor TFIIB to an acidic activating region. Nature 1991;353:569–571.

20 Sundseth R, Hansen U: Activation of RNA polymerase II transcription by the specific DNA-binding protein LSF-increased rate of binding of the basal promoter factor TFIIB. J Biol Chem 1992;267:7845–7855.

21 Hai T, Horikoshi M, Roeder R, Green M: Analysis of the role of the transcription factor ATF in the assembly of a functional preinitiation complex. Cell 1988;54:1043–1051.

22 White J, Brou C, Wu J, Lutz Y, Moncollin V, Chambon P: The acidic transcriptional activator GAL4-VP16 acts on preformed template-committed complexes. EMBO J 1992;11:2229–2240.

23 Hunter T, Karin M: The regulation of transcription by phosphorylation. Cell 1992;70:375–387.

24 Roth SY, Allis CD: Chromatin condensation: Does histone H1 phosphorylation play a role? TIBS 1992;17:93–98.

25 Bird A: The essentials of DNA methylation. Cell 1992;70:5–8.

26 Dierks P, Ooyen A, Cochran M, Dobkin C, Reiser J, Weissmann C: Three regions upstream from the cap site for efficient and accurate transcription of the rabbit β-globin gene in mouse 3T6 cells. Cell 1983;32:695–706.

27 LeBowitz JH, Kobayashi T, Staudt L, Baltimore D, Sharp PA: Octamer-binding proteins from B or HeLa cells stimulate transcription of the immunoglobulin heavy-chain promoter in vitro. Genes Dev 1988;2:1227–1237.

28 Johnson D, Carayannopoulos L, Capra J, Tucker P, Hanke JH: The ubiquitous octamer-binding protein(s) is sufficient for transcription of immunoglobulin genes. Mol Cell Biol 1990;10:982–990.

29 Pierani A, Heguy A, Fujii H, Roeder RG: Activation of octamer-containing promoters by either octamer-binding transcription factor 1 (OTF-1) or OTF-2 and requirement of an additional B-cell specific component for optimal transcription of immunoglobulin promoters. Mol Cell Biol 1990;10:6204–6215.

30 Kemler I, Bucher E, Seipel K, Müller MM, Schaffner W: Promoters with the octamer DNA motif (ATGCAAAT) can be ubiquitous or cell type-specific depending on binding affinity of the octamer site and Oct-factor concentration. Nucleic Acids Res 1991;19:237–242.

31 Yang J, Müller-Immerglück MM, Seipel K, Jansen L, Westin G, Schaffner W, Pettersson U: Both Oct-1 and Oct-2A contain domains which can activate the ubiquitously expressed U2 snRNAS genes. EMBO J 1991;10:2291–2296.

32 Zeleznik-Le NJ, Itoh-Lindstrom Y, Clarke JB, Moore TL, Ting JPY: The B-cell-specific nuclear factor OTF-2 positively regulates transcription of the human class-II transplantation gene, DRA. J Biol Chem 1992; 267:7677–7682.

33 Carey M, Leatherwood J, Ptashne M: A potent GAL4 derivative activates transcription at a distance in vitro. Nature 1990;247:710–712.

34 Inostroza JA, Mermelstein FH, Ha J, Lane WS, Reinberg D: DR1, a TATA binding protein-associated phosphoprotein and inhibitor of class II gene transcription. Cell 1992;70:477–489.

35 Meisterernst M, Roy AL, Lieu HM, Roeder R: Activation of class II gene transcription by regulatory factors is potentiated by a novel activity. Cell 1991;66:981–993.

36 Pugh BF, Tjian R: Diverse transcriptional functions of the multisubunit eukaryotic TFIID complex. J Biol Chem 1992;267:679–682.

37 Pugh BF, Tjian R: Mechanism of transcriptional activation by Sp1: evidence for coactivators. Cell 1990;61:1187–1197.

38   Zawel L, Reinberg D: Initiation of transcription by RNA polymerase II: A multi-step process. Prog Nucleic Acids Res Mol Biol 1993;45: in press.
39   Sumimoto H, Ohkuma Y, Yamamoto T, Horikoshi M, Roeder RG: Factors involved in specific transcription by mammalian RNA polyermase II: identification of general transcription factor TFIIG. Proc Natl Acad Sci USA 1990;87:9158–9162.
40   Garfinkel S, Thompson JA, Jacob WF, Cohen R, Safer B: Identification and characterization of an adenovirus 2 major late promoter cap sequence DNA-binding protein. J Biol Chem 1990;265:10309–10319.
41   Roy AL, Meisterernst M, Pognonec P, Roeder RG: Cooperative interaction of an initiator-binding transcription initiation factor and the helix-loop-helix activation domain to the TATA-box factor TFIID. Nature 1991;354:245–248.
42   Arnosti DN, Merino A, Reinberg D, Schaffner W: Oct-2 factilitates functional preinitiation complex assembly and is continuously required at the promoter for multiple rounds of transcription. EMBO J 1993;12:157–166.
43   Müller-Immerglück M, Schaffner W, Matthias P: Transcription factor Oct-2A contains functionally redundant activating domains and works selectively from a promoter but not from a remote enhancer position in non-lymphoid (HeLa) cells. EMBO J 1990;9:1625–1643.
44   Seipel K, Georgiev O, Schaffner W: Different activation domains stimulate transcription from remote (enhancer) and proximal (promoter) positions. EMBO J 1992;11:4961–4968.
45   Xu L, Thali M, Schaffner W: Upstream box/TATA box order is the major determinant of the direction of transcription. Nucleic Acid Res 1991;19:6699–6704.
46   Bäuerle P, Baltimore D: IκB: a specific inhibitor of the NF-κB transcription factor. Science 1988;242:540–545.
47   Karin M, Smeal T: Control of transcription factors by signal transduction pathways: the beginning of the end. TIBS 1992;17:418–422.
48   Ptashne M: How eukaryotic transcriptional activators work. Nature 1988;335:683–689.
49   Parthun MR, Jaehning JA: A transcriptionally active form of GAL4 is phosphorylated and associated with GAL80. MCB 1992;12:4981–4987.
50   Young RA: RNA polymerase II. Annu Rev Biochem 1991;60:689–715.

Walter Schaffner, Institute of Molecular Biology II, University of Zurich, Winterthurerstrasse 190, CH-8057, Zurich, Switzerland

Regulation of Human Erythropoietin Gene Expression in Transgenic Mice and Human Hepatoma Cells

Gregg L. Semenza

Departments of Pediatrics and Medicine, and Center for Medical Genetics, The Johns Hopkins University School of Medicine, Baltimore, Md., USA

Genes are expressed at precise levels in restricted cell types at specific developmental stages. The regulation of gene expression provides the molecular basis for development and for the maintenance of physiological homeostasis throughout life. This precise regulation is based upon the interaction of transcription factors with specific *cis*-acting DNA sequences, which determines the rate of transcription and, as a result, the level of gene expression. We have been studying human erythropoietin (EPO) gene expression as a model system for understanding the mechanisms of transcriptional regulation. EPO is the hormone that regulates erythropoiesis and, thus, blood oxygen-carrying capacity in mammals. EPO is produced primarily in the liver and kidney [1–9], and individuals with end-stage renal disease suffer anemia which is ameliorated by recombinant EPO administration [10]. Knowledge of EPO gene expression is important because of the role EPO plays in erythropoiesis, because of its cell type–specific pattern of expression, and because it represents the best-characterized example of a human gene whose expression is modulated by oxygen tension [3, 6–10, 12–20].

Localization of Sequences Regulating Cell Type–Specific
Expression of the Human EPO Gene in Transgenic Mice

In order to localize the *cis*-acting DNA sequences required for EPO gene expression in liver and kidney, we have generated mice transgenic for the human EPO gene and varying amounts of flanking DNA sequences [19, 21, 22]. The first transgene analyzed, tgEPO4, consisted of a 4 kilobase (kb) Hind III-Eco RI

fragment (Fig. 1) containing the intact human EPO gene with 0.4 kb of 5′-flank-
ing sequence (5′-FS) and 0.7 kb of 3′-flanking sequence (3′-FS). Five independent lines of mice carrying the 4 kb transgene (tgEPO4) were generated, and the
transgene was expressed in four of these lines (Table 1). Transgenic mice of
expressing lines were polycythemic with a mean hematocrit of 56%. Human
EPO RNA expression was induced by anemia or cobalt chloride administration
in the livers of tgEPO4 mice from all 4 expressing lines. However, human EPO
RNA expression was not induced in the kidney. Instead, the kidney, as well as

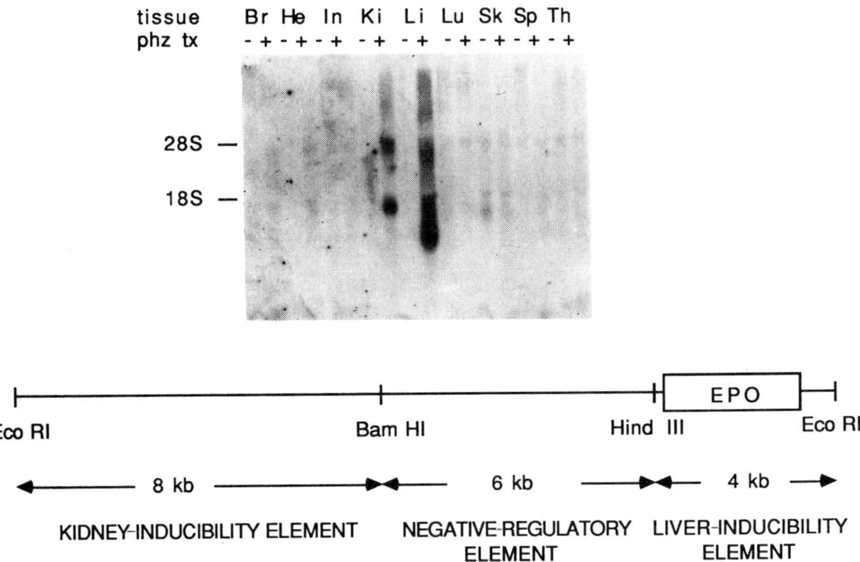

Fig. 1. Localization of *cis*-acting DNA sequences regulating human EPO gene
expression in transgenic mice. (Bottom) Line drawing depicting the human EPO gene
(box) and restriction-endonuclease sites which delimit the tgEPO4, tgEPO10, and
tgEPO18 transgenes, all of which are co-linear at their 3′ termini (Eco RI site) and extend
5′ to the Hind III, Bam HI, and Eco RI sites, respectively. The expression patterns of
these three transgene constructs allowed localization of kidney-inducibility, negative-
regulatory, and liver-inducibility elements to the indicated intervals. (Top) Autoradiograph from blot-hybridization analysis of total RNA (50 μg) extracted from brain (Br),
heart (He), intestine (In), kidney (Ki), liver (Li), lung (Lu), skin (Sk), spleen (Sp), and
thymus (Th) of tgEPO18 mice untreated (−) or treated with phenylhydrazine (phz tx) to
induce anemia (+). The Northern blot was hybridized to a ^{32}P-labeled probe specific for
human EPO RNA [19]. Positions of 18S and 28S rRNA are indicated.

Table 1. Summary of results obtained from analysis of mice transgenic for the human EPO gene and varying amounts of flanking DNA sequences

Transgene[a]	Number of lines		Human EPO RNA		Hct (%)[b]
	Total	Expression	Liver	Kidney	
tgEPO4	5	4	4	0[c]	56 (45.3–62.4)
tgEPO10	9	9	8	0	56 (47.4–78.9)
tgEPO18	8	7	7	7	80 (68.7–87.0)
tgEPO22	5	4	4	4	71 (49.4–80.0)

[a]For each transgene, the total number of transgenic mouse lines generated, the number of lines in which the transgene was expressed, the number of lines in which human EPO RNA was detected in total liver or kidney RNA of anemic mice by blot hybridization, and the mean hematocrit (Hct) of transgenic mice are shown. tgEPO4 is a 4 kb Hind III-Eco RI human genomic DNA fragment (see Fig. 1), which encompasses the EPO gene (consisting of 5 exons and 4 introns) as well as 0.4 kb of 5′-flanking sequence and 0.7 kb of 3′-flanking sequence. tgEPO10 is a 10 kb Bam HI-Eco RI fragment (see Fig. 1) with an additional 6 kb of 5′-flanking sequence relative to tgEPO4. tgEPO18 is an 18 kb Eco RI fragment (see Fig. 1) with an additional 8 kb of 5′-flanking sequence relative to tgEPO10. tgEPO22 is a 22 kb DNA fragment (not shown) with an additional 2.5 kb of 5′-flanking sequence and 1.5 kb of 3′-flanking sequence relative to tgEPO18.
[b]Grand mean hematocrit for all lines expressing each transgene is shown, with range of mean hematocrits for individual lines in parentheses.
[c]Human EPO RNA of abnormal size was constitutively expressed in kidney and other tissues in three lines.

other tissues where endogenous EPO gene expression was not detected, such as brain, constitutively expressed a human EPO RNA species of larger than normal size. These results [21] suggested that tgEPO4 contained DNA sequences necessary and sufficient for inducible expression in liver but lacked sequences required for regulated expression in kidney, the major site of synthesis in the adult.

We subsequently generated 9 lines of mice transgenic for tgEPO10, a 10 kb Bam HI-Eco RI DNA fragment (Fig. 1) which was co-linear with tgEPO4 at its 3′ end but contained an additional 6 kb of 5′-FS. Eight lines showed inducible expression in the liver and no expression in any other tissue including kidney. The mean hematocrit for tgEPO10 mice from these 8 lines was 56%. These results indicated that a negative regulatory element was located in the 6 kb Bam HI-Hind III fragment, which functioned to restrict EPO gene expression to liver and kidney [21].

Eight lines of mice transgenic for tgEPO18, an 18 kb Eco RI fragment that contained an additional 8 kb of 5'-FS relative to tgEPO10, were generated next (Fig. 1). Seven lines expressed the transgene, and these tgEPO18 mice had a mean hematocrit of 80%. Human EPO RNA levels were induced by anemia or hypoxia in both liver and kidney. The levels of human and mouse EPO RNA in transgenic mouse kidney were equivalent as determined by RNA blot-hybridization and ribonuclease-protection assays. In situ hybridization of renal cortex from tgEPO18 mice demonstrated human EPO RNA within the same peritubular interstitial cell type found to contain mouse EPO RNA. These results indicated that sequences necessary for cell type–specific and hypoxia-inducible expression of the human EPO gene in kidney are located 6–14 kb 5' to the transcription-initiation site [19].

Human EPO RNA levels in the livers of anemic tgEPO4, tgEPO10, and tgEPO18 mice were greater than the endogenous mouse EPO RNA levels by at least an order of magnitude. This increased level of expression allowed us to demonstrate by in situ hybridization that hepatic EPO RNA production in anemic mice occurs in a striking perivenous distribution [23]. Thus, even within a single cell type (hepatocytes), EPO RNA expression is specific to certain anatomical locations. The high level of human EPO RNA suggested that if EPO gene expression is down-regulated at birth (as is the case for many genes expressed in fetal liver, e.g., alpha-fetoprotein [24]), then the high level of transgene expression in adult liver might be due to the absence of *cis*-acting DNA sequences involved in postnatal hepatic EPO gene expression. To test this hypothesis, we generated 5 lines of mice transgenic for tgEPO22, which, compared to tgEPO18, included an additional 2.5 kb of 5'-FS and 1.5 kb of 3'-FS (not shown). Four lines of tgEPO22 mice expressed the transgene, which was hypoxia-inducible in liver and kidney to the same degree as tgEPO18. These results [19] suggest that if *cis*-acting sequences that repress hepatic EPO gene expression do exist, they are located quite far from the gene. An alternative explanation is that critical differences exist between humans and mice in the regulation of hepatic EPO gene expression that result in the supranormal level of human EPO gene expression in transgenic mice.

RNA blot hybridization experiments detected human EPO RNA only in liver and kidney of tgEPO18 and tgEPO22 mice. To investigate the possibility of transgene expression at lower levels in other tissues, a more sensitive ribonuclease-protection assay was employed. RNA samples from multiple tissues of transgenic mice from several tgEPO18 and tgEPO22 lines were analyzed with an antisense RNA probe specific for human EPO RNA. Several interesting observations were made from analysis of these lines (G. L. Semenza, un-published data):

1. Low levels of human EPO RNA were detected in brain, lung, testes, and thymus from transgenic mice of all lines tested.
2. In all 3 lines tested, human EPO RNA levels were greater in nonanemic than anemic lung.
3. Transgene expression was detected in spleen from 4 to 6 tgEPO18 lines but 0 of 5 tgEPO22 lines tested.

Using 250 μg of total RNA in ribonuclease-protection assays, EPO RNA has been detected in rat lung and spleen [8]; investigations of EPO gene expression in rodent brain, testes, and thymus have not been reported. Tumors of the brain (cerebellar hemangioblastoma), testes (germ cell line), and hematopoietic cells (erythroleukemia) have been reported to produce human EPO [25–28]. The presence of human EPO RNA in lung and spleen (and possibly brain, testes, and thymus) of transgenic mice may thus reflect physiological EPO gene expression. As a whole, our analysis of human EPO gene expression in transgenic mice has demonstrated that the utilization of multiple *cis*-acting regulatory elements al-lows the human EPO gene to achieve cell type-specific expression in liver and kidney which is modulated by oxygen tension.

Identification of a Hypoxia-Inducible Enhancer Element in the Human EPO Gene 3′-Flanking Sequence

The analysis of transgenic mice indicated that tgEPO4 contained DNA sequences necessary and sufficient for hypoxia-inducible EPO gene expression in liver [21, 22]. In order to identify important regulatory sequences within this 4 kb sequence, we isolated nuclei from liver, kidney, brain, and spleen of tgEPO10 mice, which express the transgene only in liver. Liver-specific DNase I–hypersensitive sites were identified in the 3′-FS of the human EPO transgene [16]. To determine whether these sequences were involved in liver-specific EPO gene expression, a 256-nucleotide (nt) fragment of 3′-FS that spanned the hypersensitive sites was cloned in either orientation 3′ to a reporter gene consist-ing of the SV40 basal promoter, *E. coli* chloramphenicol acetyltransferase coding sequences, and SV40 splice and polyadenylation signals. Recombinant plasmids were transfected into Hep 3B cells in which expression of the en-dogenous EPO gene can be induced by culturing the cells in 1% O_2. Duplicate plates of transfected cells were incubated for 48 h in 1% vs. 20% O_2, cell lysates were prepared, and CAT protein quantitated. The 256-nt EPO gene 3'-FS functioned as a hypoxia-inducible enhancer, as CAT expression was increased 5-fold in hypoxic compared to nonhypoxic cells [16, 20].

We then tested 9 different DNA sequences from within this 256-nt region and identified a 50-nt sequence which mediated 7-fold transcriptional induction in response to hypoxia [20]. Nucleotides 1–33 of this hypoxia-inducible enhancer mediated 7-fold induction of reporter gene expression when present in two tandem copies compared to 3-fold induction when present in a single copy, suggesting that nt 34–50 function to amplify the induction signal. This hypothesis was supported by the observation that a factor present in nuclear extracts from nonhypoxic and hypoxic Hep 3B cells protected nt 26–48 from digestion in DNase I footprinting studies. The sequence of nt 30–43 on the antisense strand is 5'-AGGTCGAGAGGTCA-3', which contains imperfect and perfect repeats of AGGTCA. Direct repeats of this consensus sequence separated by 1–5 nt function as selective response elements for members of the steroid-thyroid hormone receptor superfamily [29, 30], suggesting that binding of one of these transcription factors may be responsible for the DNase I footprint generated by Hep 3B nuclear extracts.

Identification of Hypoxia-Inducible Factor 1

Scanning-mutagenesis studies of the nt 1–33 sequence revealed that nt 4–12 and nt 19–23 were essential for induction, as mutations at either site eliminated hypoxia-inducible expression. Electrophoretic mobility-shift assays identified two nuclear factors which bound to a probe spanning nt 1–18 but not to a probe containing a nt 7–9 mutation which eliminated enhancer function. Binding of one factor to nt 1–18 was observed when either hypoxic or nonhypoxic Hep 3B nuclear extracts were assayed. Binding of the other factor was observed only when nuclear extracts from hypoxic Hep 3B cells were assayed. The hypoxic induction of this DNA-binding activity was blocked by treatment of cells with cycloheximide, a protein synthesis inhibitor previously shown to block hypoxic induction of EPO RNA in Hep 3B cells [13]. We have designated this DNA-binding activity hypoxia-inducible factor 1 (HIF-1). Nucleotides 1–13, which span the HIF-1–binding site (Fig. 2), are completely conserved in the homologous mouse EPO gene enhancer [18], supporting the hypothesis that HIF-1 binding is crucial for hypoxic activation of EPO gene transcription. We have not detected the binding of any hypoxia-inducible factors to nt 19–23. The binding conditions utilized may not have allowed detection of a hypoxia-inducible factor,

GAACTGAAACCACCAATATGACTCTTGGCTTTTTCTGTTTTCTGGGAACCTC

CAAATCCCCTGGCTCTGTCCCACTCCTGGCAGCAGTGCAGCAGGTCCAGGT

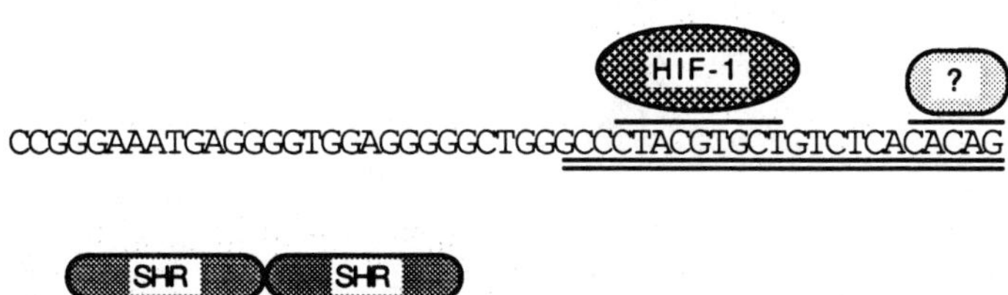

CCGGGAAATGAGGGGTGGAGGGGGCTGGGCCCTACGTGCTGTCTCACACAG

CCTGTCTGACCTCTCGACCTACCGGCCTAGGCCACAAGCTCTGCCTACGCT

GGTCAATAAGGTGTCTCCATTCAAGGCCTCACCGCAGTAAGGCAGCTGCCAA

Fig. 2. Identification of a 50-nucleotide hypoxia-inducible enhancer element in the human EPO gene 3'-flanking sequence. The 256-nt sequence first shown to function as a hypoxia-inducible enhancer [16] is shown. Underlined A, adenine residue which serves as the EPO RNA polyadenylation site [31]; underline, 50-nt sequence shown by deletion analysis to be the minimal hypoxia-inducible enhancer [20]; double underline, 33-nt sequence which, when present in two tandem copies, provides a degree of hypoxia inducibility equal to that of the 50-nt sequence; overline, binding sites for the indicated transcription factors, based upon transient-expression functional studies and protein-DNA binding assays [20]. HIF-1, hypoxia-inducible factor 1; SHR, steroid-hormone receptor superfamily member; ?, unknown.

or, alternatively, this sequence may bind a constitutive factor necessary for interaction of HIF-1 with the transcription-initiation complex. These transient-expression and DNA-binding studies [20] thus define a 50-nucleotide, functionally tripartite, hypoxia-inducible enhancer which binds several nuclear factors, one of which is induced by hypoxia via de novo protein synthesis.

References

1   Beru N, McDonald, J, Lacombe C, Goldwasser E: Expression of the erythropoietin gene. Mol Cell Biol 1986;6:2571–2575.

2   Bondurant MC, Koury MJ: Anemia induces accumulation of erythropoietin mRNA in the kidney and liver. Mol Cell Biol 1986;6:524–527.

3   Schuster SJ, Wilson JH, Erslev AJ, Caro J: Physiologic regulation and tissue localization of renal erythropoietin messenger RNA. Blood 1987;70:316–318.

4   Koury MJ, Bondurant MC, Graber SE, Sawyer ST: Erythropoietin messenger RNA levels in developing mice and transfer of ^{125}I-erythropoietin by the placenta. J Clin Invest 1988;82:154–159.

5   Koury ST, Bondurant MC, Koury MJ: Localization of erythropoietin synthesizing cells in murine kidneys by in situ hybridization. Blood 1988;71:524–527.

6   Schuster SJ, Badiavas EV, Costa-Giomi P, Weinmann R, Erslev AJ, Caro J: Stimulation of erythropoietin gene transcription during hypoxia and cobalt exposure. Blood 1989;73:13–16.

7   Ratcliffe PJ, Jones RW, Phillips RE, Nicholls LG, Bell JI: Oxygen-dependent modulation of erythropoietin mRNA levels in isolated rat kidneys studied by RNase protection. J Exp Med 1990;172:657–660.

8   Tan CC, Eckardt K-U, Ratcliffe PJ: Organ distribution of erythropoietin messenger RNA in normal and uremic rats. Kidney Int 1991;40:69–76.

9   Schuster SJ, Koury ST, Bohrer M, Salceda S, Caro J: Cellular sites of extrarenal and renal erythropoietin production in anaemic rats. Br J Haematol 1992;81:153–159.

10 Eckardt K-U, Ratcliffe PJ, Tan CC, Bauer C, Kurtz A: Age-dependent expression of the erythropoietin gene in rat liver and kidneys. J Clin Invest 1992;89:753–760.

11 Eschbach JW, Egrie JC, Downing MR, Browne JK, Adamson JW: Correction of the anemia of end-stage renal disease with recombinant human erythropoietin. N Engl J Med 1987;316:73–78.

12 Goldberg MA, Glass GA, Cunningham JM, Bunn HF: The regulated expression of erythropoietin by two human hepatoma cell lines. Proc Natl Acad Sci USA 1987;84:7972–7976.

13 Goldberg MA, Dunning SP, Bunn HF: Regulation of the erythropoietin gene: Evidence that the oxygen sensor is a heme protein. Science 1988;242:1412–1415.

14 Costa-Giomi P, Caro J, Weinmann R: Enhancement by hypoxia of human erythropoietin gene transcription *in vitro*. J Biol Chem 1990;265:10185–10188.

15 Goldberg MA, Gaut CC, Bunn HF: Erythropoietin mRNA levels are governed by both the rate of gene transcription and posttranscriptional events. Blood 1991;77:271–277.

16 Semenza GL, Nejfelt MK, Chi SM, Antonarakis SE: Hypoxia-inducible nuclear factors bind to an enhancer element located 3′ to the human erythropoietin gene. Proc Natl Acad Sci USA 1991;88:5680–5684.

17 Beck I, Ramirez S, Weinmann R, Caro J: Enhancer element at the 3′-flanking region controls transcriptional response to hypoxia in the human erythropoietin gene. J Biol Chem 1991;266:15563–15566.

18 Pugh CW, Tan CC, Jones RW, Ratcliffe PJ: Functional analysis of an oxygen-regulated transcriptional enhancer lying 3′ to the mouse erythropoietin gene. Proc Natl Acad Sci USA 1991;88:10553–10557.

19 Semenza GL, Koury ST, Nejfelt MK, Gearhart JD, Antonarakis SE: Cell type-specific and hypoxia-inducible expression of the human erythropoietin gene in transgenic mice. Proc Natl Acad Sci USA 1991;88:8725–8729.

20 Semenza GL, Wang GL: A nuclear factor induced by hypoxia via de novo protein synthesis binds to the human erythropoietin gene enhancer at a site required for transcriptional activation. Mol Cell Biol 1992;12:5447–5454.

21 Semenza GL, Dureza RD, Traystman MD, Gearhart JD, Antonarakis SE: Human erythropoietin gene expression in transgenic mice: Multiple transcription initiation sites and cis-acting regulatory elements. Mol Cell Biol 1990;10:930–938.

22 Semenza GL, Traystman MD, Gearhart JD, Antonarakis SE: Polycythemia in transgenic mice expressing the human erythropoietin gene. Proc Natl Acad Sci USA 1989;86:2301–2305.

23 Koury ST, Bondurant MC, Koury MJ, Semenza GL: Localization of cells producing erythropoietin in murine liver by in situ hybridization. Blood 1991;77:2497–2503.

24 Vacher J, Tilghman SM: Dominant negative regulation of the mouse α-fetoprotein gene in adult liver. Science 1990;250:1732–1735.

25 Trimble M, Caro J, Talalla A, Brain M: Secondary erythrocytosis due to a cerebellar hemangioblastoma: demonstration of erythropoietin mRNA in the tumor. Blood 1991;78:599–601.

26 Ascensao JL, Gaylis F, Bronson D, Fraley EE, Zanjani ED: Erythropoietin production by a human testicular germ cell line. Blood 1983;62:1132–1134.

27 Hankins WD, Schooley J, Eastment C: Erythropoietin, an autocrine regulator? Serum-free production of erythropoietin by cloned erythroid cell lines. Blood 1986;68:263–268.

28 Mitjavila M-T, Le Couedic J-P, Casadevall N, Navarro S, Villeval J-L, Dubart A, Vainchenker W: Autocrine stimulation by erythropoietin and autonomous growth of human erythroid leukemic cells in vitro. J Clin Invest 1991;88:789–797.

29 Naar AM, Boutin J-M, Lipkin SM, Yu VC, Holloway JM, Glass CK, Rosenfeld MG: The orientation and spacing of core DNA-binding motifs dictate selective transcriptional responses to three nuclear receptors. Cell 1991;65:1267–1279.

30 Umesono K, Murakami KM, Thompson CC, Evans RM: Direct repeats as selective responsive elements for the thyroid hormone, retinoic acid, and vitamin D_3 receptors. Cell 1991;65:1255–1266.

31 Jacobs K, Shoemaker C, Rudersdorf R, Neill SD, Kaufman RJ, Mufson A, Seehra J, Jones SS, Hewick R, Fritsch EF, Kawakita M, Shimizu T, Miyake T: Isolation and characterization of genomic and cDNA clones of human erythropoietin. Nature 1985;313:806–810.

Gregg L. Semenza, MD, PhD, Pediatric Genetics Unit, CMSC-1004, The Johns Hopkins Hospital, 600 N. Wolfe Street, Baltimore, MD 21205 (USA)

Discussion

to the Paper by G. L. Semenza

Gassmann (Zurich): All your transgenic animals contained the 3′ enhancer sequences as you showed us. I wonder if you ever tried to generate transgenic mice by DNA microinjection using an EPO construct lacking this enhancer?

Semenza: The prediction would be that those mice would not express the gene. The problem is that often transgenes are not expressed in the mice. For example, for the constructs that I showed you we would make anywhere from 5 to 10 lines and most of them would express the genes but some of them would not—probably because the site in which the gene had integrated, which is believed to be random, was a site from which it could not be expressed. You never know if a negative result is just because of where the transgene integrated or because you don't have the right sequences, and that's why it is important to do a number of independent lines to show that your results are reproducible. We could do that, but these experiments are extremely time-consuming and expensive, and to get a negative result I guess was not fullfilling enough for me to want to do. But that is the result we would expect to get. Another problem is: All the lines that we looked at had that 3′ element, including the lines that expressed the gene in the kidney. And one question is whether expression in the kidney requires the 3′ element or whether the element in the far 5′ flanking sequence by itself is sufficient for expression in the kidney. We don't have the answer to that question either. One of the problems with studying expression in the kidney is that there is no cell line derived from the kidney that shows regulated expression of the EPO gene and that's why it is necessary to do these very laborious experiments in transgenic mice, whereas for the characterization of the 3′ enhancer we could proceed rapidly in the tissue-culture model.

Rich (Ulm): Do you know if the HIF-1 is a heme-protein?

Semenza: No, we don't.

Fandrey (Bonn): I would like to comment and ask a question: By competitive PCR we could confirm that the EPO gene is expressed in the lung and the spleen and it amounts to about 1% of the total EPO RNA in these animals. These animals were made anemic by phenylhydrazine injection. What we could not find is this decrease by anemia in the lung; actually the signal was barely detectable in animals with normal hematocrit and it was increased by severe anemia. The same is true for the spleen. My question would be: Have you checked the bone marrow for any signs of expression of EPO gene?

Semenza: No, we have not done ribonuclease protection assays using bone marrow. I believe we have attempted experiments by in situ hybridization and those have not given a positive result.

Goldwasser (*Chicago*): Perhaps I can answer part of that question: We have detected EPO message in normal bone marrow by PCR and published it. The other thing I like to comment on is this question of inappropriate expression in tissues where we do not expect it. I think we may have to rethink all of that because, similar to the case of bone marrow, we have found it in normal brain of unstimulated animals.

Semenza: I would just make the point that expression of the first construct was inappropriate as the message was of the wrong size and it did not seem to be regulated, whereas in later data I showed low-level expression which may be physiological. But clearly much more work needs to be done on that.

Inducible Operation of the Erythropoietin 3′ Enhancer in Different Cell Lines

Evidence for a Widespread Oxygen-Sensing Mechanism
in Mammalian Cells

C. W. Pugh, P. H. Maxwell, L. G. Nicholls, O. Ebrahim,
S. M. Bartlett, P. J. Ratcliffe

Institute of Molecular Medicine, John Radcliffe Hospital, Headington,
Oxford, England

In response to severe hypoxic stimulation, levels of circulating erythropoietin can increase approximately 1000-fold [1]. This is achieved by changes in hormone production rates, which appear to be regulated principally through modulation of the level of EPO mRNA, produced by a restricted population of cells within kidney and liver [2–4]. The rapid, high amplitude induction of gene expression by an important physiological stimulus such as hypoxia has attracted interest in the regulation of erythropoietin as an example of tissue-specific and inducible gene expression.

In this paper we describe the definition of a regulatory *cis*-acting sequence lying 3′ to the erythropoietin gene and provide evidence that the oxygen-sensing system that interacts with this regulatory sequence is much more widespread than has been previously recognized.

Definition of an Oxygen-Dependent Transcriptional Enhancer Lying 3′ to the EPO Gene

Using transient transfection assays in the hepatoma cell lines Hep 3B or Hep G2, several groups including our own have recently defined a DNA sequence located approximately 120 base pairs 3′ to the poly A addition site which conveys oxygen-regulated expression on a variety of heterologous promoters [5–7].

"

Our strategy in these experiments was to couple sequence derived from the mouse erythropoietin gene to a human α_1 globin reporter gene. Recombinant plasmids containing these constructs were introduced into Hep G2 or Hep 3B cells by electroporation. After electroporation, cells were divided for parallel normoxic (21% oxygen) and hypoxic (1% oxygen) incubations. Transcripts from the α_1 globin reporter gene and co-transfected control plasmid were assayed by RNase protection. Mouse erythropoietin sequence conveyed oxygen-dependent expression on the α_1 globin gene, and an initial series of deletions localized the activity within a 123 base pair (bp) Apa I–Pvu II restriction fragment lying 3′ to the erythropoietin gene. In keeping with a functional role in erythropoietin gene regulation, this region is highly conserved between mouse and human (Fig. 1).

```
                                       polyA
MOUSE   CTGGCAACAG  CTGAAATCAC  CAACCAGACT   CCTGGCTTGT   CTCTCTTCAT
MAN     tTGaCAAgAa  CTGAAAcCAC  CAAtatGACT   CtTGGCTTtT   CTgTtTTC..


MOUSE   GACTGTACAC  ACCACACAAC  TCTCCTAGCT   GTACCTCACC   CCATCTGGTC
MAN     ..........  ..........  ..........   ..........   ..........

                                                         1 ApaI
MOUSE   GCAAGGCATC  AGATCTGGGA  AACCAGAGGT   GGAGGGGGTT   GGGCCCTACG
MAN     .........C  AGgTCcGGGA  AAtgAGgGGT   GGAGGGGGcT   GGGCCCTACG

        10          20          30           40           50
MOUSE   TGCTGCCTCG  CATGGCCCGG  CTGACCTCTT   GACCCCTCTG   GGCTTGAGGC
MAN     TGCTGtCTCa  CAcaGCCtGt  CTGACCTCTc   GACC taCcG   G CcT AGGC

        60          70          80           90           100
MOUSE   CACAATACCT  GCCCACGCTA  GTCAATAAGC   AGGCTCCATT   CAAGGCTGTC
MAN     CACAAgctCT  GCCtACGCTg  GTCAATAAGg   tGtCTCCATT   CAAGGCctca

        110         PvuII
MOUSE   TCTCAGTGGG  CAGCT
MAN     cCgCAG
```

Fig. 1.   Comparison of the human and mouse DNA sequence at the 3′ end of the erythropoietin gene. In each case the active enhancer sequence is lying approximately 120 bp 3′ to the poly A addition site (underlined). Sequence conservation is approximately 85% within the functionally defined enhancer, although the best alignment is achieved by making gaps as shown in the human sequence. The mouse sequence in this region has been numbered from the Apa I site to facilitate description of constructs containing parts of this sequence. Homology is also observed beyond the limits of enhancer activity defined in transiently transfected cells. The human sequence is represented by a dotted line in the area where no significant homology was found.

Using the polymerase chain reaction, successive deletions were generated within this area. Transfection assays using these constructs defined an area of approximately 70 bp, which was necessary and sufficient for full enhancer activity when the sequence was placed 1.5 kb 5′ to the α_1 globin promoter (Fig. 2). Deletions at the 5′ end of this sequence led to rapid loss of activity, whereas deletions at the 3′ end led to a more gradual reduction in activity. Indeed the 3′ portion of these sequences was not obligatory for mediation of hypoxic induction, since reiteration of the first 60 bp restored activity on the distant α_1 globin promoter, and in other systems shorter sequences from the 5′ end of this region were active.

When end-labeled DNA probes that included the functional enhancer were incubated with nuclear protein extract prepared from Hep G2 cells, protection

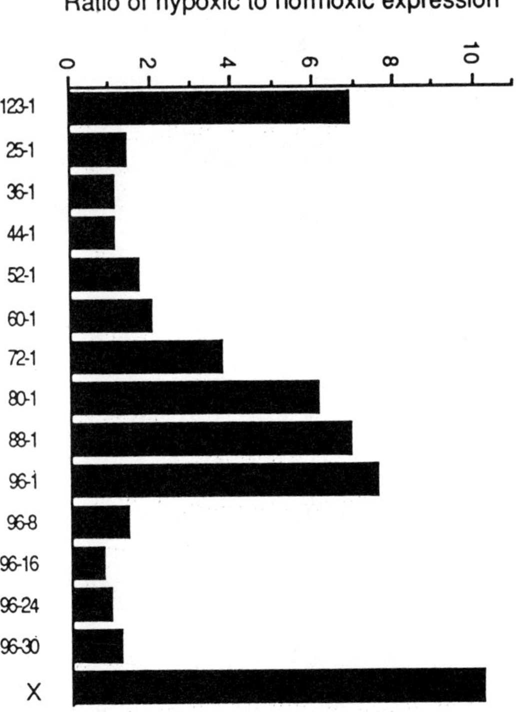

Fig. 2. Activity of constructs containing portions of the mouse erythropoietin 3′ enhancer lying 1.5 kb 5′ to an α_1 globin reporter gene. Nucleotides are numbered from the Apa I site at the 5′ end of the enhancer. The bars show the ratio of hypoxic to normoxic expression of the α_1 globin reporter after transfection into Hep G2 cells. Construct X contains two copies of nucleotides 1–60 separated by a 67 bp polylinker spacer.

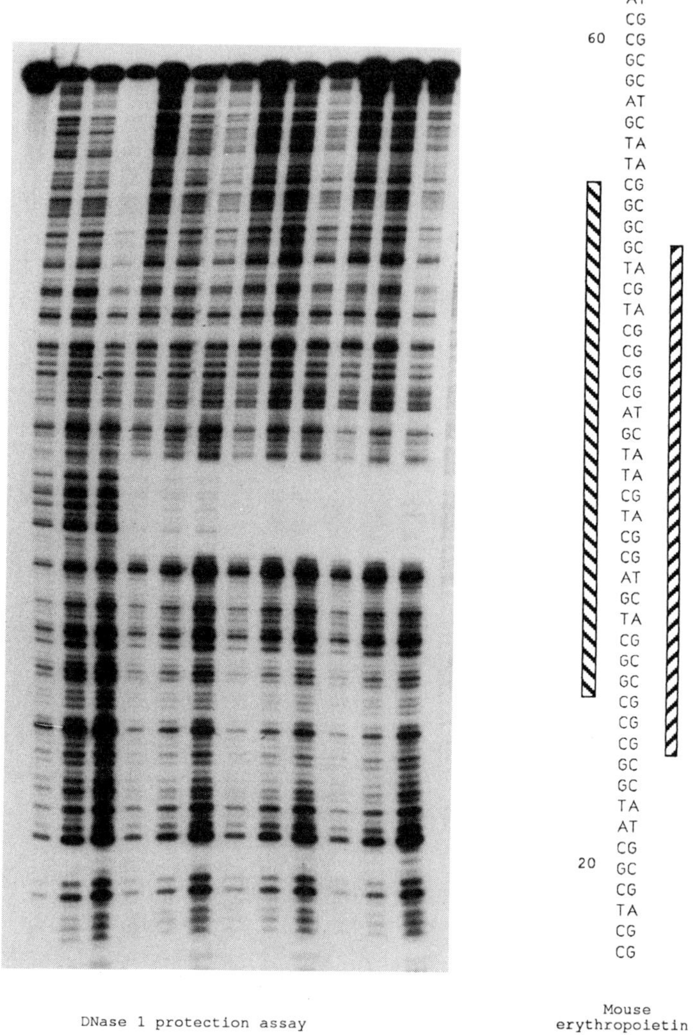

Fig. 3. An end-labeled DNA fragment containing the mouse erythropoietin 3′ enhancer was subjected to titrated digestion with DNase I. Addition of increasing amounts of nuclear extract from Hep G2 cells (last 9 lanes) resulted in protection of a stretch of DNA. The sequence corresponding to the protected fragment on the two strands is indicated by the striped bands.

from DNase I digestion was observed within the enhancer (Fig. 3). However, the most clear-cut protection was confined to the central portion of the enhancer. Bases 28–53 were protected on the 5′ strand, and bases 25–50 were protected on the 3′ strand. Similar protection patterns were observed when nuclear proteins were prepared from normoxic and hypoxic Hep G2. Since additional sequence 5′ to the footprint was required for enhancer function, it is possible that more labile binding species that interact with the 5′ region of the enhancer were not detected in these DNase I protection assays. It is equally possible that proteins bound to the protected area undergo secondary modification in hypoxia that does not alter the footprint or that Hep G2 cells, which do produce erythropoietin when incubated at 21% O_2, show some constitutive operation of this enhancer.

Oxygen-Dependent Operation of the EPO 3′ Enhancer in Many Mammalian Cell Lines

Since hypoxia induces diverse changes in gene expression in different tissues, we considered the possibility that despite tightly restricted expression of the EPO gene itself, the oxygen-sensing mechanism might be widespread. To address this question we transiently transfected multiple cell lines with recombinant plasmids containing the EPO 3′ enhancer linked to the α_1 globin reporter gene. To obtain a clear distinction of enhancer action from any other effect of hypoxia on transcript accumulation, tranfections using plasmids with or without the EPO 3′ enhancer were performed on aliquots of cells from the same pool. Cell lines tested are shown in Table 1. Hypoxic induction via the EPO 3′ enhancer was reproducibly demonstrated in all these cell lines, with the exception of MEL (mouse erythroleukemia cells). Figure 4 shows examples of transfection experiments for Hep 3B (human hepatoma), U937 (human monocyte/macrophage), MRC 5 (human fetal lung), 1BR3 (human skin fibroblast), and K1 (chinese hamster ovary). The range of cells chosen in these experiments included several not known to make EPO and several derived from organs that do not contribute importantly to EPO production in vivo.

Thus, hypoxia-inducible activity of the EPO 3′ enhancer was observed much more extensively than native gene expression [8], strongly suggesting that a physiologically relevant component of the oxygen-sensing mechanism operates widely in mammalian cells, most probably serving other purposes as well. Nuclear extracts from these cells contain proteins that bind to the EPO 3′ enhancer. Whether the nuclear protein complex is identical is the subject of continuing DNA-binding experiments. Although clear evidence of hypoxia-

Table 1.   Cell lines used in transfection experiments

Hep 3B	Human hepatoma
Hep G2	Human hepatoma
1BR3	Human skin fibroblast
MRC 5	Human fetal lung fibroblast
U937	Human monocyte/macrophage
COS 1	African green monkey renal fibroblast
COS 7	African green monkey renal fibroblast
LLC-PK1	Porcine renal epithelium
BACE	Bovine adrenal capillary endothelium
FAZA	Rat hepatoma
NRK 49F	Rat renal fibroblast
NRK 52E	Rat renal epithelium
RAEC	Rat aortic endothelium
MEL 585	Murine erythroleukemia
MEL 707	Murine erythroleukemia
RAG	Murine renal adenocarcinoma
WOP	Murine polyoma-transformed fibroblast
a23	Chinese hamster lung fibroblast
K1	Chinese hamster ovarian fibroblast

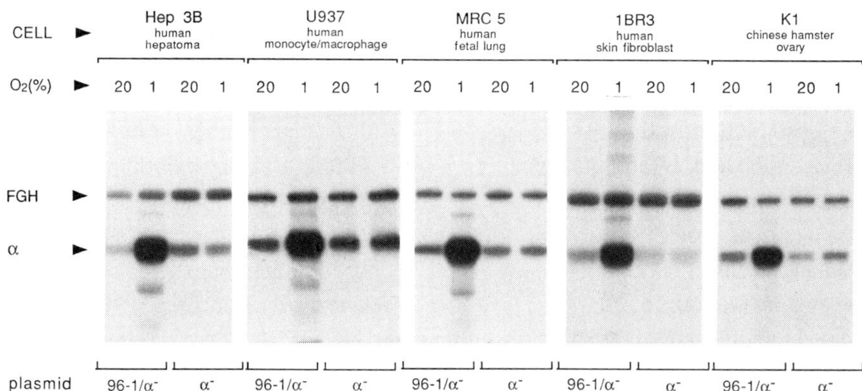

Fig. 4.   Ribonuclease protection assays of transcripts from reporter (α) and control (FGH) plasmids following normoxic and hypoxic incubation of transiently transfected cell lines. The lines used and the tissues of origin are as indicated. Alternate lanes are from normoxic and hypoxic cells. In each panel the first pair of lanes shows the results when the test plasmid contained 96 base pairs of the EPO 3' enhancer coupled to the reporter gene (96-1/α^-). The enhancer was absent from the plasmid in the second pair of lanes (α^-). Enhancer activity inducible by hypoxia was observed in all these cell lines.

inducible enhancer activity was observed, activity did vary between cell lines and in some was strongly dependent on cell density. Differences in inducibility may be intrinsic or may arise from differences in effective oxygenation with the oxygen consumption of cells at differing densities providing an important contribution to the creation of the hypoxic microenvironment.

Nevertheless, since we were unable to show inducible enhancer action in MEL cells despite extensive study of different conditions, the oxygen-sensing response does not appear to be universal in mammalian cells. Consistent with this are the findings of Beck et al. [5], who did not observe hypoxic induction of a human EPO minigene construct containing the human EPO 3′ enhancer in HeLa cells. Our previous report that the oxygen-sensing property was not seen in CHO cells [7] appears to be in error and most likely arose from the use of low cell densities in those experiments. In ongoing experiments we are testing the operation of this enhancer in more primitive eukaryotic cells. To date we have not been able to observe inducible operation of this element in *Saccharomyces cerevisiae*.

*Physiological Characteristics of EPO 3′ Enhancer Action
in the Chinese Hamster Lung Fibroblastoid Cell Line a23*

To further characterize the oxygen-sensing system interacting with the transfected EPO enhancer in cells that did not produce EPO, we performed additional experiments on the chinese hamster lung fibroblastoid line a23. In three important respects the response is identical to that governing physiological EPO production in liver and kidney. The response is activated by cobalt but not by cyanide and is abrogated by cycloheximide [9–13]. Although heat shock transcriptional induction mechanisms operate widely and anoxic exposure can activate heat shock transcription factor [14], the widespread operation of oxygen sensing we are describing appears to be quite distinct. Hypoxia at the severity used to activate the EPO 3′ enhancer in our system does not induce Hsp72, and heat does not activate the EPO 3′ enhancer.

Thus, these experiments provide strong evidence for the widespread operation in mammalian cells of a distinct oxygen-sensing system similar or identical to that controlling native EPO gene expression. For other systems, such as steroid-mediated gene expression, tissue-specific repressive influences allow only a small complement of the total number of genes bearing glucocorticoid response elements to be expressed in any one cell type [15]. In our view, it is very likely that this oxygen-sensing system acts on other genes in cells that are not specialized for the production of EPO.

Acknowledgments

This work was supported by the Wellcome Trust, the Medical Research Council (UK) (Fellowships to CWP and PHM), and the Barnes Trust (Fellowship to OE).

References

1　Jelkmann W: Erythropoietin: Structure, control of production, and function. Physiol Rev 1992;72:449–489.

2　Koury ST, Bondurant MC, Koury MJ: Localization of erythropoietin synthesizing cells in murine kidneys by *in situ* hybridization. Blood 1988;71:524–527.

3　Lacombe C, Da Silva J-L, Bruneval P, Fournier J-G, Wendling F, Casadevall N, Camilleri J-P, Bariety J, Varet B, Tambourin P: Peritubular cells are the site of erythropoietin synthesis in the murine hypoxic kidney. J Clin Invest 1988;81:620–623.

4　Koury ST, Bondurant MC, Koury MJ, Semenza GL: Localization of cells producing erythropoietin in murine liver by *in situ* hybridization. Blood 1991;77:2497–2503.

5　Beck I, Ramirez S, Weinmann R, Caro J: Enhancer element at the 3′-flanking region controls transcriptional response to hypoxia in the human erythropoietin gene. J Biol Chem 1991;266:15563–15566.

6　Semenza GL, Nejfelt MK, Chi SM, Antonarakis SE: Hypoxia-inducible nuclear factors bind to an enhancer element located 3′ to the human epo gene. Proc Natl Acad Sci USA 1991;88:5680–5684.

7　Pugh C, Tan CC, Jones RW, Ratcliffe PJ: Functional analysis of an oxygen-regulated transcriptional enhancer lying 3′ to the mouse Epo gene. Proc Natl Acad Sci USA 1991;88:10553–10557.

8　Tan CC, Eckardt K-U, Ratcliffe PJ: Organ distribution of erythropoietin messenger RNA in normal and uremic rats. Kidney Int 1991;40:69–76.

9　Goldberg MA, Glass GA, Cunningham JM, Bunn HF: The regulated expression of epo by two human hepatoma cell lines. Proc Natl Acad Sci USA 1987;84:7972–7976.

10　Goldberg MA, Dunning SP, Bunn HF: Regulation of the erythropoietin gene: Evidence that the oxygen sensor is a heme protein. Science 1988;242:1412–1415.

11　Beru N, McDonald J, Lacombe C, Goldwasser E: Expression of the erythropoietin gene. Mol Cell Biol 1986;6:2571–2575.

12　Necas E, Thorling EB: Unresponsiveness of erythropoietin–producing cells to cyanide. Am J Physiol 1972;222:1187–1190.

13　Tan CC, Ratcliffe PJ: Effects of inhibitors of oxidative phosphorylation on erythropoietin mRNA in isolated perfused rat kidneys. Am J Physiol 1991;261:F982–F987.

14　Benjamin IJ, Kroger B, Williams RS: Activation of heat shock transcription factor by hypoxia in mammalian cells. Proc Natl Acad Sci USA 1990;87:6263–6267.

15　O'Malley BW: Steroid hormone action in eucaryotic cells. J Clin Invest 1984;74:307–312.

Peter J. Ratcliffe, Room 420, Institute of Molecular Medicine, John Radcliffe Hospital, Headington, Oxford OX3 9DU, England

Discussion

to the Paper by C. W. Pugh et al.

Kurtz (Regensburg): Peter, if I try to bring yours and Gregg's findings together, would that mean that this hypoxia-inducible factor mentioned by Gregg is also expressed in cells or produced by cells which do not express the EPO gene?

Ratcliffe: We have not looked at Gregg's factor but we have looked quite extensively with footprints and retards. There are similarities in the binding of proteins by this sequence in other cells. In our provisional results they don't appear to be identical but we haven't specifically looked at the factor that Gregg has defined.

Semenza (Baltimore): Those experiments are in progress as we speak in my laboratory. Peter, I wanted to ask you about the results of the experiments at different cell densities. How do you explain those results?

Ratcliffe: One possibility is that this is an effect of cell oxygen consumption on the hypoxic microenvironment in tissue culture. In cells cultured in 1% oxygen there could be quite a variable oxygen concentration at the site of sensing, and the fact that we have an interaction between density and oxygen concentration might support that. But I think there are a great many other possible explanations for this. As you will know from the hepatoma cell work, people culture these cells in a rather particular way; they need to be healthy to optimize the response to hypoxia. I think there are a lot of permissive aspects of the way the cells are growing that allow this response to occur and I think they may be rather different in different cell types. That is why we initially made the reverse conclusion that we thought oxygen sensing was specific for hepatoma cells.

Fandrey (Bonn): I'd like to comment on the oxygen consumption or the availability of oxygen to cells in culture. We have measured the oxygen tension in the cell layer in these hepatoma cells and if you culture them under normal conditions and put them in ambient air—20.9% oxygen—within 1 hour you have an oxygen tension which is less than 1 mm Hg under what we called normal oxygen conditions. So I think we have to be very careful if we really try to compare normoxic and hypoxic cells and, regarding the oxygen consumption, these hepatoma cells—both lines—normally have a quite high oxygen consumption, which is about 8 nmol/mg of protein per minute. This oxygen consumption if you culture the cells is reduced to less than 50% within 3 days. So the cells cultured for several days might totally change their behavior and production of proteins.

Caro (Philadelphia): First, a comment regarding Dr. Kurtz's questions about the presence of this inducible factor that Dr. Semenza commented about. We have found a very similar, probably the very same, factor induced by hypoxia in Hep 3B cells which is also inducible in other hepatoma cell lines. I also have a question to you. All the cell lines that you mentioned, are they all fibroblastoid cell lines or are there parenchymal cell lines too?

Ratcliffe: No, they are not all fibroblast cells; the U937 cells are not and the LLC-PKI are of course a pig kidney epithelial line. The RAC is a mouse renal adenocarcinoma line, so although quite a few were fibroblastoid, they are not all.

Goldwasser (Chicago): I have two short questions: With regard to the concentration experiments, when you indicated the concentration of 1.0 before dilution, are those confluent cells?

Ratcliffe: In general we have used high cell densities. As for the U937 cells, they are not adherent cells; we have grown them to higher densities than are normally recommended. In the adherent cell lines we would see good responses if the cells were approaching confluence when we harvested them the morning after transfection. Obviously there is cell death after transfection, and that is another aspect that I should make clear. If the transfection voltage is very high, you will kill a lot of cells and in our hands there are some cell lines which will show a much reduced hypoxic response in that circumstance.

Goldwasser: The other question with regard to the cell lines or cells which might have a similar kind of hypoxic sensor to Hep 3B: have you done the heme kind of experiments and seen whether you inhibited it with succinylacetone?

Ratcliffe: No, we haven't done those experiments.

DNA/Protein Interactions on the Human Erythropoietin Enhancer

Anthony M. Acquaviva, Kerry L. Blanchard[a]

Brigham and Women's Hospital, Harvard Medical School, Boston, Mass., USA

Introduction

Erythropoietin (EPO) transcription is regulated by oxygen tension in Hep 3B cells, mainly at the level of transcriptional initiation [1, 2]. The rise in EPO mRNA levels induced by perfusion of kidneys with hypoxic fluid in vitro [3] or with anemic blood in vivo [4] is comparable to that of Hep 3B cells subjected to hypoxic stress. The molecular components responsible for the induction of EPO transcription by hypoxia are largely unknown, but the oxygen sensor may involve a heme protein [1]. The EPO promoter is unusual; the basal transcriptional elements present in most type II promoters are absent [5]. Canonical TATA and CAAT boxes are not present, nor are typical upstream activating regions. The promoter is highly GC rich and contains two GATA sites near the transcriptional start site.

The EPO gene has a 3′ enhancer element that confers hypoxia sensitivity on its own and heterologous promoters [6–8]. The promoter also contains elements that respond to hypoxia and that cooperate with the enhancer element to faithfully reproduce the transcriptional induction seen in vivo [9]. The regions of the promoter and enhancer that are essential for the hypoxic induction of EPO transcription contain steroid response elements (SREs), and the enhancer SREs have been shown to be necessary for the hypoxic response. The SREs in the enhancer are configured as 6 bp direct repeats with a 2 bp spacing gap (a DR-2 site) [10]. Kidney and liver extracts from anemic mice have been shown to contain EPO-specific DNA binding factors that are not present in nonanemic mice [6]. Despite extensive analysis, factors from Hep 3B cells that bind to the EPO enhancer in a hypoxia specific manner could not be demonstrated. Instead, factors that interact with the EPO enhancer are present in Hep 3B extracts

[a]*Current affiliation*: Louisiana State University Medical Center, School of Medicine in Shreveport, Shreveport, La., USA

prepared from normoxic and hypoxic cells and in extracts from cells that do not produce EPO. The major protein interactions with the enhancer are centered on the DR-2 site, and mutations in the DR-2 site that interfere with DNA binding likewise destroy the function of the EPO enhancer [10].

We present evidence that protein factors bind to the DR-2 site in the EPO enhancer whether or not the nuclear extracts are prepared from cells producing EPO. The DNA/protein contact points have been examined by methylation interference and the breadth of the contact by DNase I footprinting. The DNA/protein-binding characteristics of factors in extracts from Hep 3B, 293, and HeLa cells are similar, if not identical.

Methods

Cell Culture

Hep 3B, 293, and HeLa cells were grown in α-MEM medium supplemented with 10% defined iron-enriched calf serum and penicillin/streptomycin. Hypoxia (1% oxygen tension) was maintained in an ESPEC triple gas incubator by nitrogen washout. Carbon dioxide was maintained at 5%. Nuclear extracts were prepared as described [11, 12]. For hypoxic extracts the cells were grown in a hypoxic atmosphere for 6 hours. All buffers contained a battery of protease inhibitors and DTT.

Electrophoretic Mobility Shift Assays

Probe DNA was end-labeled on one strand by filling in staggered ends with the Klenow fragment of *E. coli* DNA polymerase I and α-^{32}P-dNTPs. Probe DNA, d(IC), and nuclear extract protein were incubated together in binding buffer for 30 min at room temperature. Electrophoresis was done in 4% polyacrylamide gels in 0.5 X TBE buffer at room temperature. The bromophenyl-blue dye front was allowed to migrate 19 cm. Gels were dried and subjected to autoradiography at $-70°C$.

DNase I Footprinting

EMSA reactions were prepared as described above but were scaled up 8-fold. The reactions were treated with DNase I and 0.5 mM $CaCl_2$ for 2 min at room temperature. The reaction was terminated by adding EGTA. The products were subjected to electrophoresis on EMSA gels, and retarded complexes and free probe were excised from the wet gel. DNA was isolated by electrophoresis onto DEAE membrane and was subjected to electrophoresis in denaturing polyacrylamide gels.

Methylation Interference

Five picomoles of DNA were methylated with dimethysulfate according to Maxam and Gilbert [13]. Preparative EMSAs and DNA isolation were performed as described for DNase I footprinting. The DNA was incubated with 1 *M* piperidine at 90°C for 30 min, purified by lyophilization, and subjected to electrophoresis in denaturing polyacrylamide gels.

The procedures for performing EMSAs, DNase I footprinting, and methylation interference analysis have been described in detail [10].

Results

The shortest fragment of the human EPO enhancer that retains function extends from the Apa I site to the HpaII site approximately 130 bp downstream of the polyadenylation site (E-43). This 43 bp fragment is necessary and sufficient for hypoxia-induced transcriptional activation [10]. A probe containing this region of the EPO enhancer was ^{32}P-end-labeled and incubated with nuclear extract from Hep 3B cells grown under hypoxic conditions. The reactions were subjected to electrophoresis on a native polyacrylamide gel followed by auto-radiography. The major DNA/protein complex migrates as a doublet approximately 50% more slowly than the free probe. The complex represents approximately 20% of the total radioactivity per reaction. To verify the specificity of DNA/protein binding, nonradioactive DNAs were added to some reactions prior to protein addition. The nonradiolabeled DNA fragments consisted of the portion of the EPO enhancer that contains the DR-2 element (E-B), the portion of the promoter that is necessary for hypoxic sensitivity (contains two SREs), and a mutated form of E-B that is missing 4 cytosine residues in the DR-2 site (Fig. 1). As shown in Figure 2, E-B efficiently displaces the complex formed on E-43, P-1 displaces the complex less efficiently, and mE-B does not compete with complex formation. Two 35 bp fragments of the enhancer that flank E-B on both ends were ineffective competitors of E-B–specific complex formation. That the complex is due to protein interacting with DNA is investigated by treating the EMSAs with ribonuclease, proteinase K, and by heat denaturation of the extract. Ribonuclease treatment leads to a minor decrease in the electrophoretic mobility of the complex but does not change the stoichiometry of the interactions. Proteinase K and thermal denaturation completely disrupted complex formation. When extracts were incubated at 37°C, endogenous nuclease activity degraded a substantial portion of the free and bound probe. Whether the cells were grown under normoxia or hypoxia, nuclear extracts contained protein factors that interacted with the DR-2 region of the EPO enhancer. No hypoxia-specific DNA/protein interactions were detected in any portion of the enhancer (data not shown).

The DNA/protein interactions formed between Hep 3B extracts and the DR-2 region of the EPO enhancer co-migrated with complexes formed in nuclear

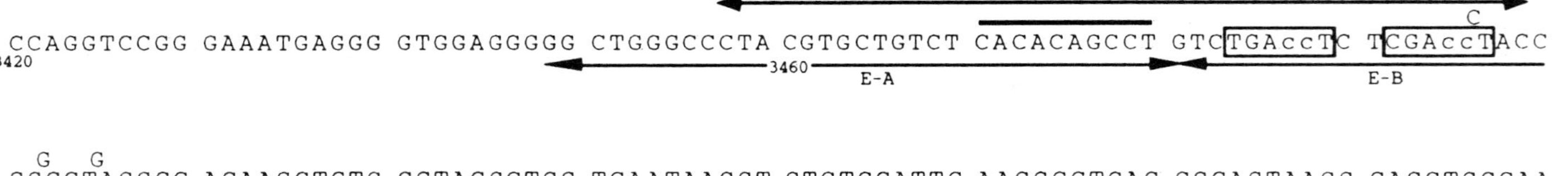

Fig. 1. The sequence of the human EPO promoter and enhancer is shown. The top two lines are promoter sequence and the bottom two lines are enhancer sequence. Arrows indicate probes and competitors created by chemical synthesis or restriction enzyme digestion. Boxes indicate SRE half-sites. The bent arrow represents an artibrary transcriptional start site. The solid blunt line over the sequence demonstrates areas of homology between the promoter and the enhancer. The dashed line identifies a repeat sequence in the promoter. The lowercase letter in the SRE sites of the enhancer represent the deleted cytosine residues in the mutated form of E-B, mE-B. The nucleotides above the sequence line in the enhancer are sequence polymorphisms present in this clone. Sequence coordinates are identical to those in the GenBank file: HUMERPA. A similar map has been previously presented [10].

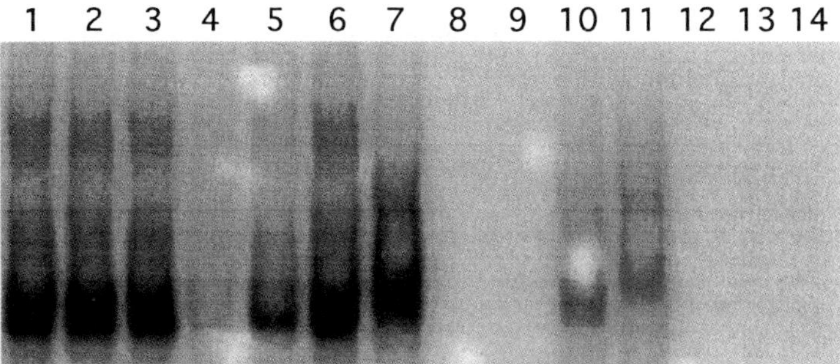

Fig. 2. Electrophoretic mobility shift assays with E-B and Hep 3B nuclear extract. Nuclear extract from hypoxic Hep 3B cells was incubated with radiolabeled E-43 probe and subjected to EMSAs. The major complex is comprised of a doublet. Competitor DNAs were added at a 50-fold molar excess, RNase A at 10 units/reaction, proteinase K at 10 μg/reaction, when added. Lanes: 1, E-A competitor; 2, mE-B competitor; 3, E-C competitor; 4, E-B competitor; 5, P-1 competitor; 6, no additions; 7, RNase A; 8, proteinase K; 9, RNase A and proteinase K; 10, no additions; 11, RNase A; 12, proteinase K, 13, RNase A and proteinase K; 14, extract heated to 70°C for 15 min. All reactions were incubated at room temperature for 20 min prior to addition of RNase A or proteinase K. In lanes 1–9 and 14 the reactions were incubated for an additional 60 min at room temperature, while in lanes 10–13 the reactions were incubated at 37°C for 60 min after additions. The position of the free probe is not shown.

extracts from 293, HeLa, and K562 cells [10]. None of these cell lines except Hep 3B produce EPO. The major complex did not form in reactions containing nuclear extract from MOLT-4, a T-lymphocyte cell line. Detailed studies of the DNA/protein interactions in nuclear extracts from cell lines that do not produce EPO have been undertaken. Nuclear extracts prepared from normoxic 293 and hypoxic Hep 3B cells were incubated with end-labeled E-B probe, treated with a dilute solution of DNase I, and subjected to electrophoresis in a native poly-acrylamide gel. Free probe and probe involved in specific DNA/protein complexes were isolated and subjected to electrophoresis on a denaturing poly-acrylamide gel. Figure 3 shows the extent of the DNase I footprint of protein factors in Hep 3B and 293 nuclear extracts on E-B. The individual components of the doublet complex formed during EMSAs with 293 and Hep 3B (only one shown) extracts have similar footprints. The footprints of the DNA/protein interactions from 293 extract extend 2 nucleotides farther toward the 5′ end of the enhancer than does the Hep 3B footprint. These footprints extend slightly into the polylinker portion of the probe in this direction.

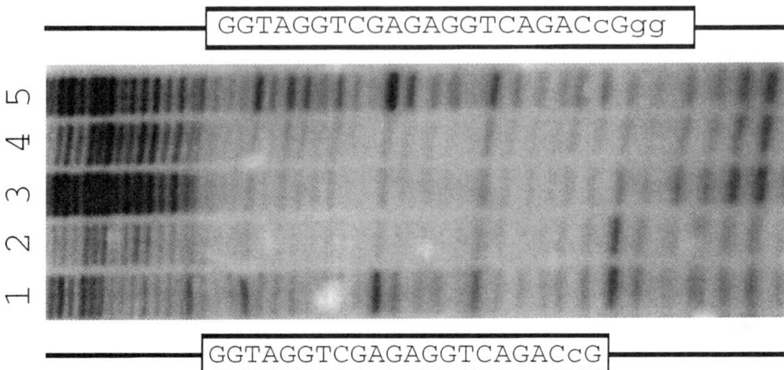

Fig. 3.   DNase I footprint of E-B/nuclear extract interactions. Preparative EMSA with nuclear extract from hypoxic Hep 3B or normoxic 293 cells and end-labeled E-B probe were incubated with dilute DNase I. The DNA in the specific complexes was isolated and electrophoresed under denaturing conditions. Lanes: 1, free probe from Hep 3B reactions; 2, lower specific complex from Hep 3B reaction; 3, upper specific complex from 293 reaction; 4, lower specific complex from 293 reaction; 5, free probe from 293 reaction. Boxes represent the extent of the footprint, nucleotide sequence in capital letters is from the EPO enhancer, and lower case letters indicate polylinker sequence.

The DNA/protein contact points between the DR-2 element and proteins from crude nuclear extracts were examined by methylation interference. Radio-labeled E-B probe was methylated prior to incubation with nuclear extracts from normoxic and hypoxic Hep 3B cells and from normoxic 293 and HeLa cells. After preparative EMSAs, free probe and probe involved in specific DNA/protein complexes were isolated. The DNA was cleaved with piperidine and subjected to electrophoresis on a denaturing polyacrylamide gel. Figure 4 shows that methylation of the paired guanines in the SRE half-sites of the DR-2 element interfered with protein binding in all extracts. The pattern of methylation interference is indistinguishable between extracts made from EPO-producing and nonproducing cell lines. The methylation interference pattern of DNA/protein interactions from normoxic and hypoxic Hep 3B cells are identical.

Discussion

The shortest functional human EPO enhancer contains a direct repeat of SRE half-sites separated by a 2 bp gap. This repeat sequence is necessary for the activity of the enhancer [10]. We demonstrate binding of a protein factor from nuclear extracts of normoxic and hypoxic Hep 3B cells and from nuclear extracts of cells that do not produce EPO. The DNase I footprint and methylation interference pattern of the DNA/protein interactions formed on end-labeled E-B in nuclear extracts from EPO-producing and nonproducing cells are essentially

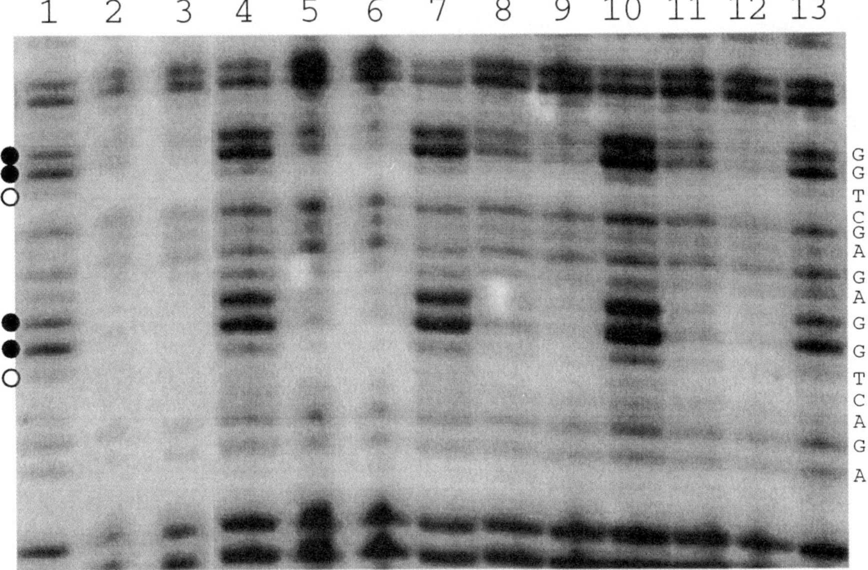

Fig. 4. Methylation interference analysis of Hep 3B, 293, and HeLa nuclear extracts with E-B probe. The loading pattern of the gel was: free probe, upper specific complex, and lower specific complex in a repeated motif. Lanes: 1–3, normoxic Hep 3B extract; 4–6, hypoxic Hep 3B extract; 7–9, normoxic 293 extract; 10–12, normoxic HeLa extract; 13, G reaction of naked probe. Filled circles indicate guanosines that interfere with protein binding when methylated. Open circles indicate thymidine residues that are modified in an unknown fashion and interfere with protein binding to E-B.

identical. The identities of the protein factors that bind to the DR-2 element are unknown. The similarity of the *cis*-acting element to a steroid receptor response element and the characteristic methylation interference pattern suggest that steroid hormone receptors or superfamily members are involved in the regulation of EPO production.

The simplest model for the regulation of EPO posits the production of a cell-specific transcriptional factor that activates the EPO gene only during hypoxia. Against this model is the observation that normoxic Hep 3B cells, hypoxic Hep 3B cells, and cells that do not produce EPO have DNA-binding proteins that interact with the EPO enhancer in vitro in an identical manner. Possible tissue-specific mechanisms for the hypoxic induction of transcription by steroid receptor superfamily members include posttranslational modification of the receptor, the presence of a hypoxia or cell-specific ligand for activation, and/or the production of an auxiliary protein that modifies the activity of the DR-2–binding protein. Phosphorylation [14, 15], novel ligand production [16, 17], and hetero-dimer formation [18] have been shown to play a role in the regulation of transcription by steroid hormone receptors.

The presence of SRE half-sites in the promoter and a DR-2 site in the enhancer of the human EPO gene suggests that the functional cooperativity between the promoter and enhancer may derive from interactions between similar *cis*-elements. This contention is buttressed by the observation that the SRE half-sites in the promoter are able to compete in EMSAs with the DR-2 element in the enhancer (see Fig. 2 and [10]). Recently, evidence has been presented that estrogen receptor can recognize widely spaced estrogen response element (ERE) half-sites in the far upstream region of the ovalbumin gene and act synergistically with palindromic EREs in the near promoter, presumably through a DNA looping mechanism [19]. EPO regulation by steroid receptor superfamily members through the promoter and enhancer SREs could involve a similar mechanism.

Acknowledgment

KLB was supported by a Damon Runyon-Walter Winchell Cancer Research Fund Fellowship, DR-055, and an American Cancer Society Junior Investigator Research Award.

References

1   Goldberg MA, Glass GA, Cunningham JM, Bunn HF: The regulated expression of erythropoietin by two human hepatoma cell lines. Proc Natl Acad Sci USA 1987;84:7972–7976.

2 Goldberg MA, Dunning SD, Bunn HF: Regulation of the erythropoietin gene: Evidence that the oxygen sensor is a heme protein. Science 1988;242:1412–1415.

3 Ratcliffe PJ, Jones RW, Phillips RE, Nicholls LG, Bell JI: Oxygen-dependent modulation of erythropoietin mRNA levels in isolated rat kidneys studied by RNase protection. J Exp Med 1990;172:657–660.

4 Fandrey J, Bunn HF: Physiologic regulation of erythropoietin mRNA in vitro and in vivo: Accurate measurement by competitive polymerase chain reaction. Clin Res 1992;40:211A.

5 Jacobs K, Shoemaker C, Rudersdorf R, Neill SD, Kaufman RJ, Mufson A, Seehra J, Jones SS, Hewick R, Fritsch EF, Kawakita M, Shimizu T, Miyake T: Isolation and characterization of genomic and cDNA clones of human erythropoietin. Nature (London) 1985;313:806–810.

6 Semenza GL, Nejfelt MK, Chi SM, Antonarakis SE: Hypoxia-induced nuclear factors bind to an enhancer element located 3' to the human erythropoietin gene. Proc Natl Acad Sci USA 1991;88:5680–5684.

7 Pugh CW, Tan CC, Jones RW, Ratcliffe PJ: Functional analysis of an oxygen-regulated transcriptional enhancer lying 3' to the mouse erythropoietin gene. Proc Natl Acad Sci USA 1991;88:10553–10557.

8 Beck I, Ramirez S, Weinmann R, Caro J: Enhancer element at the 3'-flanking region controls transcriptional response to hypoxia in the human erythropoietin gene. J Biol Chem 1991;266:15563–15566.

9 Blanchard KL, Acquaviva AM, Bunn HF: Analysis of the promoter region necessary for regulated expression of human erythropoietin in Hep3B cells. 33rd meeting of the American Society of Hematology. Denver, Colorado, Blood 1991;78 (Suppl 1):375a, abstrt 1491.

10 Blanchard KL, Acquaviva AM, Galson DA, Bunn HF: Hypoxic induction of the human erythropoietin gene: Cooperation between the promoter and enhancer, each containing steroid receptor response elements. Mol Cell Biol 1992;11.

11 Dignam JD, Lebovitz RM, Roeder RG: Accurate transcription initiation by RNA polymerase II in a soluble extract from isolated mammalian nuclei. Nucleic Acids Res 1983;11:1475–1489.

12 Shapiro DJ, Sharp PA, Wahli WW, Keller MJ: A high-efficiency HeLa cell nuclear transcription extract. DNA 1988;7:47–55.

13 Maxam AM, Gilbert W: Sequencing end-labelled DNA with base specific chemical cleavages. Meth Enzymol 1980;65:499–560.

14 Denner LA, Weigel NL, Maxwell BL, Schrader WT, O'Malley BW: Regulation of progesterone receptor-mediated transcription by phosphorylation. Science 1990;250:1740–1743.

15 Power RF, Mani SK, Codina J, Conneely OM, O'Malley BW: Dopaminergic and ligand-independent activation of steroid hormone receptors. Science 1991;254:1636–1639.

16 Kliewer SA, Umesono K, Noonan DJ, Heyman RA, Evans RM: Convergence of 9-*cis* retinoic acid and peroxisome proliferator signalling pathways through hetero-dimer formation of their receptors. Nature (London) 1992;358:771–774.

17 Zhang X-K, Lehmann J, Hoffmann B, Dawson MI, Cameron J, Graupner G, Hermann T, Tran P, Pfahl M: Homodimer formation of retinoid X receptor induced by 9-*cis* retinoic acid. Nature (London) 1992;358:587–591.

18 Widom RL, Ladias JAA, Kouidou S, Karathanasis SK: Synergistic interactions between transcription factors control expression of the apolipoprotein AI gene in liver cells. Mol Cell Biol 1991;11:677–687.

19 Kato S, Tora L, Yamauchi J, Masushige S, Bellard M, Chambon P: A far upstream estrogen response element of the ovalbumin gene contains several half-palindromic 5'-TGACC-3' motifs acting synergistically. Cell 1992;68:731–742.

Kerry L. Blanchard, PhD, MD, Section of Hematology/Oncology, Louisiana State University, 1501 Kings Highway, Shreveport, LA 71130 (USA)

Discussion

to the Paper by A. M. Acquaviva and K. L. Blanchard

Kurtz (Regensburg): Dr. Blanchard, probably I have missed it. What happens to EPO gene expression and EPO protein synthesis in intact Hep 3B cells if you add steroids to the cells?

Blanchard: I did not do that because I'm not much of a cell biologist, so what I did was use a reporter system and, using a TK promoter and the enhancer from the EPO gene, I transfected cells and I treated them with a lot of different ligands that all recognize the site. And it has no effect. The stippled columns represent the inducible activity. Now these are difficult experiments: you have to use stripped serum; you have to be certain that you don't have these hormones present. These hormones are placed in variable concentration down in the nanomolar-range concentrations. The basal expression is flat and I don't think there is any real difference between any of these numbers. So I don't think that any of these ligands have any effect. I can say that in using the EPO promotor and using the enhancer in front of the EPO promotor, I see responsiveness to thyroid hormones, thyroxin. The responsiveness is about threefold, so if you add it you get a threefold induction without hypoxia over basal activity, and when I strip the serum with Dowex and with charcoal the basal activity falls and that is totally recovered plus some extra with adding thyroxin. And that is using the short EPO promotor, the 117 base-pair promotor.

Caro (Philadelphia): It is interesting to note that testosterone is a well-known stimulator of EPO production in animals and in humans. It was originally used to stimulate EPO production in patients with renal disease; however, you don't find any effects with it. The results you showed were with the enhancer. What about if you just use the promotor region and look for changes in basal activity?

Blanchard: That is a very good question and I have not done that experiment. I think if there were steroid people in the audience they would scream and cringe at the way I have done these experiments. I have not used necessarily physiological hormones and I don't know whether or not Hep 3B cells can modulate those hormones and make them physiologic, so that is an unanswerable question by me right now.

Semenza (Baltimore): Dr. Blanchard, can you comment on exactly what role you think the promoter plays in the transcription of the EPO gene—whether you consider it a positive element, a negative element, or something else?

Blanchard: I will try. I consider it a positive element in the very unrealistic situation I placed it. I think that the exact role of the promoter can really only be addressed through the types of experiments that you are doing and transgenics, which are very difficult with a very weak promotor without the enhancer. I think that chromatin structure probably is very important, and if we could make homologous recombinants of the EPO gene with promotor mutants that would be very interesting.

Semenza: The comment I would like to make is that if you compare the TK promoter with the 126-nucleotide enhancer to the p117 EPO promoter with the 126-nucleotide enhancer, you showed that the TK promoter gave 900 units and an 11-fold induction whereas the EPO promoter gave 250 units and 45-fold induction. So it appears that the EPO promoter is increasing the fold of induction by lowering the level of activity and lowering the basal level more than it does the induced. That is my interpretation of your data.

Blanchard: I think that is absolutely true, since it is impossible to compare promotor strength in cells in a transient transfection system when it is not in the context of a chromatin structure. I have a hard time deciding that you can compare basal activity of two different promotors and make anything of it. I think if I mutated the promotor—the EPO promotor—which we are in the process of doing, this would answer the question more directly, but you are absolutely right that we are looking at fold induction, we are not looking at basal activity. The other experiment would be to place it in front of another weak promotor and see if there is an effect, and there may well be.

Semenza: Could you also comment about that interpretation with respect to Dr. Goldwasser's results regarding the binding factor that has been localized in the 5′ flanking sequence in kidney cells?

Blanchard: I think it is in the same region as what Dr. Goldwasser showed. We did some ribonuclease treatments of our extracts, and ribonuclease treatment does not destroy the complex formation in either the promotor or the enhancer. I guess I really cannot address whether or not there are negative regions in the promotor that are turning off basal transcription. As with most promotor bashing, as you delete the promotor you get to the point where you don't have activity anymore with the EPO promotor, and I did not find a region 5′ of the HindIII site that leads to great repression of the basal activity. But, as you know, it is a very inactive promotor alone, and it is difficult to make a lot out of small numbers.

Fandrey (Bonn): I would like to comment on the effect of thyroid hormones on EPO production. We have performed studies in Hep G2 cells, and we see a three-fold stimulation on the RNA level by thyroid hormones without an increase in oxygen consumption. This direct stimulation of EPO production by thyroid hormones could also be confirmed in isolated perfused rat kidneys by Horst Pagel.

Localization of Erythropoietin-Producing Cells in the Livers and Kidneys of Transgenic Mice

Stephen T. Koury,[a] Gregg L. Semenza[b]

[a]Department of Medical Technology, State University of New York at Buffalo, Buffalo, N.Y. and [b]Center for Medical Genetics, Departments of Pediatrics and Medicine, The Johns Hopkins University School of Medicine, Baltimore, Md., USA

The kidneys and liver are the major organs responsible for the production of erythropoietin in adults [reviewed in 1]. In situ hybridization was used to identify cortical peritubular cells as the source of EPO within the kidney [2, 3]. We have previously used a combination of in situ hybridization, Northern blot analysis, and measurement of serum EPO concentration to demonstrate that the kidney increases its output of EPO by recruiting additional peritubular cells to produce EPO, rather than by inducing a set number of EPO-producing peritubular cells to increase their individual output of EPO [4]. We also determined that the EPO-producing peritubular cells represented a small subset of the total number of cortical interstitial cells [4].

Semenza et al. [5–7] have generated a series of transgenic mice carrying the human erythropoietin (EPO) gene and varying amounts of 5'- and 3'-flanking sequences for use in the identification of *cis*-acting DNA sequences involved in the regulation of EPO production. Four transgenes have been analyzed thus far. Mice carrying a 4 kilobase (kb) transgene consisting of the human EPO gene, 0.7 kb of 3'-flanking sequence, and 0.4 kb of 5'-flanking sequence (tgEPO4) were polycythemic, and human EPO mRNA was constituitively expressed in all tissues examined [5]. There was a slight increase of EPO mRNA in the liver, but not in the kidney, when mice carrying this transgene were made anemic. The second transgene analyzed (tgEPO10) was identical to tgEPO4, but contained an additional 5.6 kb of 5'-flanking sequence [6]. Mice carrying this transgene were also polycythemic, but human EPO mRNA was only detectable in the liver. There was a several hundred-fold increase in human EPO mRNA in the livers of these mice when they were made severely anemic by blood loss [6]. The third transgene (tgEPO18) contained an additional 8 kb of 5′-flanking sequence compared to tgEPO10 [7]. The fourth transgene (tgEPO22) contained a total of 16.5 kb of 5′-flanking sequence and 2.2 kb of 3′-flanking sequence [7]. Mice carrying either of these transgenes were polycythemic but exhibited inducible expression of human EPO mRNA in kidney as well as liver. The pattern of human EPO gene expression in the kidneys and livers of mice carrying these transgenes led to the following conclusions concerning sequences which flank the human EPO gene:

1. An element responsible for inducing hepatic EPO expression resides in the first 300 base pairs of 3′-flanking sequence.
2. A negative regulatory element that restricts EPO expression to kidney and liver resides between 0.4 and 5 kb 5′ to the gene.
3. The element responsible for the induction of EPO expression in the kidney lies between 6 and 14 kb 5′ to the gene.

Tissue specificity of the expression of human EPO mRNA in these transgenic mice was initially determined by Northern blot analysis. However, it was not possible using Northern analysis to determine which types of cells in these tissues were responsible for the expression of human EPO mRNA. We therefore employed the technique of in situ hybridization to identify cells in liver and kidney that expressed human EPO mRNA and to determine how these cells differed from those expressing endogenous murine EPO mRNA.

Methods and Materials

Transgenic Mice and Induction of Anemia

The generation of lines of mice containing each of the transgenes has been described elsewhere [5–7]. Mice carrying the tgEPO10 transgene were made anemic by removal of blood from the retro-orbital sinus while they were under ether anesthesia followed by volume repletion with isotonic saline. Unbled mice had a hematocrit of 55% and were bled to either a hematocrit of 20 or 10% [8]. Mice carrying the tgEPO18 or tgEPO22 transgenes were made anemic by intraperitoneal injection of 60 μg of phenylhydrazine per gram of body weight at 12-h intervals starting 36 h prior to sacrifice. Hematocrits ranged from 13–28% after this treatment [7]. Unbled mice had hematocrits of ~70%, due to low level contituative expression of the human EPO transgene in kidney and liver [7].

In Situ Hybridization

Kidneys and livers were fixed in 4.0% paraformaldehyde and embedded in paraffin. Sections 3 μm in thickness were subjected to in situ hybridization using ^{35}S-labeled cRNA probes specific for either human or mouse EPO mRNA as previously described [8].

Results and Discussion

When transgenic mice containing the tgEPO10 transgene were made severely anemic (hematocrit 10%), human EPO mRNA was strongly expressed in the liver, but not expressed in any other tissue tested [6]. Furthermore, human EPO mRNA was expressed at supranormal levels in the liver compared to endogenous murine EPO mRNA [6, 8]. This supranormal level of expression greatly facilitated identification of cells producing human EPO in the livers of transgenic mice.

Figure 1 is a photomicrograph of an in situ autoradiogram in which cells expressing human EPO mRNA were localized. Cells containing hybridized mRNA in autoradiograms are overlaid with silver grains. One striking finding consistently observed in livers of severely anemic tgEPO10 mice was that cells producing human EPO were preferentially found in the vicinity of central veins

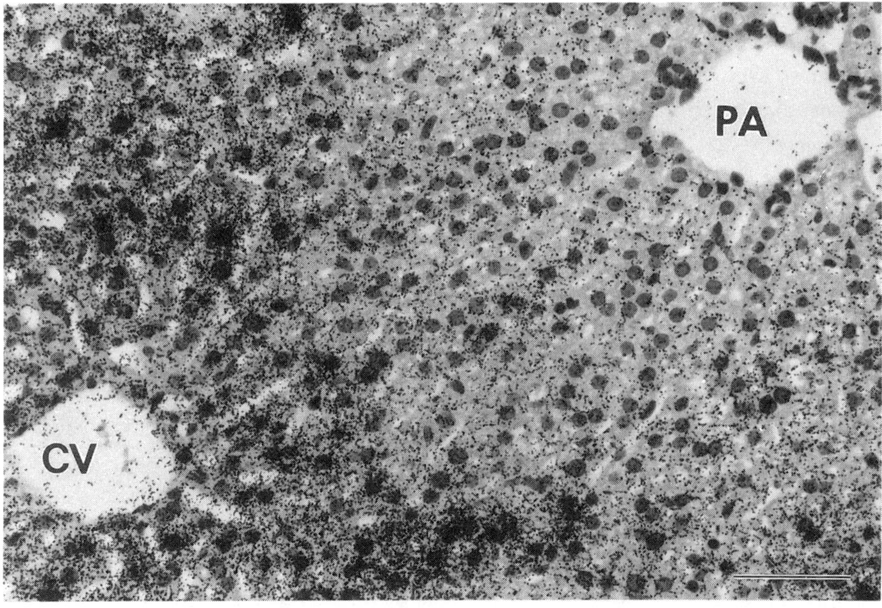

Fig. 1. Localization of human EPO mRNA in the liver of a severely anemic tgEPO10 mouse by in situ hybridization. CV, central vein; PA, portal area. Bar = 50 μm.

and were generally absent from portal areas. Central veins are easily distinguished from portal veins in histological sections in that the latter have hepatic arteries and bile ducts as companion structures. We used a technique that removes the silver grains from the autoradiographic emulsion in order to identify the cell types expressing human EPO mRNA [2, 8]. All of the cells that were heavily overlaid with silver grains were hepatocytes. The distribution of EPO-producing cells illustrated in Figure 1 follows the pattern of known oxygen gradients within the liver, with the portal area having the highest oxygen concentration and the central vein the lowest [9]. These results are consistent with the notion that EPO-producing cells must reach a threshold level of hypoxia before EPO gene expression is induced and that induction of EPO gene expression occurs in an all or none manner [4].

In order to determine if an all-or-none recruitment of cells producing human EPO mRNA occurred, we performed in situ hybridization to localize human EPO mRNA in livers of unbled tgEPO10 mice as well as tgEPO10 mice bled to hematocrits of 20 and 10%. We reasoned that the size of the zone of human EPO-producing cells would vary with hematocrit if recruitment of hepatocytes to produce human EPO mRNA was the mechanism by which these transgenic mice increased their hepatic output of human EPO. The results of this experiment are shown in Figure 2, which is composed of photomicrographs of in situ autoradiograms taken of the same area with either darkfield (Fig. 2 A, C, E) or brightfield optics (Fig. 2 B, D, F). In the darkfield photomicrographs, areas of liver containing EPO mRNA appear bright. Figures 2A and 2B illustrate the distribution of human EPO mRNA-producing cells in the liver of a tgEPO10 mouse bled to a hematocrit of 10%. This is very similar to what was shown at a higher magnification in Figure 1. Human EPO mRNA-containing cells are found preferentially around central veins and contain abundant EPO mRNA. Figures 2C and D illustrate the distribution of human EPO mRNA-producing cells in the liver of a tgEPO10 mouse bled to a hematocrit of 20%. Northern blot analysis confirmed that livers taken from transgenic mice bled to this hematocrit had only a small fraction of the amount of human EPO mRNA present in livers from transgenic mice bled to a hematocrit of 10% [8]. As can be seen in the darkfield photomicrograph (Fig. 2C), the distribution pattern of cells producing human EPO is remarkably similar to that seen in livers of tgEPO10 mice bled to a hematocrit of 10% (Fig. 2A). However, fewer silver grains were found over human EPO-producing cells at the 20% hematocrit as compared to the 10% hematocrit. Figures 2E and F demonstrate the silver grain pattern seen over livers of unbled tgEPO10 mice (hematocrit 55%). While not ruling out cell recruitment entirely, these results indicate that increased human EPO production per cell is the primary mechanism by which the amount of human EPO mRNA is increased

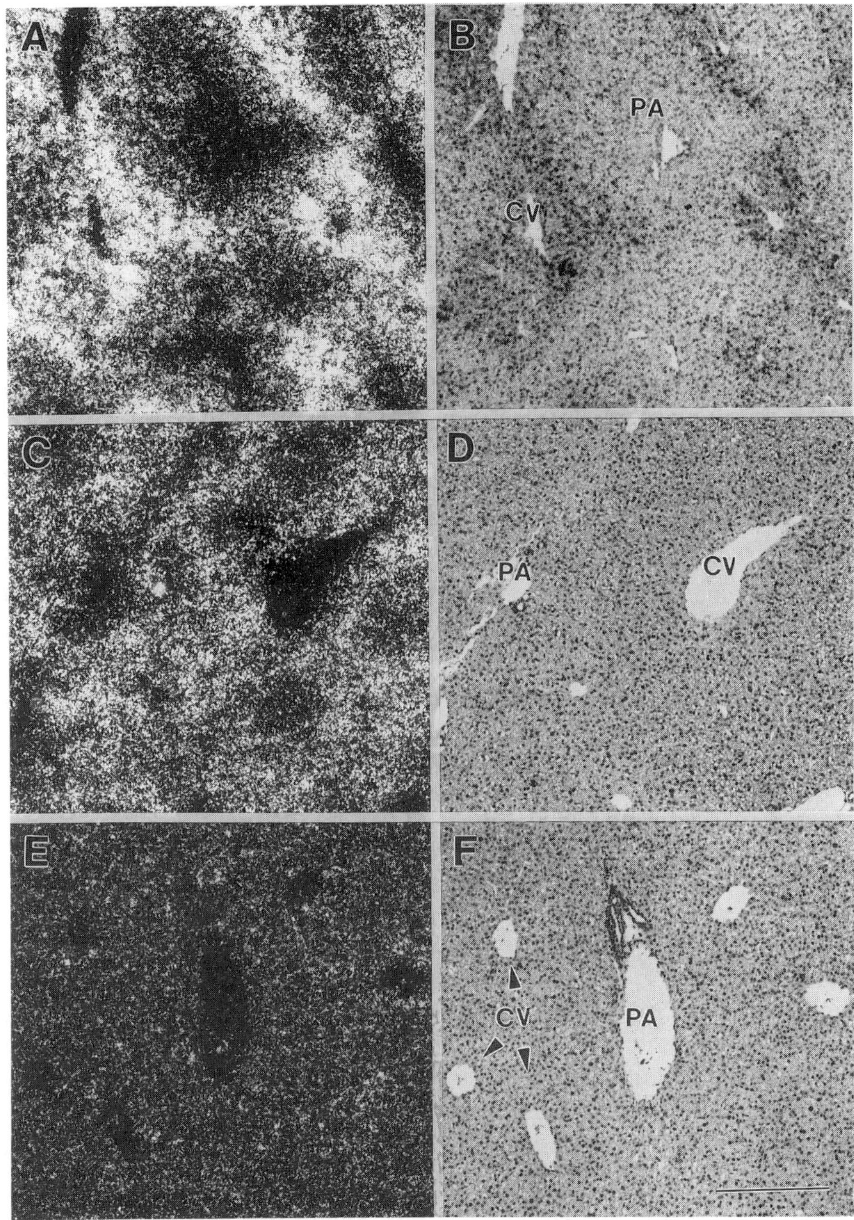

Fig. 2. Localization of human EPO mRNA in the livers of transgenic mice bled to a hematocrit of 10% (A, B), bled to a hematocrit of 20% (C, D), or unbled (hematocrit 55%) (E, F). CV, central vein; PA, portal area. Photomicrographs A, C, and E taken with darkfield optics and B, D, and F with brightfield optics. Bar = 250 μm.

in response to increasing severity of anemia in these transgenic mice. The results also indicate that different regulatory mechanisms control the response of human EPO-producing cells in transgenic liver and in cells expressing the endogenous murine EPO gene in the kidney.

When we localized the cells that produce murine EPO mRNA in the livers of nontransgenic mice, two EPO-producing cell types were identified. The majority (80%) were hepatocytes, and the remainder were a subset of nonepithelial cells found in the periphery of venous sinusoids (not shown) [8]. Since severe anemia was required to detect significant numbers of EPO-producing cells in the livers of nontransgenic mice, we were unable to perform experiments to determine whether recruitment or increased production per cell is the mechanism whereby EPO production is modulated in the livers of nontransgenic mice. Similar results were recently obtained when EPO-producing cells were localized in the livers of anemic rats using a cRNA probe specific for rat EPO mRNA [10].

As stated above, no human EPO mRNA was detected in the kidneys of even severely anemic tgEPO10 mice using Northern analysis. We performed in situ hybridization on kidneys from tgEPO10 mice to confirm this observation. As illustrated in Figure 3A, cells expressing the endogenous murine EPO gene were detected in the normal peritubular location. Figure 3B is an in situ autoradiogram of a section from the same kidney as in 3A, but hybridized with the human EPO mRNA-specific probe, demonstrating that human EPO mRNA was absent from peritubular cells. The following conclusions were reached as a result of this experiment:

1. The mouse and human EPO cRNA probes were specific for their respective target EPO mRNA under the conditions used for our in situ hybridization experiments.
2. Expression of the endogenous murine EPO gene in the kidney was independent of that of the human EPO transgene.

When human EPO mRNA-producing cells were localized in the livers of either tgEPO18 or tgEPO22 mice, a similar pattern to that described above for tgEPO10 mice was observed (not shown). Mice carrying either of these transgenes also exhibited inducible expression of human EPO in the kidney, so we therefore used in situ hybridization to localize cells that expressed the human EPO mRNA. We also localized the cells expressing the endogenous murine EPO gene on sections cut from the same piece of kidney. Figures 3C and D illustrate the results of in situ hybridization experiments using kidney from an anemic mouse carrying the tgEPO18 transgene. Human EPO mRNA–producing cells were found in the peritubular spaces (Fig. 3C) just as were cells expressing the

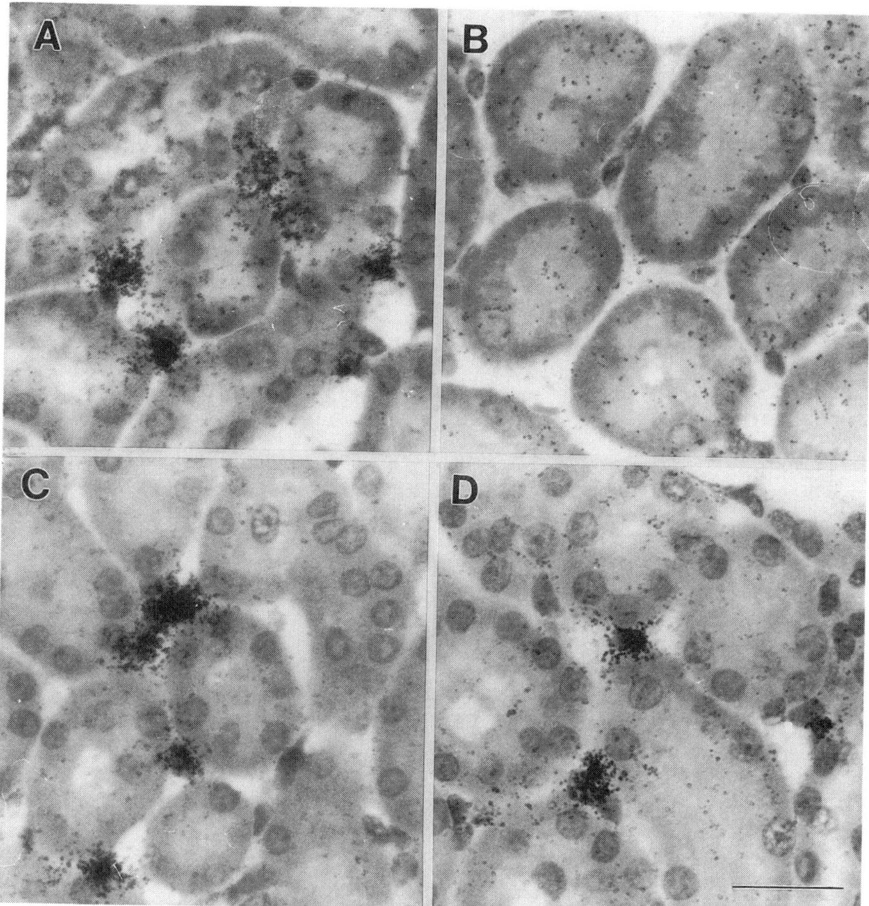

Fig. 3. In situ autoradiograms of kidney sections from anemic tgEPO10 (A and B) and tgEPO18 (C and D) mice hybridized with the murine EPO mRNA-specific probe (A and C) or with the human EPO mRNA-specific probe (B and D). Bar = 50 μm.

endogenous murine EPO gene (Fig. 3D). Similar results were obtained using tgEPO22 mice (not shown) [7]. We quantitated the number of cells producing either human EPO mRNA or murine EPO mRNA in the kidney of a tgEPO18 mouse by counting the total number of positive cells in sections hybridized with the probe specific for either human EPO mRNA or for murine EPO mRNA. The number of positive cells detected with each probe was expressed relative to the number of square centimeters of renal cortex contained in the sections [4, 7]. Figure 4 illustrates that there was no statistically significant difference in the number of positive cells per square centimeter when comparing means using Student's *t*-test (p = 0.606) [7]. These results demonstrate that the tgEPO18 and tgEPO22 transgenes were induced in both a tissue- and cell-specific manner in the kidney and suggest that the tgEPO18 transgene and the endogenous murine EPO gene were expressed in the same peritubular cells in kidneys of tgEPO18 mice.

We are currently using tgEPO18 and tgEPO22 transgenic mice to study EPO production during mid to late gestation. The fetal liver has been reported to be the organ responsible for the production of the majority of EPO in the fetus [11], but there appears to be species variation in the timing and extent of EPO production in the fetal liver [12, 13]. Previous studies using RNase protection

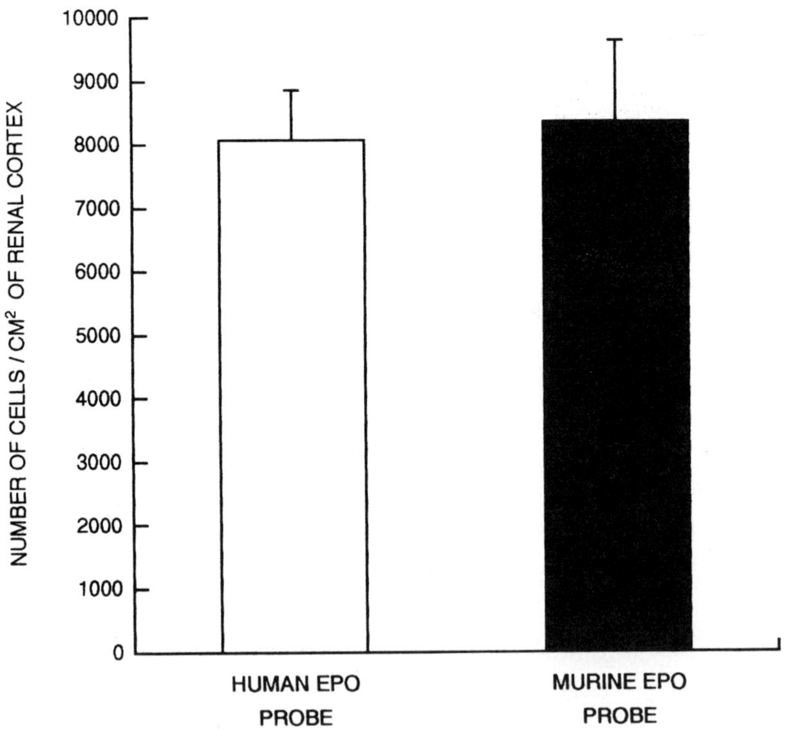

Fig. 4. Quantitation of the number (mean + 1 standard deviation) of EPO-producing cells detected in sections of the kidney cortex of a tgEPO18 mouse using either the human or murine EPO mRNA–specific probes [7].

assays on RNA isolated from organs dissected from murine fetuses indicated that the endogenous murine EPO gene is barely detectable in the liver at 14 days postcoitum (p.c.) and is undetectable thereafter [12]. The same study demonstrated that fetal kidney could be induced to produce EPO as early as day 19 p.c. Semenza et al. [7] have also documented expression of human EPO mRNA by Northern analysis in pooled isolated livers from fetuses carrying the tgEPO22 transgene at 14 days p.c. The use of in situ hybridization obviates the need for isolating fetal kidney and liver, while permitting determination of the cell types responsible for EPO production in each of these organs.

References

1 Krantz SB: Erythropoietin. Blood 1991;77:419–434.
2 Koury ST, Bondurant MC, Koury MJ: Localization of erythropoietin synthesizing cells in murine kidneys by in situ hybridization. Blood 1988;71:524–527.
3 Lacombe C, Da Silva J-L, Bruneval P, Fournier J-G, Wendling F, Casadevall N, Camilleri J-P, Bariety J, Varet B, Tambourin P: Peritubular cells are the site of erythropoietin synthesis in murine hypoxic kidney. J Clin Invest 1988;81:620–623.
4 Koury ST, Koury MJ, Bondurant MC, Caro J, Graber SE: Quantitation of erythropoietin-producing cells in kidneys of mice by in situ hybridization: Correlation with hematocrit, renal erythropoietin messenger RNA and serum erythropoietin concentration. Blood 1989;74:645–651.
5 Semenza GL, Traystman MD, Gearhart JD, Antonarakis SE: Polycythemia in transgenic mice expressing the human erythropoietin gene. Proc Natl Acad Sci USA 1989;86:2301–2305.
6 Semenza GL, Dureza RC, Traystman MD, Gearhart JD, Antonarakis SE: Human erythropoietin gene expression in transgenic mice: Multiple transcription initiation sites and cis-acting regulatory elements. Mol Cell Biol 1990;10:930–938.
7 Semenza GL, Koury ST, Nejfelt MK, Gearhart JD, Antonarakis SE: Cell-type-specific and hypoxia-inducible expression of the human erythropoietin gene in transgenic mice. Proc Natl Acad Sci USA 1991;88:8725–8729.
8 Koury ST, Bondurant MC, Koury MJ, Semenza GL: Localization of cells producing erythropoietin in murine liver by in situ hybridization. Blood 1991;77:2497–2503.
9 Maxwell AP, MacManus MP, Gardiner TA: Misonidazole binding in murine liver: A marker for cellular hypoxia in vivo. Gasteroenterology 1989;97:1300–1303.
10 Schuster SJ, Koury ST, Bohrer M, Salceda S, Caro J: Cellular sites of extrarenal and renal erythropoietin production in anemic rats. Br J Hematol 1992;81:153–159.
11 Zanjani ED, Poster J, Burlington H, Mann LI, Wasserman LR: Liver as the primary site of erythropoietin formation in the fetus. J Lab Clin Med 1977;89:640–644.
12 Eckardt KU, Ratcliffe PJ, Tan CC, Bauer C, Kurtz A: Age-dependent expression of the erythropoietin gene in rat liver and kidneys. J Clin Invest 1992;89:753–760.

Stephen T. Koury, PhD, Department of Medical Technology, The University at Buffalo Clinical Center, Building AA, Room 107, 462 Grider Street, Buffalo, NY 14215 (USA)

Discussion

to the Paper by S. T. Koury and G. L. Semenza

Eckardt (Regensburg): If I remember correctly, in those transgenic mice of Dr. Semenza that did only express in liver you reported that positive cells were only hepatocytes whereas in normal mice you found a small percentage of nonparenchymal cells also positive. Could you comment if this is also true in those lines tg EPO 18 and 22 which show expression in the kidney as well?

Koury: In the experiments I have done so far it appears that by far the majority of cells are hepatocytes. The problem is if the nonparenchymal cells which make EPO are regulated in a similar fashion to those that are expressing the endogenous murine EPO gene, then they will not express very much EPO mRNA and be a minority of the total number of cells expressing EPO mRNA. It may therefore take very long exposures in order for those to be seen. The enhanced production by hepatocytes is just so pronounced that it is hard to pick those cells out. I have not really seriously done a lot of destaining experiments to try to match up the aggregations of grains with specific cells, but so far it appears that it's all hepatocytes even in those lines that express the human gene in the kidney as well as the liver.

Wardrop (Cardiff): I was very interested in your demonstration of EPO-gene expression in fetal kidney. Have you any examination of fetal liver or other tissues during this period of active erythropoesis?

Koury: Yes, we are doing some in situ hybridizations using the transgenic mice that showed the nice Northern blot signal from Dr. Semenza on day 14 of gestation. One experiment had very nice results showing grains that were over cells in a day-14 mouse liver. On day 14 the liver contains red-cell precursors as well as hepatocytes, and the red-cell precursors were completely devoid of grains. We could see grains over very large cells with a lot of cytoplasm, a morphology which would be consistent with being hepatocytes. We do not get this result consistently and I am working on making the technique more stringent in our laboratory to try to get a more consistent result.

Rich (Ulm): I think it is important for this audience to realize that the peritubular cell is not the only cell in the kidney that is producing erythropoietin. The tubular cell has also been postulated.

Koury: The tubular cell has been *postulated* to produce erythropoietin.

Rich (Ulm): I would say both are postulated, actually, but I think an interesting point is what P. Ratcliffe has told us today—that if different cells are capable of sensing oxygen then it is quite possible that in the kidney more than one cell is also capable of sensing oxygen and producing erythropoietin. There are many pieces of evidence that would also suggest that the proximal tubular cell is capable of producing erythropoietin. So I would not be so dogmatic in saying that just the peritubular cell is the site of EPO production.

Koury: Well, I disagree with that. I do not think tubular cells produce erythropoietin, and I do not think there is any good evidence that normal tubular cells can make erythropoietin.

Rich: The evidence is just as good as yours.

Koury: What is the evidence?

Rich: In situ hybridization.

Koury: You are talking about P. Maxwell's work?

Rich: I am indeed, and our own. My question has never been answered as to why you obtain silver grains concentrated over the nucleus in your in situ hybridization results.

Koury: I have gone over this many times, and you and I exchanged letters in *Blood* discussing this. I think I expressed our opinion about what happened with P. Maxwell's work. He had specific hybridization, but in using 32p as the isotope for detection there is no way to resolve the production to a cellular level. I would also like to point out that peritubular cells have been identified as producing EPO in the rat as well as in the mouse. Dr. Eckhardt in collaboration with Dr. Bachmann in Zurich has recently used digoxigenin-labeled probes and also found that peritubular cells make EPO there. So it has nothing to do with radioactivity. Dr. Schuster at the Cardeza Foundation has also recently published a paper in which peritubular cells were found to produce EPO in rat kidney.

Caro (Philadelphia): I would like to intervene. We cannot continue with this interesting discussion because we are running out of time. I give Dr. Ratcliffe the last word.

Ratcliffe (Oxford): As you say, we have shown that in addition to hepatoma cells, many other non-EPO-producing cells can sense oxygen. I think, however, that this can neither confirm nor refute arguments as to which cell makes EPO in kidney. I would like to ask you a separate question: I am going to ask you about the difference between liver and kidney because that could be relevant to our findings. As I understand it, the physiologists have driven microelectrodes through kidney and one of the findings they report is that kidney cells in juxtaposition have very different oxygen tensions. So I wonder whether very steep oxygen gradients is the reason for your all-or-none phenomena in kidney, and I wonder therefore if you know anything as to what the oxygen tension gradients are in liver in comparison to kidney, and whether this may give a physiological reason for the phenomenon you so nicely demonstrated.

Koury: I really don't know. Perhaps Dr. Eckardt may be more familiar with the literature on that. But I don't know the absolute values for oxygen in either of those locations.

Accumulation of Erythropoietin mRNA in Rat Liver and Kidneys

Kai-Uwe Eckardt,[a] Chorh C. Tan,[b] Peter J. Ratcliffe,[b] Armin Kurtz[a]

[a]Institute of Physiology, University of Regensburg, Germany, and [b]Institute of Molecular Medicine, John Radcliffe Hospital, Headington, Oxford, England

Although the first successful attempt to define the important role of liver and kidneys in erythropoietin (EPO) formation date back more than 30 years [1], the question about the organs contributing to EPO production and their relative importance under different conditions is still not completely resolved. While the sites of EPO production were originally deduced from the results of organ ablation studies, demonstration of EPO mRNA nowadays provides a more direct way to assess tissue specific expression of the EPO gene. Using a sensitive RNAse protection assay, we have recently studied the accumulation of EPO mRNA in rats at different ages and under different conditions of reduced oxygen availability. Our results, summarized in this contribution, indicate that liver and kidneys are the major but not the sole site of EPO mRNA accumulation in the rat, that the contribution of the liver to the total EPO mRNA varies with age and the severity of hypoxic stimulation, and that under severe hypoxia it is more significant than previously recognized.

Role of Liver and Kidneys in EPO Formation

Organ ablation studies performed by several investigators have revealed that in adult animals the increase in serum EPO levels in response to hypobaric hypoxia is reduced by ~80–90% after bilateral nephrectomy [1–3], the remaining EPO formation being abolished when nephrectomy is combined with subtotal hepatectomy [4]. The conclusion drawn form these experiments was that during adulthood the kidneys play the predominant role in EPO formation, whereas the liver is responsible for some 10–15% of the total hormone production. The question, however, whether EPO is directly synthesized by liver and kidneys remained controversial until EPO mRNA was demonstrated in both organs of hypoxic rats by Northern blotting [5, 6]. Using more sensitive techniques, such as RNase protection, it became possible to detect EPO mRNA not only under hypoxic conditions, but also in kidneys and liver of normoxic animals [7–10]. Furthermore, using this technique we found low levels of EPO mRNA in addition in brain, testis, lung, and spleen [8, 9]. No EPO mRNA was detectable in the gastrointestinal system, heart, skeletal muscle, bone marrow, and salivary glands [8, 9]. Although studies with negative results using RNase protection cannot exclude the presence of small quantities of EPO mRNA in these tissues, these findings do not support the concepts proposed by others that EPO mRNA is expressed in substantial numbers of bone marrow macrophages [11] or that the salivary glands play an important role in EPO formation [12]. Interestingly, in all organs in which EPO mRNA was demonstrable, with the exception only of lung, hypoxia was found to increase EPO mRNA levels [8, 9], indicating that oxygen-sensing mechanisms controlling EPO mRNA levels may be widely distributed and do not essentially rely on specific organ functions. However, in order to judge the physiological importance of EPO mRNA expression in different organs, it appears essential to consider their quantitative contribution. Such estimation in adult hypoxic rats reveals that the liver is clearly the major extrarenal site of EPO mRNA accumulation, whereas even the combined contribution of extrarenal organs apart form liver is quantitatively insignificant [9]. Whether this is also true in the basal state is less certain, because under this condition quantification of the low levels of EPO mRNA in extrarenal organs is imprecise [9]. Furthermore, in the case of brain and testis it remains questionable whether, due to diffusion barriers, EPO produced in these organs can enter the systemic circulation.

Thus, in conclusion, although expression of EPO mRNA is more widespread, at least under hypoxic conditions liver and kidneys appear to be the major sites of EPO mRNA accumulation, and the question of their relative contribution under different conditions therefore arises.

EPO mRNA Accumulation in Liver and Kidneys during Postnatal Development

In contrast to the situation in adults, in fetal and neonatal animals bilateral nephrectomy was found to have little or no effect on EPO formation, whereas hepatectomy alone almost completely prevented an increase in serum EPO concentrations under hypoxia [2, 13–15]. These observations led to the proposal that EPO formation "shifts" from liver to kidneys during development. In order to assess age-dependent changes in the production site of EPO in intact animals, we have quantified the expression of EPO mRNA in rat liver and kidneys during postnatal development [10].

When relating EPO mRNA to tissue weight to assess the responsiveness of EPO gene expression in liver and kidney tissue, we found that tissue concentrations of EPO mRNA in liver under both normoxic and hypoxic conditions are maximal within the first week of life and thereafter decline during development (Fig. 1). Also in kidneys of unstimulated animals EPO mRNA concentrations were maximal immediately after birth. In contrast to the situation in liver, however, under stimulation renal EPO mRNA concentrations increased with age and in adult rats were up to 7-fold higher than in newborns. As a consequence of these opposite changes with age in liver and kidneys, the relative contribution of both organs to the total EPO mRNA differed markedly at different stages of

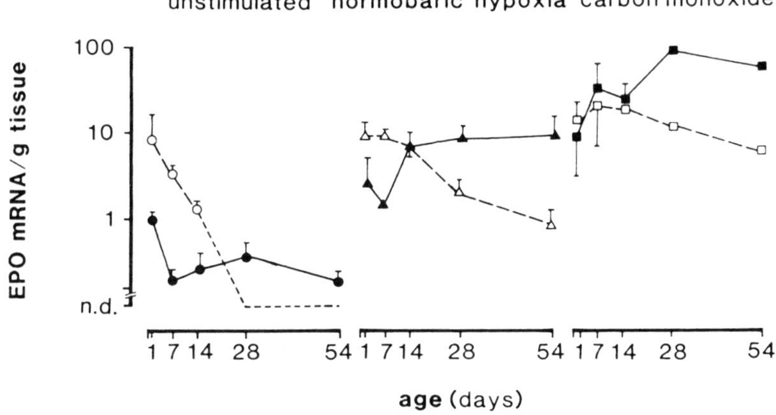

Fig. 1. Changes with development in the concentration of EPO mRNA per gram tissue in liver (open symbols) and kidneys (closed symbols) of rats studied under unstimulated conditions (○, ●) or after exposure to normobaric hypoxia (4 h) (△, ▲) or carbon monoxide (4 h) (□, ■). EPO mRNA was measured by RNase protection and quantified by scintillation counting of protected EPO mRNA bands. Values are expressed in arbitrary units, derived from comparison with the EPO mRNA signal of an external standard that was coanalyzed on each gel. (Values are means ± SD, n = 3–8.) [Adapted from Ref. 10.]

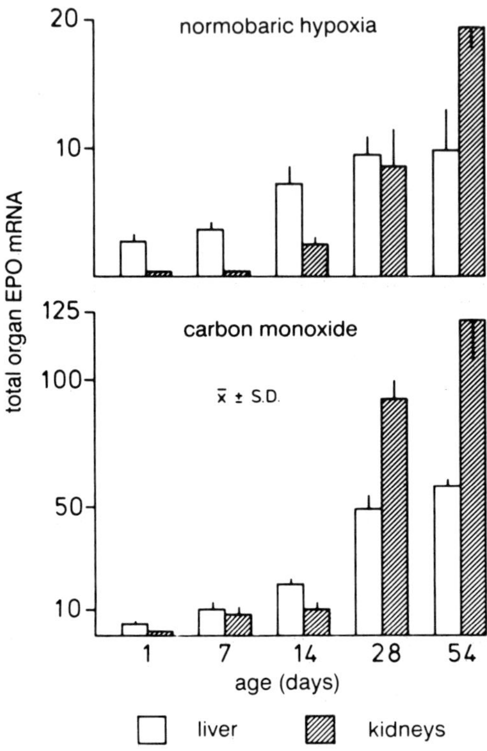

Fig. 2.   Changes with development in the total amount of EPO mRNA in liver and kidneys of rats exposed for 4 h to normobaric hypoxia or carbon monoxide. Values were calculated from the concentration of EPO mRNA per gram wet weight of tissue (Fig. 1) and the weight of liver and both kidneys. [Adapted from Ref. 10.]

development. Thus, when organ weight was taken into consideration, the liver was found to contain 85–91% of the total EPO mRNA in newborns (Fig. 2). Although during the first weeks of life the total amount of EPO mRNA increased in both organs under hypoxic stimulation, the increase in kidneys was more pronounced than in liver, so that the hepatic contribution to the total EPO mRNA decreased to 50% within 2–4 weeks. Thereafter the total amount of EPO mRNA in the liver remained almost constant, whereas the amount of EPO mRNA in the kidneys increased progressively with development and thus accounted for an increasingly greater proportion of the total. The mechanisms underlying this ontogeny of EPO formation have not been resolved. The observation that the contribution of liver and kidneys changes gradually during postnatal development indicates, however, that the "shift" in their predominance is not directly related to the changes in hemodynamics and oxygenation that occur at birth. This conclusion is also supported by another study by Koury et al., who found that in mice the kidneys contain the majority of EPO mRNA already during late gestation [16].

EPO mRNA Accumulation in Liver and Kidneys of Adult Animals

Despite the age-dependent decline in the hepatic contribution to the total EPO mRNA, we found that in adult rats under severe hypoxic stimulation the liver still contains about the same amount of EPO mRNA as one kidney and accounts for about 30–40% of the total EPO mRNA (Fig. 2). This proportion is surprisingly high in view of the experiments in anephric animals, which indicate a much lower extrarenal potential for EPO formation [1–3]. Our experiments showed, however, that hepatic expression of EPO mRNA is reduced by about 50% after bilateral nephrectomy [10]. Although the reason for this supression remains unknown, we believe that due to this reduction in hepatic EPO mRNA accumulation, studies in nephrectomized animals may so far have underestimated the contribution of the liver to EPO formation.

The relatively high contribution of the liver to the total renal EPO mRNA in severly hypoxic rats was found independent of whether EPO formation was stimulated by normobaric hypoxia [8–10], carbon monoxide [10] (Fig. 2), or blood loss [9, 10], and therefore the sensitivity of liver and kidneys towards reductions in oxygen carrying capacity or arterial oxygen tension appears to be similar. Furthermore, the duration of hypoxic exposure was also not found to be a principal determinant of the relative contribution of both organs. Thus in severely anemic rats studied 8 h after acute bleeding [9] or after 4 days of repetitive phlebotomies [10], the liver contained on average 34 and 37% of the total EPO mRNA.

While these experiments indicate that many of the characteristics of EPO mRNA expression in liver and kidneys are similar and that overall the hepatic potential for EPO mRNA accumulation is quite significant, we found, however, that the sensitivity of the liver towards mild and moderate hypoxic stimulation is less than that of the kidneys. In rats studied 8 h after graded acute hemorrhage, both liver and kidneys were found to respond over a wide range of reductions in hematocrit values, but the feedback characteristic in both organs was somewhat different, and the liver accounted for less than 20% of the total EPO mRNA in mildely anemic animals (Fig. 3). Similarly, under mild degrees of normobaric hypoxia, the hepatic EPO mRNA response was much lower than at more severe

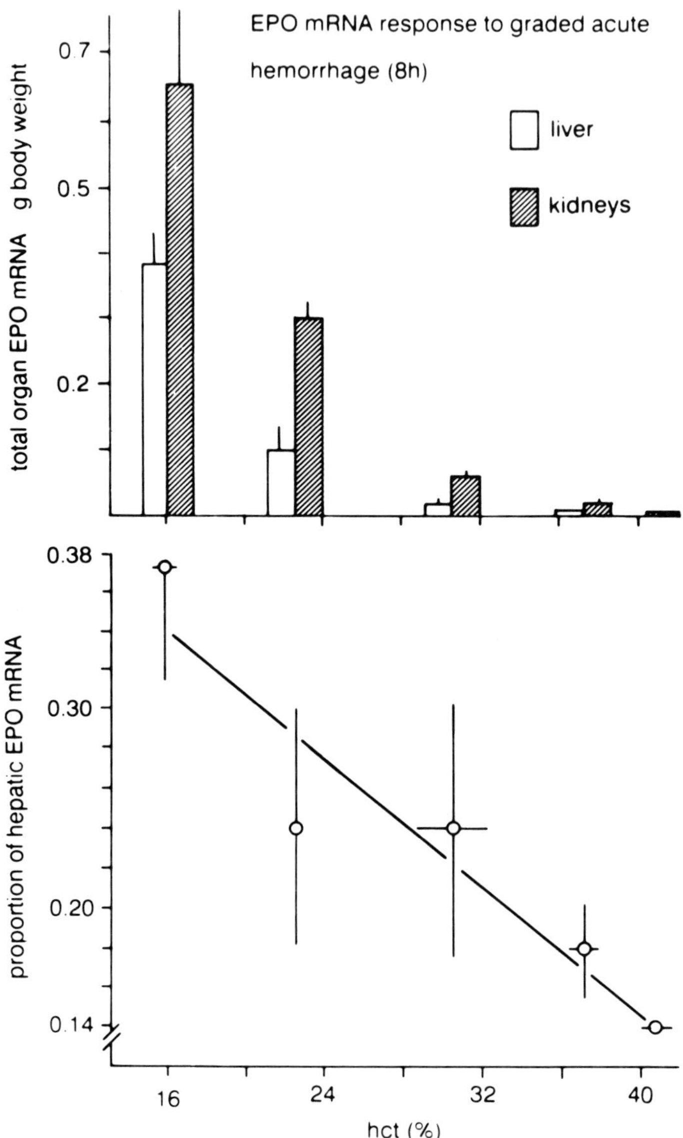

Fig. 3. Total amount of EPO mRNA in liver and kidneys (upper panel) and proportion of hepatic EPO mRNA to the total (liver + kidney) EPO mRNA (lower panel) in adult rats exposed to graded acute hemorrhage with saline replacement. EPO mRNA was quantified by RNase protection and is expressed in arbitrary units, except for the value of the hepatic proportion in control animals, which was estimated by densitometry. Values are mean ± SE, n = 5–7. Values of the hepatic proportion of EPO mRNA fitted the regression line: hepatic proportion of EPO mRNA = 46.8 − 0.80 × hct (%); r^2 = 86.9, p < 0.02. The proportion of hepatic EPO mRNA at a mean hematocrit of 15.8% was significantly higher than in animals with a mean hematocrit of 37.2%. [Adapted from Ref. 9.]

72

intensities of hypoxic stimulation [9], and also in unstimulated animals we have estimated that the liver contains only about 16% of the amount of EPO mRNA in both kidneys [9].

Correlation between EPO mRNA and Serum Hormone Levels

When considering the significance of the accumulation of EPO mRNA, an important question arises with regard to the efficiency with which EPO mRNA in liver and kidneys is translated to achieve a rise in serum hormone concentrations under different stimuli and at different stages of development. We have not measured hormone production rates directly, and thus changes or differences in translation rate cannot be excluded. Several indirect lines of evidence indicate, however, that the amount of EPO mRNA in liver and kidneys is the major determinant of EPO production rates in both organs. Thus, during the course of hypoxic exposure, changes in EPO mRNA levels in liver and kidneys precede and parallel changes in serum hormone concentrations [6, 9]. Second, when animals of a certain age are exposed for constant time periods to hypoxic stimuli of varying severity, a close correlation can be found between the sum of renal and hepatic EPO mRNA and the serum hormone concentrations [9, 10] (Fig. 4). Finally, the increase in EPO mRNA in bilaterally nephrectomized animals indicates that the relationship between EPO and mRNA and hormone production rates in liver and kidneys is comparable, if one takes into account that hepatic EPO mRNA is reduced under this condition, as mentioned above.

However, when the rise in serum EPO during acute hypoxic exposure was compared with EPO mRNA in developing rats, the slope of the regression line relating serum EPO on the ordinate to EPO mRNA on the abscissa, increased 9-fold between day 1 and day 54 [10]. This finding would be compatible with an age-dependent increase in translational efficacy. It could, however, also be due to age-dependent alterations in EPO metabolism. In fact, Widness and coworkers have recently reported that in fetal and neonatal sheep clearance and distribution of EPO are significantly increased as compared to adult animals [17], which supports the latter explanation.

Role of Hepatic EPO mRNA Accumulation in Chronic Renal Failure

The findings, indicating a substantial production capacity for EPO in the liver, also raise the question of the pathophysiological significance of hepatic EPO formation in patients with chronic renal failure, in whom inappropriately low EPO levels are considered to be the primary course of their anemia.

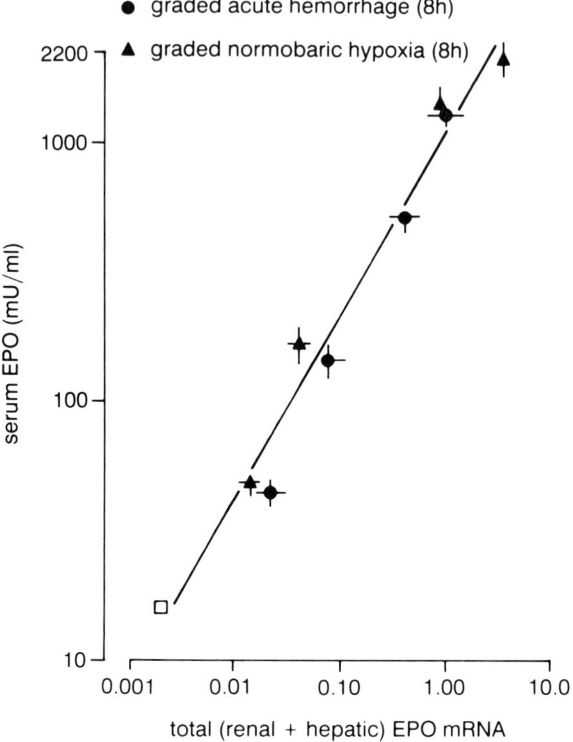

Fig. 4.   Correlation between the sum of renal and hepatic EPO mRNA per gram body weight and serum hormone levels in adult rats exposed to graded acute hemorrhage (see Fig. 3) or graded normobaric hypoxia (7.5, 9, 11, 14% oxygen). Values are mean ± SE, n = 3–7. Values fitted the regression line: log serum EPO (mU/ml) = 3.03 + 0.71 × log EPO mRNA/g body weight; r^2 = 0.97, p < 1 × 10^{-5}. [Adapted from Ref. 9.]

Presently no information is available about extrarenal production capacity for EPO in humans, and studies in mice indicate, in comparison with our findings, that significant species-dependent differences may exist [16]. However, rats rendered chronically uremic by subtotal nephrectomy were found to develop an anemia that is accompanied by inappropriately low serum EPO levels [8]. When these uremic rats were exposed to normobaric hypoxia, however, serum EPO concentrations increased 10-fold, and the accumulation of EPO mRNA in their livers was unchanged as compared to controls (Fig. 5). Thus, at least in this model of chronic renal failure, anemia develops despite a substantial hepatic potential for EPO formation. It is of interest that in humans with chronic renal failure, marked increases in serum EPO levels were found when intercurrent illness or exposure to high altitude led to hypoxia [18–20].

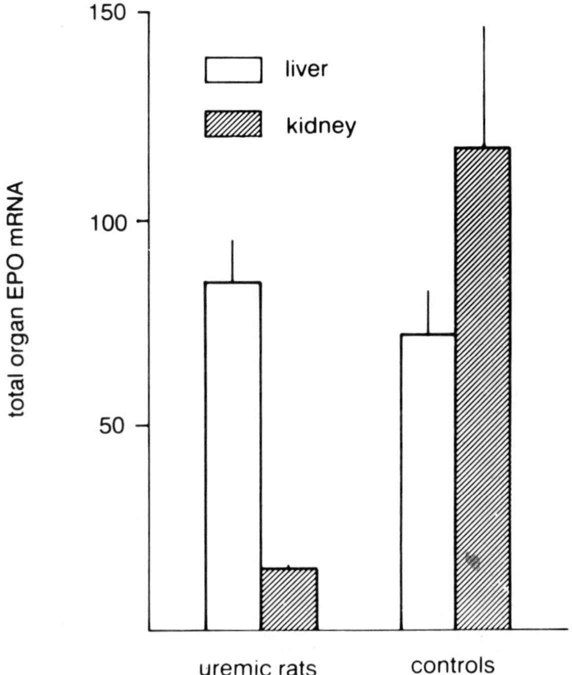

Fig. 5. Total amount of EPO mRNA in liver and kidneys of adult rats rendered uremic by subtotal nephrectomy and control animals under normobaric hypoxia (7% oxygen for 4 h). EPO mRNA was quantified by RNase protection and is expressed in arbitrary units; values are mean ± SE, n = 4. Under hypoxic exposure serum EPO rose from 32 ± 4 mU/ml to 349 ± 41 mU/ml in uremic rats and from 24 ± 3 mU/ml to 1009 ± 119 mU/ml in control animals (mean ± SE, n = 4–5). In hypoxic uremic rats EPO mRNA increased in both remnant renal tissue and liver, and hepatic EPO mRNA accumulation was not different from that in control animals.

References

1 Jacobson LO, Goldwasser E, Fried W, Plzak L: Role of the kidney in erythropoiesis. Nature 1957;179:633–634.

2 Wang F, Fried W: Renal and extrarenal erythropoietin production in male and female rats of various ages. J Lab Clin Med 1972;79:181–186.

3 Schooley JC, Mahlmann LJ: Erythropoietin production in the anephric rat. I. Relationship between nephrectomy, time of hypoxic exposure, and erythropoietin production. Blood 1972;39:31–38.

4 Fried W: The liver as a source of extrarenal erythropoietin production. Blood 1972;40:671–677.

5 Bondurant MC, Koury MJ: Anemia induces accumulation of erythropoietin mRNA in the kidney and liver. Mol Cell Biol 1986;6:2731–2733.

6   Schuster SJ, Wilson JH, Erslev AJ, Caro J: Physiologic regulation and tissue localization of renal erythropoietin messenger RNA. Blood 1987;70:316–318.

7   Koury ST, Koury MJ, Bondurant MC, Caro J, Graber SE: Quantitation of erythropoietin-producing cells in kidneys of mice by in situ hybridization: correlation with hematocrit, renal erythropoietin mRNA, and serum erythropoietin concentration. Blood 1989;74:645–651.

8   Tan CC, Eckardt K-U, Ratcliffe PJ: Organ distribution of erythropoietin messenger RNA in normal and uremic rats. Kidney Int 1991;40:69–76.

9   Tan CC, Eckardt K-U, Firth J, Ratcliffe PJ: Feedback modulation of renal and hepatic erythropoietin messenger RNA in response to graded anemia and hypoxia. Am J Physiol 1992;263:F474–F481.

10 Eckardt K-U, Ratcliffe PJ, Tan CC, Bauer C, Kurtz A: Age dependent expression of the erythropoietin gene in rat liver and kidneys. J Clin Invest 1992;89:753–760.

11 Vogt C, Pentz S, Rich IN: A role for the macrophage in normal hemopoiesis: III. In vitro and in vivo erythropoietin gene expression in macrophages detected by in situ hybridization. Exp Hematol 1989;17:391–397.

12 Clemons GK, De Mannicor D, Fitzsimmons SL, Garcia JF: Immunoreactive erythropoietin studies in hypoxic rats and the role of the salvary glands. Exp Hematol 1987;15:18–23.

13 Carmena AO, Howard D, Stohlman F: Regulation of erythropoiesis XXII. Erythropoietin production in the newborn animal. Blood 1968;32:376–382.

14 Zanjani ED, Poster J, Burlington H, Mann LI, Wasserman LR: Liver as the primary site of erythropoietin formation in the fetus. J Lab Clin Med 1977;89:640–644.

15 Gruber DF, Zucali JR, Wleklinski J, LaRussa V, Mirand EA: Temporal transition in the site of rat erythropoietin production. Exp Hematol 1977;5:399–407.

16 Koury MJ, Bondurant MC, Graber SE, Sawyer ST: Erythropoietin messenger RNA levels in developing mice and transfer of 125I-erythropoietin by the placenta. J Clin Invest 1988;82:154–159.

17 Widness JA, Veng-Pedersen P, Modi NB, Schmidt RL, Chestnut DH: Developmental differences in erythropoietin pharmacokinetics: Increased clearance and distribution in fetal and neonatal sheep. J Pharmacol Exp Ther 1992;261:977–984.

18 Chandra M, Clemons GK, McVicar M: Relation of serum erythropoietin levels to renal excretory function: Evidence for lowered set point for erythropoietin production in chronic renal failure. J. Pediatr 1988;113:1015–1021.

19 Walle AJ, Wong GY, Clemons GK, Garcia JF, Niedermayer W: Erythropoietin-hematocrit feedback circuit in the anemia of end-stage renal disease. Kidney Int 1987;31:1205–1209.

20 Blumberg A, Keller H, Marti HR: Effect of altitude on erythropoiesis and oxygen affinity in anaemic patients on maintenance dialysis. Eur J Clin Invest 1973;3:93–97.

K.-U. Eckardt, MD, Physiologisches Institut der Universität Regensburg, Universitätsstrasse 31, 93053 Regensburg, Germany

Discussion

to the Paper by K.-U. Eckardt et al.

Caro (Philadelphia): Let me just clarify something, the studies in the kidney. Were they simultaneously done in the same preparation, the immunohistochemistry and the in situ hybridization?

Eckardt: Yes, on the same tissue section nonradioactive in situ hybridization and immunofluorescence against the enzyme.

Caro: And endothelial cells do not contain these 5′ nucleotidase?

Eckardt: No.

Rich (Ulm): You know that unstimulated macrophages contain very high concentrations of 5′ nucleotidase?

Eckardt: There is another indirect evidence that macrophages are not the production site of erythropoietin in the kidney, and this is that if you irradiate the animals you lose the macrophages within a short time. However, the production capacity for erythropoietin in the kidney is not altered after whole-body irradiation. So I think there is good evidence that macrophages are not the production site.

Rich: I was not suggesting that macrophages were involved in EPO production in the kidney. However, small numbers of macrophages are present in the peritubular region. I am only pointing out that the ectoenzyme 5′-nucleotidase has been used as a marker for macrophages since in unstimulated macrophages high concentrations are present, while in stimulated macrophages low concentrations of the enzymes are found. The marker can therefore be used for subpopulations of macrophages. Furthermore, macrophages are not affected by such doses of irradiation; that is, they are not lost at all. And whole-body irradiation would not affect the kidney since there are few if any proliferating cells.

Breymann (Zürich): With increasing severity of anemia you have increasing recruitment of hepatocytes. Do you think you have also a limited recruitment in the kidney? That you have [something] like an exhaustion of producing kidney peritubular cells, that they have a limited production?

Eckardt: The implication of your question is probably a misunderstanding of what I said. I have not looked at the expression of erythropoietin mRNA in single hepatocytes, but as Steven Koury mentioned there is obviously no recruitment in the liver. In the kidney, even under a very severe stimulation, only a small subset of the total interstitial population and also only a small subset of the population of peritubular fibroblasts produce erythropoietin. So, from this point of view, I would say it does not look as if there is limitation simply because no more cells are available.

Semenza (Baltimore): Have you quantitated the number of cells that are producing EPO and 5′ nucleotidase—are they identical or are they just an overlapping subset of cells?

Eckardt: It is an overlapping subset of cells. It is clearly a minority of the peritubular fibroblasts and they have some particularities. For example, in a cooperative study with Steven Koury, we looked very carefully at the distribution of peritubular cells' expression of erythropoietin, and—in addition to what he found previously, that they are only present in the cortex—we furthermore saw that they are only present in the cortical labyrinth and not the medullary rays. So there are some characteristics, and he also quantified some time ago these cells and found that they are predominantly present around proximal tubules.

Blanchard (Shreveport): In the early '70s, Gordon and Dornfest looked at organ-specific EPO production in rats after phenylhydrazine treatment. They looked for up to a month, I believe. Their assay system was nowhere as specific as yours, but they did demonstrate that EPO produced in the kidneys fell with time. Their kidney levels approached normal levels in anemic animals at 3 weeks, while the liver production increased throughout the entire phenylhydrazine treatment. Do you have any comments on that?

Eckardt: I cannot really comment on this because the data that I showed you with 4 days of anemia was the longest period we have investigated so far. It may be that beyond this period there are further changes. The experiment is very difficult—it is tremendously difficult to keep a rat continuously anemic. They have so high a regenerative potency that you have to bleed them again and again, and then you have fluctuations of the hematocrit—so it is very difficult to interpret, I would say.

Halpérin (Geneva): If I understood correctly, you suggested that the oxygen sensor mechanism in the hepatocytes is less sensitive than in the kidney. As a matter of fact, in your in vitro studies on hepatocytes submitted to different conditions of oxygenation, the EPO mRNA production really increased significantly only at a F_iO_2 of 3%; is that correct? Do you have parallel experiments on peritubular cells in the kidney showing that there is really a difference in sensitivity?

Eckardt: No, we don't have parallel experiments. I think nobody has at present data about expression of erythropoietin in kidney cells in vitro. And when I say the sensitivity is somewhat lower, I can only say that this is true for the whole organ, and of course the sensitivity of the whole organ is determined by several factors, including molecular factors of oxygen sensing—but also including, for instance, hemodynamics and oxygen consumption—which may all influence the production if you consider the whole organ.

Bondurant: In earlier studies, Dr. Koury and I looked in the mouse after bleeding and never found the lowering of erythropoietin after a period of time. In fact, in the slide that Steve Koury showed, it always correlated exactly with the hematocrit regardless of how long after the bleeding it took place. Do you have any idea what the discrepancy is—is it species, is it mode of induction of hypoxia, or do you have any ideas?

Eckardt: That is a very fascinating point, which I do not think anybody understands yet. It seems to depend on the stimulus; I do not think it is a matter of species. We see down-regulation of EPO production and down-regulation of messenger RNA in liver and kidneys in rats exposed to hypoxic hypoxia. With anemia it seems to be different because EPO levels will stay continuously high. On the other hand, if you bleed animals acutely or if you bleed humans acutely and investigate the time course of erythropoietin levels, you can also see some kind of overshoot in the erythropoietin levels and there is a slight down-regulation. Why this is not as pronounced in chronic anemias as in chronic hypoxia I do not know.

Wideroe (Norway): I would like to give a couple of clinical observations. I can support some of your findings and your discussion. It is an observation from many groups that patients with renal anemia, with virus hepatitis, have increased erythropoiesis. This can support some of your findings concerning the liver-related erythropoiesis in adult patients. Another observation is that anephric patients transferred from hemodialysis to continuous peritoneal dialysis polytransfused and, with iron overload, showed a significant increase in erythropoiesis during the first weeks on peritoneal dialysis. Some years ago we measured the erythropoietin activity on colony-forming unit cells and found a significant increase in this stimulation in the blood and in the peritoneal dialysate. We suggested that the erythropoiesis-stimulating activity in the peritoneal fluid could be explained by activated macrophages, stimulated by the cycling of peritoneal dialysis fluid. Transport of erythropoietin from blood into the peritoneal cavity is not a possible explanation.

Eckardt: I can only say that we have also got some evidence confirming this in studies where we measured immunoactive erythropoietin under certain conditions. As I said, we do not really know what the production capacity of the liver is in humans, but there is evidence that there may be considerable extrarenal production capacities. So I think one of the main questions regarding the pathophysiology of the system is why this extrarenal production capacity is not used in chronic renal failure. In this respect, it may be interesting that Steven Tan in Oxford showed in a study we performed together that also in the rat, where the production capacity is proven to be high, anemia develops after subtotal nephrectomy. However, when you then expose these uremic rats to hypoxia they produce a lot of erythropoietin and they have an unchanged production capacity in their liver.

Lacombe (Paris): Did you try to do your double-labeling experiments on the liver of anemic mice, nontransgenic?

Eckardt: No, we have not done any studies on the liver yet, because I thought the topic of the liver is more or less solved after the observation that the majority of cells are hepatocytes.

Lacombe: But you have also a population of small cells; probably this population may be the same population as the interstitial cell in the kidney, so it would be interesting to do this experiment.

N.N.: Let me clarify again: your double-labeling was not on the transgenic mice?

Eckardt: It was not in mice at all; it was in anemic rats.

Ratcliffe (Oxford): I will, in fact, introduce the topic of transgenic mice, since we have some data which strongly support Dr. Eckardt's observations. We have made transgenic mice which bear an EPO-SV40 T antigen fusion gene and express T antigen in renal interstitial cells when the animals are made anemic. It is possible to detect T antigen by immunohistological means and perform double labeling with other antibodies on the same section. Dr. Eckardt arranged for Dr. Kaissling to make the ectonucleotidase antibody available to us, and my colleagues Drs. Maxwell and Pugh have been able to demonstrate double-labeling of interstitial cells with antibodies to T antigen and ecto-nucleotidase.

Measurement of Quality of Life in International Trials Involving Dialysis Patients and the Use of Recombinant Human Erythropoietin

R. M. Lindsay, A. P. Heidenheim

Artificial Kidney Research Centre, Victoria Hospital, and the University of Western Ontario, London, Ontario, Canada

Introduction

The patient with end-stage renal failure (ESRD) being treated by dialysis faces a stressful and disruptive chronic illness with a complex and demanding treatment regime. This has an impact on the quality of life of both patients and their families, changing the distribution of responsibility with regard to decision making, employment, and housework as well as affecting diet, recreation, and social activity [1–3]. Members of the nephrological team should, therefore, be concerned not only with the biological and physiological but also with the psychological and social functioning of their patients. Knowledge of the latter can aid in treatment decisions, improve patient compliance, and supplement morbidity and mortality measures in evaluative research. Consequently, there is a need for assessment tools that address the multidimensional nature of patient quality of life in clinical research settings. For such tools to be of value, they must be reliable, valid, and sensitive to change over time and to the impact of alternative treatment interventions. Such assessment tools usually take the form of questionnaires. These should be straightforward, easy to understand, short, and easy to complete in order to maximize return rates and minimize missing data. The tools should also provide for flexible combinations of scales and indices adaptable to different clinical research questions. Given that sample size requirement will often necessitate multicenter research designs and that large-scale studies are frequently international in scope, quality-of-life instrumentation should be suitable for multicultural applications and sensible in a variety of languages [4, 5]. This paper describes the performance of 7 quality-of-life scales in research carried out in 8 countries in 6 languages from Europe and North

America. The focus of the study is on the response rates, reliability, validity, and sensitivity of the instruments.

Methods

Quality-of-Life Instrumentation

There are two approaches to the measurement of patient quality of life: global and disease-specific. Global assessments tend to rate levels of overall function and satisfaction in general abstract domains. Disease-specific tools focus on concrete symptoms, stressors, dysfunctions, and discomfort related to a particular disease and its treatment. The global method is most useful for assessments of large heterogeneous populations or when comparing different illnesses (e.g., cancer vs. diabetes) but is usually insensitive to small clinically significant differences. Disease-specific assessment is more suitable for clinical trials of alternative interventions (e.g., the impact of erythropoeitin) as the questionnaire items have been chosen specifically to fit the illness and treatment of interest. On the other hand, disease-specific instruments will have a narrow range of applicability limited to the illness and treatment for which they were designed [4].

With the exception of scale 7, Basic Personality Inventory, the assessment tools reported here are disease and treatment specific. They have been assembled over several years within applied renal research settings. Other than the Physiological Index (scale 1), which is compiled by the medical staff from records, the questionnaires are patient completed.

1. Physiological index: This index was originally described by one of the authors [6], was in turn evaluated by Strauch et al. [7], and consists of 18 weighted measures selected for their relevance to an ESRD population: hepatitis, renal osteodystrophy, urine volume, serum urea, serum creatinine, blood pressure, hematocrit, weight increment between dialysis, serum potassium, diabetes, myocardial infarct, fundi, congestive heart failure, angina pectoris, pericarditis, GI ulcers, anephric. Original items and weights were validated through feedback from nephrologists from 100 West German dialysis centers [7]. Physiological Index scores range from 7 to 94, with higher values indicating poorer physiological functioning.

2. Psychosocial Stress Scale: This 9-item index measures the amount of stress experienced in day-to-day personal and family life related to the symptoms of ESRD and the demands of dialysis: financial problems, marriage strain, dependency, altered sexuality, interference with vacations, vocations, child care, and social life, and loss of family role. The scale yields a stressor count (range 0–9) of the number of individual stressors experienced and a total stress score (0–81). An average per-item stress score can also be computed by dividing the total stress by the number of stressors.

3. Disease Stress Scale: This is a 14-item scale of distress experienced due to the symptoms of chronic uremia: weakness, tiredness, shortness of breath, blood pressure problems, up/down health, headaches, physical illness, fluid retention,

cramps, itch, fear of death, inability to sleep, dizziness, sexual problems, and nausea. Additional items can be included for individual research projects. For example, in the clinical trial involving erythropoeitin, three additional symptoms were addressed: feeling cold or chilly, inability to perspire, and aching in arms/legs. The stressor count (0–14 or 0–17) indicates the number of items affecting the person, and the total stress score (0–126 or 0–153) represents the sum total of disease-related stress from all 14 sources. Average per-item stress can also be computed.

4. Sleep Adequacy: The sleep questionnaire contains 4 subscales, computed by summing the component items: interference with sleep (range 0–27), sleep disruptions (range 0–27), fatigue upon awakening (range 0–24), and fatigue during the day (range 0–30).

5. Dialysis Somatic Symptoms Distress Scale: This is an index of 11 physical symptoms that commonly occur during hemodialysis: nausea, vomiting, headache, muscle cramps, dizziness, tingling of extremities, itching, shivering, back pain, chest pain, and hypotension. Five additional items were included for the EPO project: dyspnea, wheezing, perspiration, hives, and rash. Patients are scored via a Symptom Count (0–11 or 0–15) of the total number of incidents that occurred during the dialysis session and via a Total Discomfort score (0–99 or 0–135) equaling the sum total of distress reported from all items. Average per-item stress can also be computed.

6. Fatigue Rating Scale: This scale measures the mean level of fatigue experienced by patients in the time period between dialysis sessions. Scores range from 0 to 9.

7. Basic Personal Inventory: The full Basic Personality Inventory is a psychological profile composed of 12 scales, each consisting of 20 true/false items, with a corresponding score range of 0 to 20 [8]. While the orientation of the inventory as a whole is toward the measurement of psychopathology, we have found 6 of the scales—depression, denial, anxiety, social introversion, self-depreciation, and hypochondriasis—to be appropriate for use with psychologically normal populations such as dialysis patients.

Analysis

This analysis is an assessment of the psychometric properties of the 7 quality-of-life measures under the following areas:

1. Missing data rates: the proportion of unanswered composite items expressed as a percentage of the number of items in the scale multiplied by the number of times the scale was administered.

2. Reliability: refers to its consistency both internally and over time. In a scale with internal consistency, all component items tap slightly different aspects of the same underlying phenomenon and are highly interrelated. Cronbach's alpha, a conservative measure of internal consistency/reliability, can be interpreted as the overall intercorrelation between component items; it ranges from 0 to 1, with 0.6 taken by convention as the minimum level for research purposes. Stability over time is evaluated by test-retest reliability using the correlation between scores

obtained over a short period of time during which the measured phenomenon is assumed not to have changed [9, 10]. All scales were administered twice, 2–4 weeks apart, to cohorts of patients.

3. Validity: centers on the question of whether a scale actually measures the underlying theoretical concept, here a specific domain of quality of life. Generally this is demonstrated by showing that the scale scores correlate in logical directions with other variables.

4. Sensitivity: demonstrated by an ability to discriminate between treatment groups in the expected directions at statistically significant levels.

Patients

A total of 300 hemodialysis patients from 27 dialysis centers were pooled from 2 separate recently completed clinical trials. The trials were coordinated by the authors. The trials were: (a) A Multi-Centre Study on Short Hours versus Conventional Dialysis [11], which hypothesized that short-hours, high-flux dialysis would improve patient acceptance and quality of life (Study I) and (b) The Haemodialysis/Haemoglobulin Quality of Life Study (data as yet unpublished), which examined the influence of dialyzer geometry before and after the elevation of hemoglobin by rhEPO on patient quality of life (Study II). Table 1 shows the distribution of patients by country. The distribution of age, sex, risk, etc. was similar across countries and represents that currently seen in clinical practice. More details of this patient base will soon be published.

Results

Missing Data Rates

Figure 1 shows the percentage of missing items for each of the scales. It can be seen that all of the scales had relatively low rates of missing data ranging from a high of 2.45% of items (fatigue awakening) to a low of 0.06% (somatic

Table 1.   Hemodialysis patients participating in clinical trials

Participating countries	Number of patients	Percentage of sample
Italy	72	24.0
Germany	33	11.0
England	30	10.0
France	21	7.0
Denmark	5	1.7
Sweden	26	8.7
Canada	69	23.0
United States	44	14.7
TOTAL	300	100.0

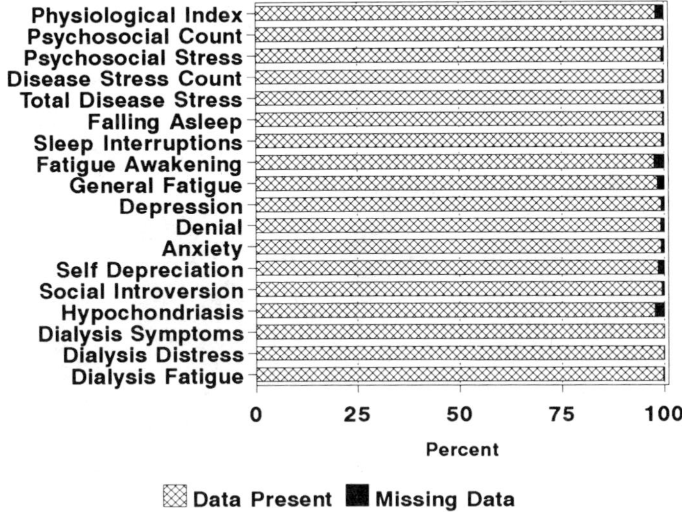

Fig. 1.   Missing data rates for quality-of-life scales and their indicators.

symptoms count). No particular country or language had an influence on missing data rates. In summary, the 18 scales are composed of a total of 245 individual items, which generated 409,560 data points over the course of both studies. Of these, only 2870 (0.7%) were missing. In other words, 99.3% of the quality-of-life data was forthcoming from the respondents and available for analysis.

Reliabilities

Table 2 shows the scale reliabilities. The Cronbach's alpha coefficients of internal consistency exceeded the minimum standard for all scales except the physiological index. This was to be expected, as this index consists of items involving different physiological systems, each important to the health of the dialysis patient but not expected to co-vary to any great extent. Test-retest correlation coefficients all show moderate to high correlations indicating stability over time.

Validity

Table 3 shows the moderate interscore correlation for 5 of the quality-of-life scales. The physiological index is not included in construct validity as it measures pathophysiological status and has already demonstrated to be of proven value [7]. The Basic Personality Inventory was fully evaluated outside this particular study [8]. The authors have found this scale to be of value in predicting

Table 2. Reliabilities for the quality-of-life scales and their indicators

Scale	Internal consistency		Test-Retest		
	alpha	n	r	p	n
Physiological index	0.3983	769	.9195	.000	146
Psychosocial stressor count	0.6931	1051	.7580	.000	72
Total psychosocial stress	0.7105	1034	.7072	.000	71
Disease stressor count	0.7001	1044	.3754	.000	73
Total disease stress	0.7704	1025	.8366	.000	70
Difficulty falling asleep	0.7378	1059	.7886	.000	72
Sleep interruptions	0.6031	630	.6884	.000	72
Fatigue awakening	0.7037	1043	.8018	.000	66
General fatigue	0.7160	1035	.7476	.000	72
Depression	0.8791	975	.8375	.000	76
Denial	0.6800	976	.8650	.000	77
Anxiety	0.8393	992	.7069	.000	77
Social introversion	0.7685	928	.6378	.000	77
Self-depreciation	0.8068	1003	.7877	.000	74
Hypochondriasis	0.7589	665	.7677	.000	77
Somatic symptoms count	0.6090	6921	.4730	.000	74
Total somatic distress	0.6644	6863	.3881	.000	74
Interdialysis fatigue	0.6958	6906	.6710	.000	74

Table 3. Evidence for construct validity for quality-of-life scales

Scale	Variable	r	p
Pindex	Hypochondriasis	0.17	0.01
Psychosocial stress	Anxiety	0.31	0.001
	Depression	0.36	0.001
	Social readjustment	0.52	0.001
Disease	Anxiety	0.32	0.001
Stress	Depression	0.31	0.001
	Coping	0.39	0.001
Sleep scales	Depression	0.25–0.35	0.0001
	Fatigue	0.29–0.42	0.0001
Somatic symptoms	Treatment stress	0.34–0.41	0.001
Fatigue	Somatic symptoms	0.53	0.001
	Disease stress	0.48	0.001
	Psychosocial stress	0.31	0.001
	Treatment stress	0.24	0.001

survivors and nonsurvivors on dialysis [12] and success or failure of home hemodialysis programs [13].

Sensitivity

1. Physiological Index: In past research, the index successfully discriminated between survivors (n = 168; mean score = 11.98) and subsequent deaths (n = 20; mean score = 15.20) in a home dialysis population (p < 0.001) [14].

2. Psychosocial Stress Scale: The instrument was sensitive enough to register a significant (p < 0.05) reduction in stressor count (2.05 to 1.03) and total stress scores (7.48 to 3.81) accompanying the transition from 4-h cellulosic haemodialysis to 3-h high flux dialysis membrane (Study I). Likewise, a decrease in total psychosocial stress was noted accompanying treatment with erythropoietin, from 10.90 to 7.51 (p < 0.001) (Study II; Fig. 2).

3. Disease Stress Scale: The scale was able to measure the reduction in Disease Stressor Count (2.35 to 1.30) and Total Disease Stress (8.50 to 4.96) during the crossover from conventional to high-flux dialysis (Study I). Likewise there was a statistically significant reduction in the

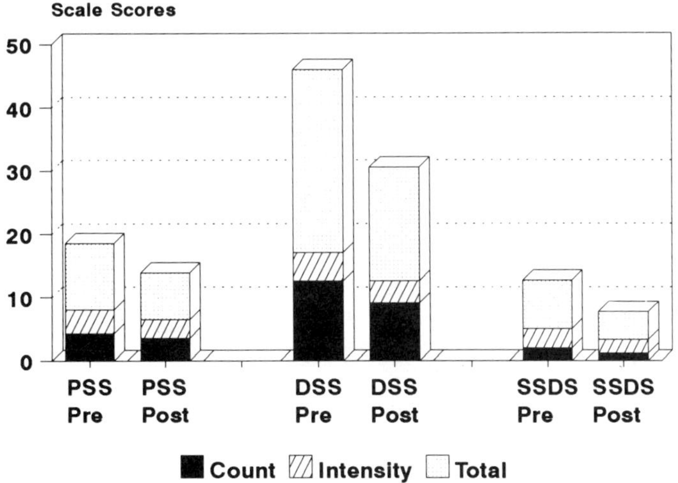

Fig. 2. Psychological stress scales before (Pre) and after (Post) EPO therapy. PSS, psychosocial stress; DSS, disease stress; SSDS, somatic symptoms distress.

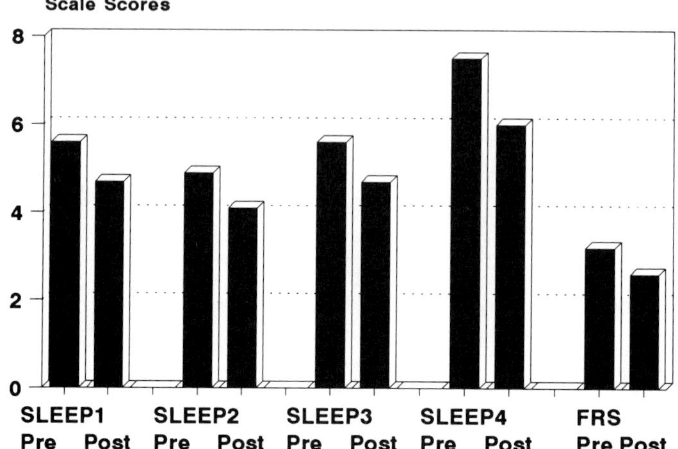

Fig. 3. Sleep scales before (Pre) and after (Post) EPO therapy. SLEEP1, falling asleep; SLEEP2, interruptions; SLEEP3, awakening; SLEEP4, general fatigue; FRS, fatigue rating scale.

Stressor Count (6.36 to 4.67; $p < 0.0001$) and in Total Stress (30.69 to 18.56; $p < 0.0001$) from preerythropoietin to posterythropoeitin (Study II; Fig. 2).

4. Sleep Scales: The sleep scales were sensitive enough to show an erythropoeitin treatment effect: Interference Falling Asleep was reduced from 5.58 to 4.85 ($p < 0.05$), Sleep interruptions went from 5.09 to 4.06 ($p < 0.0001$), Fatigue Awakening declined from 5.91 to 4.85 ($p < 0.01$), and General Fatigue dropped from 7.65 to 6.19 ($p < 0.001$) (Study II; Fig. 3).

5. Somatic Symptoms Distress Scale: The instrument was sufficiently sensitive to register a reduction in both the Symptom Count score (1.63 to 1.21; $p = 0.01$) and the Total Distress Score (4.25 to 3.11; $p = 0.002$) during the crossover from conventional to high-flux dialysis (Study I). Likewise, the preerythropoietin to posterythropoeitin contrast shows a reduction in Symptom Count from 2.09 to 1.25 accompanied by a drop in Total Distress from 8.15 to 4.55 ($p < 0.0001$) (Study II; Fig. 2).

6. Interdialysis Fatigue Rating Scale: Prior to erythropoietin, patients registered a mean score of 3.27, which dropped to 2.62 ($p < 0.0001$) after treatment (Study II).

7. Basic Personality Inventory: Statistically significant changes from pre-erythropoietin to posterythropoeitin were obtained for depression (8.20 to 7.19; p = 0.044), self-depreciation (4.62 to 3.69; p = 0.003) and social introversion (6.91 to 5.84; p = 0.008) (Study II).

Discussion

The scales[1] described can be used alone or in combination to provide a flexible and comprehensive quality-of-life assessment for hemodialysis patients. The addition of the physiological index provides a further outcome measurement, which, in addition, can be used as a controlling parameter for the quality-of-life measures (it being likely that sicker patients have reduced quality of life). The low missing-data rates from all countries and languages attest to the clarity of the instructions, the constituent items, and the layout of the forms and indicates that patients themselves regard the questions as relevant to their predicament. The present analysis confirms the reliability of internal consistency and the test-retest reliability of the battery; the scales are sufficiently free of random error to furnish an accurate estimate of a magnitude of stresses, symptoms, discomfort, and psychological side effects associated with ESRD and dialysis. The patterns of statistically significant interrelations in expected directions confirm the face validity of the scales and support the claim that they are tapping into meaningful quality-of-life domains. Finally, the ability of the scales to register statistically significant treatment effects testifies to the sensitivity and suitability of their use in evaluation research. Overall, the scales appear suited for use in multinational clinical trials involving ESRD patients treated by dialysis.

Acknowledgments

The authors wish to acknowledge the collaboration of, for Study I: Dr. P. Shandran, Dialysis P.C., Des Moines, Iowa; Dr. K. P. Anderson, Iowa Lutheran Hospital, Des Moines, Iowa; Drs. B. Haberstroh and T. Liu, Kitchener-Waterloo Hospital, Kitchener, Ontario; Dr. R. Manning, Hotel Dieu Hospital, St. Catherines, Ontario; Drs. R. Lindsay, W. Clark, A. L. Linton, Victoria Hospital, London, Ontario; Dr. J. MacAnally, Medical Center East, Elizabeth, New Jersey; Drs. C. Saiphoo and A. Manuel, Sunnybrook Medical Centre,

[1]The scales are available for research use by contacting the authors.

Toronto, Ontario; Dr. W. McCready, McKellar General Hospital, Thunder Bay, Ontario; Dr. B. Conly, Plummer Memorial Hospital, Sault Ste. Marie, Ontario; Dr. J. Price, Vancouver General Hospital, Vancouver, British Columbia. For Study II: Prof. K. Koch, Medizinische Hochschule, Hannover, Germany; Prof. K. Schaefer, St. Joseph Krankenhaus, Berlin, Germany; Prof. G. Stein, Nephrologische Abteilung, Jena Lobedea, Germany; Dr. M. J. Goggin, Kent and Canterbury Hospital, Canterbury, England; Dr. G. Degremont, Centre Hospitalier, Cambrai Cedex, France; Dr. M. Tolani, Polyclinique St. Come, Compiegne, France; Dr. J. Brasseur, Centre Hospitalier, St. Quentin Cedex, France; Dr. G. Fournier, Association IR Beauce et Perche, Chartres, France; Dr. C. Ogg, St. Guy's Hospital, London, England; Dr. Manno, Casa di Cura, Bari, Italy; Prof. Romagnoli, Ospedale Regionale, Padova, Italy; Prof. Saporiti, Ospedale Regionale, Venezia, Italy; Dr. C. Cascone, Ospedale Provinciale, Castelfranco Veneto, Italy; Dr. B. Agazia, Ospedale Provinciale Civile, Adria, Italy; Dr. L. Weiss, Central Jukhuset, Karlstad, Sweden; Dr. T. Lindholm, University Hospital, Lund, Sweden; Dr. P. O. Andersson, Lasarettet i Norrkoping, Norrkoping, Sweden; Dr. J. Wallis, Leicester General Hospital, Leicester, England. The authors also wish to thank Miss J. Elphee for the preparation of this manuscript.

References

1 Kaplan Denour A: An overview of psychological problems in haemodialysis patients; in Levy NB (ed): Psychonephrology: Psychological Problems in Kidney Failure and Their Treatment. New York, Plenum, 1983, vol 2, pp 3–14.
2 Evans RW, Manninen DL, Garrison Jr LP: The quality of life of patients with end-stage renal disease. N Engl J Med 1985;312:553–559.
3 Kutner NG, Brogan D, Kutner MH: End-stage renal disease treatment modality and patients' quality of life. Am J Nephrol 1986;6:396–402.
4 Guyatt GH, Bomardier C, Tugwell PX: Measuring disease-specific quality of life in clinical trials. CMAJ 1986;134:889–885.
5 Spilker B: Introduction; in Spilker B (ed): Quality of Life Assessments in Clinical Trials. New York, Raven Press, 1990, p 3.
6 Kennedy AC, Lindsay RM, Murphy AV, Allison MEM, McLeod O: A scoring system for assessing patients on regular dialysis. Lancet 1969;1:701–702.
7 Strauch MR, Lipke R, Schafheutle R, Nachbauer B, Stauch-Rahauser G: A standardized list of somatic criteria for comparative assessment of regular dialysis therapy patients. Artif Organs 1978;2(suppl):370–372.
8 Jackson DJ: The Basic Personality Inventory. Port Huron, Mich., Research Psychologists Press, 1976.

9   Sellitz C, Wrightsman LS, Cook SW: Research methods in social relations. New York, Holt, Rinehart, Winston, 1976, 3rd ed.

10 Helmstadter GC: Principles of Psychological Measurement. Chicago, Rand McNally, 1976.

11 Lindsay RM, Heidenheim AP, Spanner E, Burton H, Lindsay S, LeFebvre JMJ: A multi-centre study of short hours (SH) dialysis using AN69S—preliminary results. ASAIO Trans 1991:37(3):M465-M467.

12 Wai L, Richmond J, Burton H, Lindsay RM: The influence of psychosocial factors on survival of home dialysis patients. Lancet 1981;2:1155–1156.

13 Richmond JM, Lindsay RM, Burton HJ, Conley J, Wai L: Psychological and physiological factors predicting the outcome on home haemodialysis. Clin Nephrol 1982;17(3):109–113.

14 Burton HJ, Canzona L, Lindsay RM, Palmer S: Adaptation to home dialysis: The Ontario experience. Final report. London, Canada, University of Western Ontario Press, 1985.

R. M. Lindsay, Victoria Hospital, 375 South Street, London, Ontario, Canada N6A 4G5

Discussion

to the Paper by R. M. Lindsay and A. P. Heidenheim

Bergström (Stockholm): When you use these instruments, don't you have to do placebo-controlled studies? Otherwise I think the results will not be meaningful.

Lindsay: It is very difficult to do placebo-controlled studies in those, such as a change from high-flux dialysis to conventional dialysis. All you can do is to do prospective randomized ones and to make sure that the groups are all properly cohorted, which we have done in both of the studies for age, sex, risk factor, and buffer. Certainly you can do it if you look at a specific drug. We have done this as well, out of the renal field, and we have got involved in looking at antihypertensive agents and lipid-lowering agents. In a lipid study, placebo-controlled, just completed, significant differences were detected by the quality-of-life instruments.

Anemia and the Heart

M. Leschke, F. Schoebel, B. E. Strauer

Department of Cardiology, Pneumology, and Angiology, Heinrich-Heine-
Universität Düsseldorf, Düsseldorf, Germany

Introduction

Anemia is a common cause of increased cardiac output and when extremely
severe may result in heart failure due to a high-output state even in the absence of
underlying heart disease [1]. In this review article, clinical, epidemiological, as
well as pathophysiological aspects of anemia emphasizing vascular hemodynamics will be considered. Although anemia is a frequent clinical complication associated with a reduction of oxygen transport capacity, it is common
clinical experience that cardiovascular events such as angina pectoris and myocardial infarction and cerebrovascular events are quite rare. This is a consequence of apparently metabolically induced peripheral vasodilation and improved rheological flow properties resulting in an increased cardiac output as
compensatory mechanisms of reduced oxygen transport capacity [2].

The characteristic compensatory cardiovascular mechanisms and hemodynamic adaptions to anemia leading to a new balance of oxygen supply and
demand will be reviewed. Furthermore, the interrelation between myocardial
perfusion and oxygen transport capacity under different rheological circumstances will be demonstrated.

Clinical and Epidemiological Aspects

The severity of cardiac symptoms such as fatigue, exertional dyspnea, and
edema depend on the severity of anemia, the rapidity with which anemia
develops, and the presence of an underlying cardiac disease, such as coronary
artery, myocardial, or valvular heart disease. Even severely anemic patients
without underlying cardiac disease have few if any cardiac symptoms, whereas

in the presence of coronary artery disease, anemia lowers the threshold for development of angina pectoris. In the absence of underlying cardiac disease, congestive heart failure as a result of severe anemia (hemoglobin < 4 g/dl) occurs rarely in previously stable patients and is usually the result of rapid progression of anemia [3].

According to epidemiological data from the Honolulu Heart Program [4], hemotocrit is significantly correlated with the 10-year mortality rate due to coronary artery disease. Significantly higher baseline hematocrit levels were found in men who subsequently died of coronary artery disease compared to the total population. This relationship, however, lost its statistical significance when blood pressure, age, cholesterol level, smoking, and alcohol were taken into account. In the Puerto Rico Heart Health Program [5], the initial hematocrit was related to the cardiac risk in 8700 men between the age of 45 and 64 years. The incidence of cardiovascular events in the group with high hematocrit levels was nearly twice as high as in the group with the lowest hematocrit values.

In a retrospective study, hematocrit values of 100 patients with acute myocardial infarction (48.6 ± 4.05%) were significantly higher compared to 100 age-matched control subjects (44.7 ± 3.5%) [6]. These data suggest that the incidence of myocardial infarction may be influenced by rheological mechanisms, such as sludge phenomenon, and thereby by an alleviated predisposition to intravascular thrombosis subsequent to elevated hematocrit levels. These clinical and epidemiological data, however, underline the tolerance of the myocardium to a reduced oxygen-transport capacity due to different cardiovascular compensatory mechanisms in coronary and systemic circulation.

Compensatory Cardiovascular Mechanisms

The compensation of acute and chronic anemia and hence reduced oxygen content of arterial blood critically depends upon cardiorespiratory function and circulating blood volume. Tissue hypoxia and reduced blood viscosity in anemia lead to reduced systemic vascular resistance, which is associated with increased cardiac output [1, 7, 8]. Furthermore, chronic anemia enhances formation of intercoronary collaterals and causes increases in preload and a reduction in afterload [1]. A slow development of anemia is associated with cardiac hypertrophy and general vasodilation, which increases venous return (preload) and reduces peripheral resistance (afterload). The improved venous return is partly due to enhanced blood fluidity in anemia. Increased left ventricular end-diastolic volume is demonstrated in anemic patients. Another mechanism of enhanced left ventricular function in chronic anemia has been attributed to increased levels of catecholamines and a noncatecholamine inotropic factor in plasma [9]. Experimental data from papillary muscles placed in serum obtained from patients with chronic anemia exhibit increased contractility even though plasma catecholamine levels were within the normal range. The cardiac enlargement that develops with severe, chronic anemia usually results from dilation and eccentric hypertrophy with a normal ratio of wall thickness to cavity diameter, thus providing for unchanged systolic stress and oxygen demand [10].

In Figure 1 the compensatory mechanisms in anemia are exhibited as a flow chart. Anemia leads to a significant fall in hematocrit and, thus, blood viscosity resulting in a reduced oxygen-transport capacity of blood. The resultant tissue hypoxia evokes several compensatory mechanisms, such as hypoxic peripheral vascular dilation, which is associated with increased blood flow to the periphery. Tissue hypoxia is furthermore compensated by an increased oxygen extraction due to a shift to the right in the oxygen dissociation curve mediated by an increase in red cell 2,3-DPG [1, 7].

Hemodynamic Adaptions to Anemia

The central hemodynamic change in chronic anemia is an increased cardiac output indicating the existence of a hyperkinetic state. It has been postulated that this hyperkinetic response to anemia only occurs when hemoglobin levels fall below 7 g/100 ml [7]. Several mechanisms for these hemodynamic changes have been proposed, including a decreased systemic vascular resistance, an adaption to increased filling pressure due to increased venous return, a reduction of blood

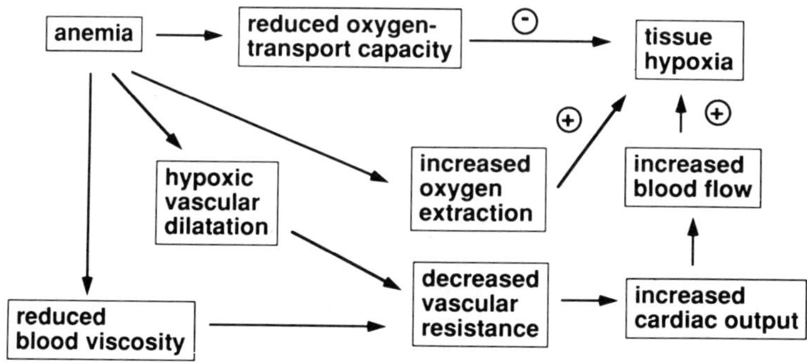

Fig. 1. Compensatory circulatory mechanisms in anemia.

viscosity, resulting in an increase in cardiac stroke volume, the shift of the oxyhemoglobin dissociation curve to the right, and finally some humoral mechanisms. Analysis by Duke and Abelmann [7] revealed that the severity of anemia did not correlate with the level of cardiac output and that at the same level of hemoglobin, the lowest cardiac output was usually present in the older age group. The authors found an inverse relationship between age and cardiac index before and after correction of anemia. Following transfusion therapy the ejection fraction fell significantly by an average of nearly 40% [7]. The authors suggest that the immediate reversal of the high output state by orthostatic stress or by a vasoconstrictor drug indicates that the increased blood flow is primarily mediated by lowered peripheral resistance due to vasodilation rather than to lowered blood viscosity. According to these data the primary change in hemodynamic response to anemia seems to be the peripheral vasodilation induced by metabolic mechanisms such as local tissue hypoxia, increased lactate production, local acidemia, and an accumulation of vasoactive substances, such as adenosine and bradykinin, with rheological aspects being of secondary importance.

In patients with chronic anemia as opposed to patients with polyglobulia, characteristic hemodynamic alterations in the coronary microcirculation were found (Fig. 2 and 3). Previous studies of our working group were performed with regard to disturbances of coronary microcirculation in patients with hematological alterations. These patients with anemia (n = 6) and polyglobulia and polycythemia (n = 4) had typical angina pectoris despite macroscopically normal coronary arteries. In both groups, coronary resistance and coronary flow were measured by the argon-inert gas method. Details of this study [11], including the exact method, have been previously described [12].

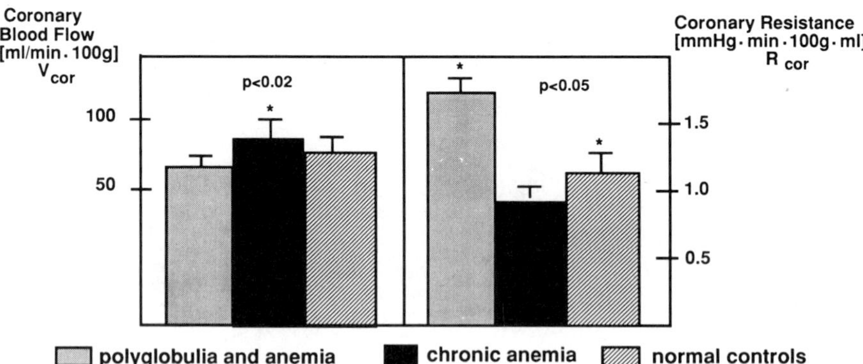

Fig. 2. Coronary blood flow and coronary resistance in polyglobulia, polycythemia (n = 4; hemoglobin < 18 g/dl), and anemia (n = 6; hemoglobin < 10 g/dl).

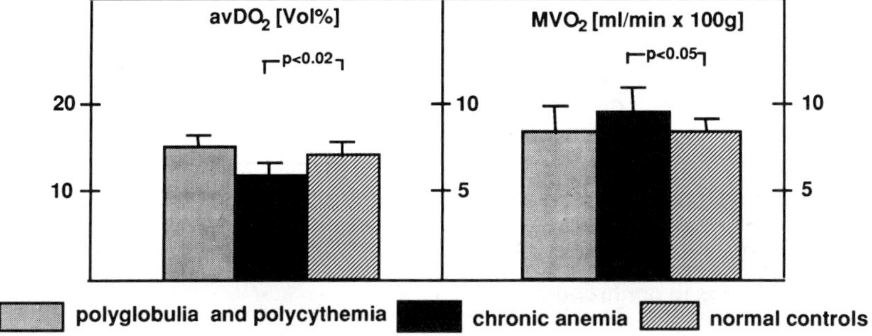

Fig. 3. Left ventricular oxygen consumption (MVO$_2$) and arterial-coronary venous oxygen difference (avDO$_2$) in polyglobulia, polycythemia (n = 4; Hb > 18 g/dl), and anemia (n = 6; Hb < 10 g/dl).

Patients with chronic anemia show a significant increase in coronary blood flow as compared to normal subjects, accordingly coronary resistance is significantly lower in normal control subjects than in patients with polyglobulia. Due to the higher red cell mass and the abnormally elevated whole blood viscosity in patients with polyglobulia and polycythemia, coronary blood flow at rest was significantly decreased, whereas coronary resistance was increased nearly 50% in comparison to normal subjects. The coronary oxygen extraction was reduced in anemia due to a proportionally greater increase of coronary blood flow, whereas the myocardial oxygen consumption due to increased coronary flow and relatively low coronary oxygen extraction was significantly higher than in control subjects.

In general, anemia is associated with characteristic hemodynamic conditions such as (a) elevated cardiac output, (b) decreased vascular resistance, and, in terms of coronary microcirculation, (c) elevated coronary blood flow and (d) reduced coronary resistance.

Rheological Considerations, Oxygen Transport, and Myocardial Perfusion

The oxygen transport capacity is determined by hematocrit levels and rheological flow properties [13]. Furthermore, blood rheology influences oxygen delivery to different tissues, although hematocrit changes have minor effects on oxygen delivery in comparison to an elevation of plasma viscosity and increased fibrinogen levels [14–16]. The determinants of oxygen delivery are shown in Figure 4. A different distribution of blood flow maintains oxygenation of vital organs.

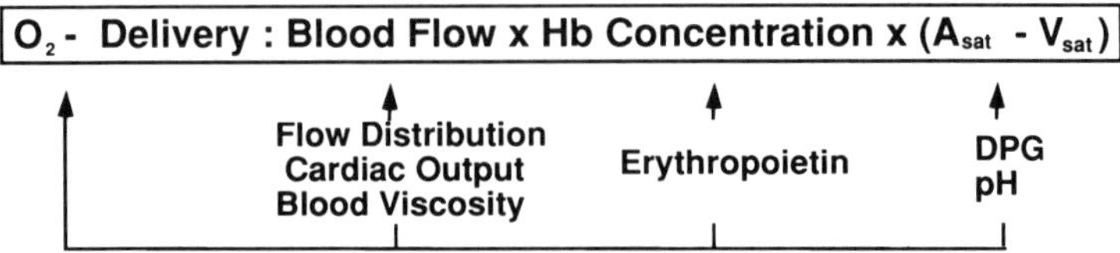

Mechanisms of compensation of hypoxia:

(1) Distribution of blood flow maintains oxygenation of vital organs
(2) Increase of total cardiac output
(3) Increased erythropoietin production
(4) Oxygen unloading is enhanced by a shift to the right in the oxygen
dissociation curve due to an increase of 2,3-DPG

Fig. 4.   Determinants of oxygen delivery.

Focusing on coronary circulation, coronary blood flow is determined by several factors, such as driving pressure, coronary vessel geometry, and coronary resistance [17]. This basic relationship of fluid characteristics to blood flow is defined in approximation by the law of Hagen-Poiseuille [15], in which the blood viscosity is inversely related to blood flow. A decrease in blood viscosity, as in chronic anemia, therefore, is associated with increased blood flow. Beside rheological properties, coronary resistance is further determined by a vascular component, e.g., macroscopic stenosis in coronary artery disease and disturbed coronary autoregulation, as well as by a myocardial component, e.g., left ventricular hypertrophy in hypertensive heart disease. For further considerations, a normal coronary autoregulation is assumed.

In a defined state of anemia, for instance, the increase of blood flow is proportionally larger in the coronary bed than in the renal, mesenteric, or femoral bed [18]. Most tissues, e.g., the working muscle, can increase oxygen delivery by extracting a larger proportion of oxygen from the supply transported to the capillaries. In contrast, the myocardium normally works at near maximum oxygen extraction and must increase its oxygen delivery to satisfy higher demands either by an increase in the amount of oxygen transported to the coronary capillaries or by an increase in flow. Secondary metabolic compensatory mechanisms in chronic anemia are increased erythropoietin production and shift to the right in the oxygen dissociation curve due to an increase of 2,3-DPG. Considering the pathophysiological relationship between anemia and the heart, it is therefore essential to understand the determinants of myocardial oxygen transport and how myocardial oxygen transport is affected by hematocrit changes.

Studies in anesthetized dogs [19] have shown that maximal oxygen delivery far exceeds the supply at all hematocrit levels (Fig. 5). When hematocrit is

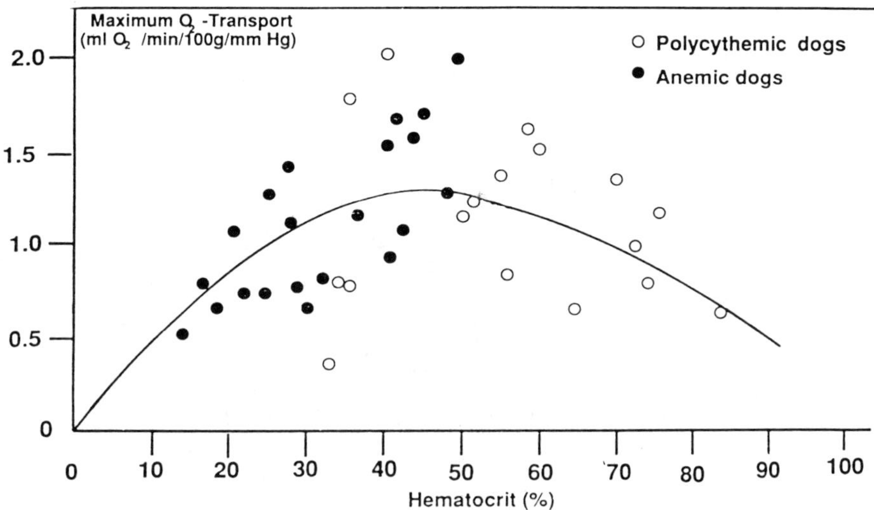

Fig. 5. Maximum oxygen transport adjusted per unit perfusion pressure as a function of hematocrit in anemic and polycythemic dogs [19].

plotted against maximum oxygen transport, an inverted U-shaped relationship results. This finding is only defined at physical rest conditions with normal vascular regulation. In other words, these data prove that in otherwise normal subjects, the occurrence of severe anemia rarely if ever results in myocardial hypoxia because of several compensatory mechanisms (Fig. 1). However, when myocardial oxygen demands increase, e.g., during exercise, maximum oxygen transport exceeds demand only over a limited range of hematocrit, especially in states of flow-limiting conditions as in hemodynamically relevant vascular stenoses. Further studies from Jan and Chien [13] could demonstrate that the range of "optimum hematocrit" for maximum oxygen transport was much wider in coronary (hematocrit 20–60%) than in systemic circulation (hematocrit 40–60%). The oxygen extraction ratio in coronary circulation was constant over a wide range of hematocrit levels between 10 and 70%, suggesting that the myocardial oxygen consumption was primarily determined by the coronary oxygen transport.

As discussed above, delivery of oxygen to different types of tissue is directly proportional to blood flow, hemoglobin concentration, and the difference in arterio-venous oxygen saturation. In anemic patients, an increase in blood flow induced by reduced blood viscosity and enhanced oxygen delivery compensate for the reduced oxygen transport capacity. In conditions, however, with elevated

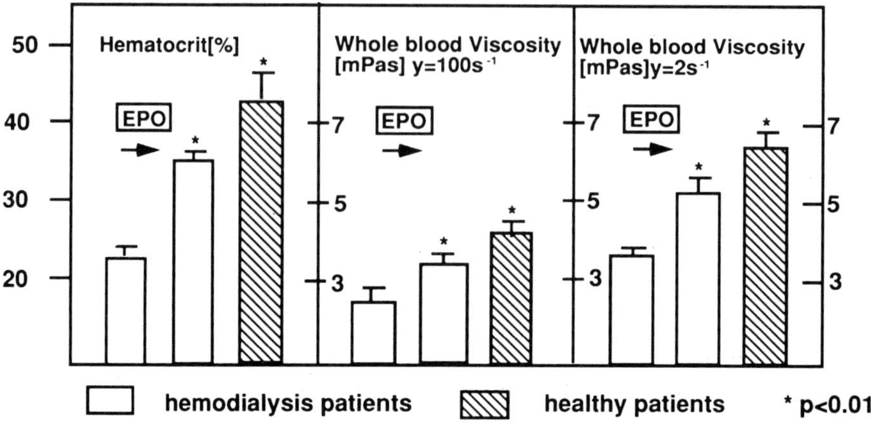

Fig. 6. Hemorheological parameters in healthy subjects (n = 15) and hemodialysis patients (n = 8) prior to and during treatment with rhEPO.

blood viscosity, e.g., polyglobulia and polycythemia, an increase in coronary resistance and a reduction in coronary blood flow result (Fig. 2 and 3). Blood viscosity, due to its non-Newtonian behavior, increases exponentially with increased hematocrit levels [15]. Blood flow decreases as an essentially linear function of hematocrit. Therefore, oxygen transport decreases significantly at hematocrit values just above 40% [20] because of increased blood viscosity.

As an example of rheological changes in anemia, hematocrit levels and whole blood viscosity at high and low shear rates are exhibited in hemodialysis patients before and during treatment with human erythropoietin and in healthy subjects (Fig. 6) [21]. Whole blood viscosity and hematocrit are significantly reduced in hemodialysis patients with renal anemia. During treatment with erythropoietin, whole blood viscosity is significantly increased due to elevated hematocrit values by about 42% at low shear rates and 32% at high shear rates. From these data, the hemodynamic consequences of correction of anemia can be derived. From a rheological point of view, the formerly "optimal" microcirculatory flow conditions in extreme anemia have changed to an unfavorable condition due to elevated whole blood viscosity. The correction of anemia is associated with a rise in peripheral resistance and with a decrease in cardiac output. The increase in total peripheral resistance is induced by an enhanced viscous resistance of blood to flow and an increased degree of arteriolar vasoconstriction [19, 21].

Hemodilution and Myocardial Ischemia

Still a matter of debate is whether therapeutically induced hemodilution leads to coronary flow improvement or to a deterioration in coronary flow, especially in patients with coronary artery disease in whom a reduction of coronary vascular reserve, e.g., the capacity to enhance coronary blood flow in the poststenotic segments depending on the degree of the stenosis, has to be expected. In experiments on dogs undergoing strictly isovolemic blood exchange for dextran 60 or packed red cells, respectively, Sunder-Plassmann et al. [23] were able to confirm that maximum oxygen transport did not coincide with the animals' control hematocrit but with a hematocrit of about 30%. The increase in oxygen transport was explained by the enhanced cardiac output being proportionally greater than the corresponding fall in arterial oxygen content of blood. During normovolemic hemodilution, an increase in flow to all layers of myocardium in epicardium, endocardium, and the papillary muscle could be shown [23]. Review of studies on coronary flow and myocardial oxygen supply leads to the conclusion that, in the absence of coronary artery disease and in the absence of higher work demands, the myocardial oxygen supply is sufficiently maintained due to enhanced coronary flow at even lower hematocrit levels with slightly increased oxygen extraction [23].

Contrary to these results, Restorff et al. [24] showed that already at rest coronary flow increased more than 7-fold with diminished hematocrit levels in order to cover myocardial oxygen consumption. The coronary dilation capacity estimated by measurement of the reactive hyperemia fell from 600% at control hematocrit to 45% at lowest hematocrit levels. During exercise coronary blood flow and myocardial oxygen consumption increased further, leading to a complete exhaustion of coronary dilation capacity at low hematocrit values between 16 and 22%. These data clearly indicate that hemodilution is tolerated in healthy subjects with normal coronary reserve, whereas hemodilution is of limited value in coronary artery disease with reduced coronary reserve. Some previous studies, however, demonstrated a significant increase of collateral blood flow in ischemic myocardium [25] and in the "border zone" of myocardial infarction [26].

In conclusion, in subjects with normal coronary arteries, a wide range of hematocrit changes (20–60%) is clinically well tolerated without incidence of myocardial ischemia. According to epidemiological data, elevated hematocrit levels tend to provoke a higher incidence of cardiovascular events in patients with coronary artery disease due to abnormal blood rheology and, thus, disturbed myocardial microcirculation. Conversely, it can be postulated that anemia unmasks myocardial ischemia by decreasing the threshold for angina pectoris and apparently reduces the incidence of cardiovascular events in coronary artery disease due to increased blood fluidity assuming an adequate left ventricular function and coronary reserve are maintained. In general, it cannot be concluded from these data to what extent patients with severe coronary artery disease and therefore severely reduced coronary reserve would benefit from therapeutically induced "anemia," e.g., hemodilution or whether they would profit at all in terms of improved myocardial perfusion.

References

1 Varat MA, Adolph RJ, Fowler NO: Cardiovascular effects of anemia. Am Heart J 1972;83:415–426.

2 Schmid-Schönbein H: Blood rheology and cardiac microcirculation: Is there a place for hemodilution in coronary insufficiency?; in Schmid-Schönbein H, Messmer K, Rieger H (eds): Hemodilution and Flow Improvement. Basel, S. Karger, 1981, pp 325–339.

3 Rosenthal DS, Braunwald E: Hematological-oncological disorders and heart disease; in Braundwald E (ed): Heart Disease. Philadelphia, WB Saunders Company, 1988, pp 1734–1753.

4 Carter C, McGee D, Reed D, Yano K, Stemmermann G: Hematocrit and the risk of coronary heart disease: The Honolulu Heart Program. Am Heart J 1993;105:674–679.

5 Sorlie PD, Garcia-Palmieri MR, Costas R, Havlik RJ: Hematocrit and risk of coronary heart disease: The Puerto Rico Heart Health Program. Am Heart J 1981;101:456–461.

6 Burch GE, De Pasquale NP: The hematocrit in patients with myocardial infarction. JAMA 1962;180:63–65.

7 Duke M, Abelmann WH: The hemodynamic response to chronic anemia. Circulation 1969;39:503–515.

8 Denenberg BS, Conier G, Jones R, Spann JF: Cardiac function in sickle cell anemia. Am J Cardiol 1983;51:1674–1678.

9 Florenzano F, Diaz G, Regonesi C, Escobar E: Left ventricular function in chronic anemia. Evidence of noncatecholamine positive inotropic factors in the serum. Am J Cardiol 1984;54:638–645.

10 Grassman W, Jones D, McLaurin LP: Wall stress and patterns of hypertrophy in the human left ventricle. J Clin Invest 1975;56:56–64.

11 Strauer BE, Böhme H, Samtleben W, Schulte S, Volger E: Clinical approach to disturbances in microcirculation of the heart. Clin Hemorheology 1984;4:45–66.

12 Strauer BE: Ventricular function and coronary hemodynamics in hypertensive heart disease. Am J Cardiol 1979;44:999–1006.

13 Jan KM, Chien S: Effect of hematocrit variations on coronary hemodynamics and oxygen utilization. Am J Physiol 1977;233:H106–H113.

14 Gordon RJ, Snyder GK, Tritel H, Taylor WJ: Potential significance of plasma

viscosity and hematocrit variations in myocardial ischemia. Am Heart J 1974;87:175–182.

15 Schmid-Schönbein H, Rieger H, Fischer T: Blood fluidity as a consequence of red cell fluidity: Flow properties of blood and flow behaviour of blood vascular diseases. Angiology 1980;31:301–319.

16 Leschke M, Strauer BE: Hemorheologic profile and precursors in myocardial ischemia; in von Arnim Th, Maseri A (eds): Predisposing Conditions for Acute Ischemic Syndromes. Darmstadt, Steinkopff Verlag, 1989, pp 85–95.

17 Strauer BE: The significance of coronary artery reserve in clinical heart disease. Am J Cardiol 1990;15:775–783.

18 Finch CA, Lenfant C: Oxygen transport in man. N Engl J Med 1972;286:407–419.

19 Baer RW, Vlahakes GJ, Uhlig PN, Hoffman JIE: Maximum myocardium oxygen transport during anemia and polycythemia in dogs. Am J Physiol 1987;252:H1086–H1095.

20 Williams WJ (ed): Hematology, 2nd ed. New York, McGraw-Hill, 1977, p 256.

21 Schäfer RM, Leschke M, Strauer BE, Heidland A: Blood rheology and hypertension in hemodialysis patients treated with erythropoietin. Am J Nephrol 1988;8:449–453.

22 Grassman W, Jansen D, McLaurin P: Wall stress and patterns of hypertrophy in man in the human left ventricle. J Clin Invest 1975;56:56–64.

23 Sunder-Plassmann L, Klövekorn WP, Holper K, Hase U, Messmer K: The physiological significance of acutely induced hemodilution; in Proc 6th Eur Conf Microcirculation, Aalburg. Basel, Karger, 1970, p 23.

24 Messmer K: Compensatory mechanisms for acute dilutional anemia. Bibl Haematol 1981;47:31–42.

25 Yoshikawa H, Powell WJ, Bland JHL, Lowenstein E: Effect of acute anemia on experimental myocardial ischemia. Am J Cardiol 1973;32:670–678.

26 Sjöquist POB, Kareld L, Wahlmund GC, Holmberg S: Moderate normovolaemic haemodilution increases regional myocardial blood flow but has no effect on experimental infarct size. Scand J Clin Lab Invest 1986;46:677–683.

Matthias Leschke, Medizinische Klinik und Poliklinik B, Abteilung für Kardiologie, Pneumologie und Angiologie, Heinrich-Heine-Universität Düsseldorf, Moorenstrasse 5, 40225 Düsseldorf 1, Germany

Discussion

to the Paper by M. Leschke et al.

Koch (*Hannover*): Do you consider the myocardial hypertrophy induced by anemia to be risk factor or not?

Leschke: Several studies, including the Framingham study, could show that left ventricular hypertrophy is an independent cardiovascular risk factor. The same is true for the constellation of renal anemia in association with arterial hypertension due to renal dysfunction leading to left ventricular hypertrophy. Left ventricular hypertrophy induced by anemia without arterial hypertension presents a different situation and, according to my knowledge, there are no valid data on the incidence of cardiovascular events, especially regarding this constellation. I suppose that we should consider the myocardial hypertrophy induced by anemia as a risk factor.

Koch: You said, as far as I recall your slides, that this type of hypertrophy was rather mild, isn't it? And you gave a specific description of it. Is there a difference between the hypertrophy caused by anemia and that by pressure work?

Leschke: Indeed, there does exist a different pattern of myocardial hypertrophy due to volume overload in anemia and due to increased pressure load in arterial hypertension. Volume overload leads to an eccentric left ventricular hypertrophy with normal myocardial contents of collagen and no microvascular changes in contrast to increased content of collagen and microvascular changes in concentric left ventricular hypertrophy due to arterial hypertension. This form of hypertrophy induced by anemia is also associated with slightly elevated oxygen consumption and slightly elevated systolic wall stress.

Winearls (*Oxford*): Does your presentation help us to balance the advantages and risks, in a hemodialysis patient, of having a hematocrit of 40% or 30%? You showed that between 30% and 40% there is a linear increase in systemic oxygen delivery. However, you also showed that in normal individuals the risk of cardiovascular events increases as the hematocrit increases between 40% and 50%. Is there any evidence of a difference of cardiovascular events between 30% and 40%?

Leschke: There does exist epidemiological data which indicate that individuals with lower hematocrit levels have a minor risk of cardiovascular events in respect to individuals with higher hematocrit levels in patients with coronary artery disease. On one hand, low hematocrit levels may detect ischemia of viable myocardium; on the other hand, lower hematocrit levels may improve rheological blood properties and therefore diminish the risk of development of cardiovascular events, meaning thrombosis and myocardial infarction.

Gaehtgens (Berlin): I am referring to the data that you showed from the literature discussing the problem of optimal hematocrit, in particular with reference to the myocardial circulation. There seems to be substantial conflict in the literature between results that have been derived from various sources. Some papers that you quoted—e.g., by Jan and Chien—show a rather wide range of optimal hematocrit, between 40 and 60, and, on the other hand, there are conflicting data, also from clinical studies, that clearly indicate that subnormal hematocrits are optimal. What are the reasons for these discrepancies?

Leschke: One reason for the discrepancy between experimental data and clinical data might be the fact that clinical situations with anemia are often associated with a decreased blood volume, which leads to reduced perfusion and possibly increased ischemia. Maybe the reduction of the intravascular blood volume is one factor for the observed discrepancy between experimental and clinical data.

Recombinant Human Erythropoietin Therapy: Benefits for the Heart and Physical Performance

K. M. L. Leunissen, J. J. J. M. Wirtz, W. van Kuijk, J. P. van Hooff

Department of Nephrology, University Hospital Maastricht, Maastricht,
The Netherlands

Introduction

Anemia is a common finding in patients with chronic renal failure. In most patients hematocrit falls as renal disease progresses, but it eventually tends to stabilize at 15–25%. The major factor in anemia due to chronic renal failure is diminished bone marrow red cell production, secondary to reduced secretion of recombinant human erythropoietin (rhEPO).

Previously, anemia due to renal failure was only treated if patients developed severe symptoms, such as extreme fatigue, shortness of breath, heart failure, and increased frequency of angina pectoris. Increasing hematocrit by transfusion often relieved the patient's complaints for a certain period of time. The risks of a blood transfusion (like hepatitis, iron overload, immunological sensitization) limited the use of this therapy, leaving chronic renal failure patients with average hematocrit levels of 20–25%.

Hemoglobin concentration is certainly one of the most important determinants of maximal aerobic power and thus of performance in many types of physical activities. The introduction of rhEPO, while increasing the hemoglobin level of dialysis patients, could be expected to improve physical performance in these patients and to reduce exertional dyspnea, thereby improving the quality of life. Furthermore, the correction of anemia with rhEPO could normalize functional and structural cardiovascular abnormalities related to chronic anemia.

In this article we will initially discuss the functional and structural cardiovascular changes caused by chronic anemia, including effects on physical performance. Furthermore, we will discuss the short- and long-term effects of rhEPO therapy in correcting the anemic state. Finally we will give some data concerning physical performance from quality-of-life questionnaires filled out by patients undergoing rhEPO treatment.

Hemodynamic Response to Chronic Anemia

In many patients with chronic anemia, rapid circulation time and increased cardiac output indicate the existence of a hyperkinetic state, usually accompanied by increased tissue extraction of oxygen [1]. The increase in cardiac output during chronic anemia depends upon the age of the patient. Several mechanisms for these changes have been postulated. The reduced blood viscosity decreases the resistance to blood flow in the peripheral vessels, increases the venous return, and consequently increases the cardiac output [2]. Moreover, hypoxemia due to a diminished transport of oxygen by the blood causes a vasodilatation of the tissue vessels, thereby increasing venous return and cardiac output. The decreased arterial pressure in chronic anemia might be related to a generalized vasodilatation and a reduced blood volume [1], whereas venoconstriction maintains central blood volume and venous pressure [1]. One of the major effects of anemia is a greatly increased workload for the heart. Myocardial oxygen consumption, indirectly assessed by tension time and pressure rate indices, appears to be increased in dialysis patients [3].

Cardiac hemodynamics were assessed by heart catheterization in 9 anemic hemodialysis patients by Capelli et al. [3]. They showed increased stroke work index and left ventricular work indices. Left ventricular end-diastolic pressure was elevated in all patients and did not fall with the occlusion of the arteriovenous fistulas. Myocardial mass increased and resulted in an increased myocardial oxygen demand. However, the increased oxygen requirements may not be reached because of reduced erythrocyte mass. Persistence of pressure volume overload and severe anemia are conducive to myocardial failure in these patients.

Chronic anemia not only induces functional changes in the cardiovascular state but also proves to have effects on structural changes. The increased venous return will lead to increased left ventricular dimensions, especially of the end-diastolic left ventricular diameter [4]. Silberberg et al. studied left ventricular mass index determined by echocardiography in 78 patients treated by dialysis for at least 3 months [5]. A significant relationship was found between anemia and left ventricular hypertrophy. The mean left ventricular mass index was 158 ± 6 g/m^2 in patients in the lowest quartile of serum hemoglobin and 140 ± 10, 132 ± 7, and 120 ± 8 in the second, third, and uppermost quartiles, respectively ($p = 0.005$). This relationship persisted after adjusting for systolic blood pressure, treatment mode, and suspected coronary artery disease. These data indicate that anemia may contribute to the development of left ventricular hypertrophy in patients with end-stage renal disease. Florenzano et al. also found some evidence for the existence of a non–catecholamine-positive inotropic factor in the serum of chronic anemic patients [6]. It is likely that the development of hypertrophy allows tissue oxygen needs to be met by increasing stroke volume while normalizing systolic wall stress. However, we have to realize that left ventricular hypertrophy in patients with end-stage renal disease is certainly multifactorial.

Microvascular structural changes have been described in hemodialysis patients [7]. Light and electron microscopic investigations of skin biopsies revealed thickening of the basement membrane, endothelial activation, and chronic inflammatory cell infiltration with participation of mast cells [8–10]. There was no relation to creatinine level, hemodialysis status, or known duration of renal failure. Intravital microscopy revealed microvascular rarefaction, reduction in number of arterioles, and structural changes in hypertensive patients. The same was true in hemodialysis patients, especially in the hypertensive dialysis patients. The percentage of tortuous capillaries was 35.5% in nonhypertensive and 61.8% in hypertensive patients (Fig. 1). In normal controls this percentage is

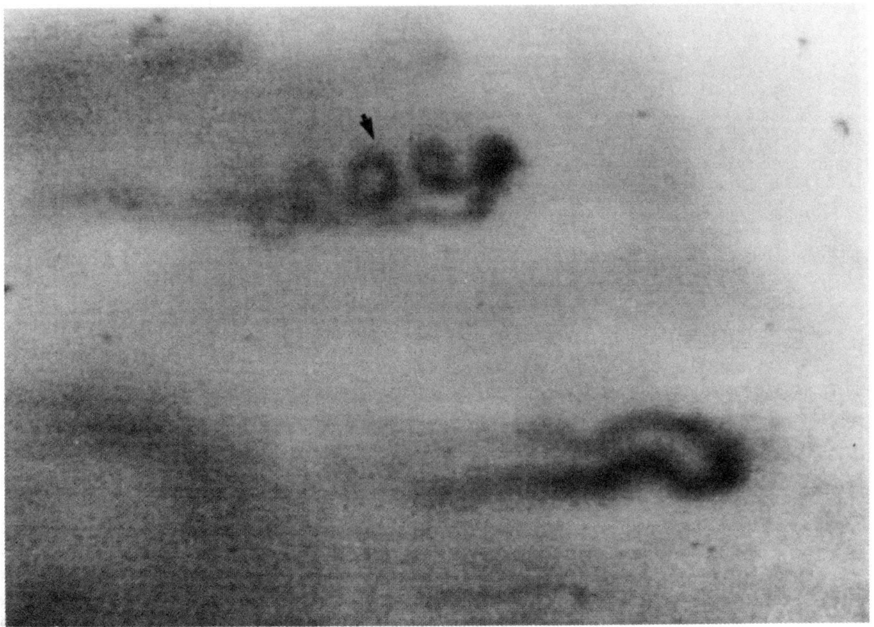

Fig. 1. Pathological capillary loop with arterial tortuosity (arrow), generally accompanied by venous vasodilatation. [From Ref. 7, with permission.]

about 10% [7]. The cause of the abnormal microvascularity in hemodialysis patients is multifactorial: hypertension, uremic toxins, and anemia could be responsible. Gilchrest et al. reported that microangiopathy was much less severe in the transplant recipients and that changes regressed from severe to moderate within 2 months after transplantation [10].

Hemodynamic Effects of Correcting Anemia

Duke and Abelmann studied the effect of gradual correction of anemia by specific therapy in patients with chronic anemia. They found a significant decrease in heart rate, stroke index, and cardiac index, while peripheral resistance increased significantly. Rapid blood transfusions resulted in a rise in cardiac output, venous pressure, and blood volume [1].

Neff et al. [11] studied the effect of correction of anemia in chronic renal failure patients. Forty patients were hemodynamically studied before and during a 6- to 12-week period during which the patients were transfused with red blood cells to a normal hematocrit. The cardiac index decreased, reaching a normal level at a hematocrit of 30%. Diastolic blood pressure rose progressively (± 20 mm Hg) to a hematocrit of 40%, at which level peripheral vascular resistance increased by 80% (Fig. 2). There was a significant inverse correlation between cardiac index and hematocrit ($r = -0.76$; $p < 0.01$) and a positive correlation between peripheral resistance and hematocrit ($r = 0.675$; $p < 0.01$).

Hematocrit is an important determinant of blood viscosity. The increase in cardiac output at a lower hematocrit is related to an increase in venous return and a decrease in outflow impedance, in part related to decreased blood viscosity. In a study by Murray et al. [2], mean cardiac output was plotted against mean hematocrit ratios obtained during control periods and after isovolumic exchange with dextran solutions of three different molecular weights. Recipients of low molecular weight dextran had higher cardiac outputs at comparable hematocrits. The authors concluded that reduction in outflow impedance in anemic patients is probably largely determined by changes in whole blood viscosity. The increase of whole blood viscosity due to the increasing hematocrit [12, 13] is in part responsible for the increase of peripheral vascular resistance, especially in cases of structural microvascular changes [7].

Chronic Anemia and Exercise Capacity

The importance of lowered blood hemoglobin levels in limiting exercise capacity and peripheral maximum oxygen uptake (VO_2) has been shown. In 9 healthy male subjects chronic anemia was induced by repeated venesections at 8–

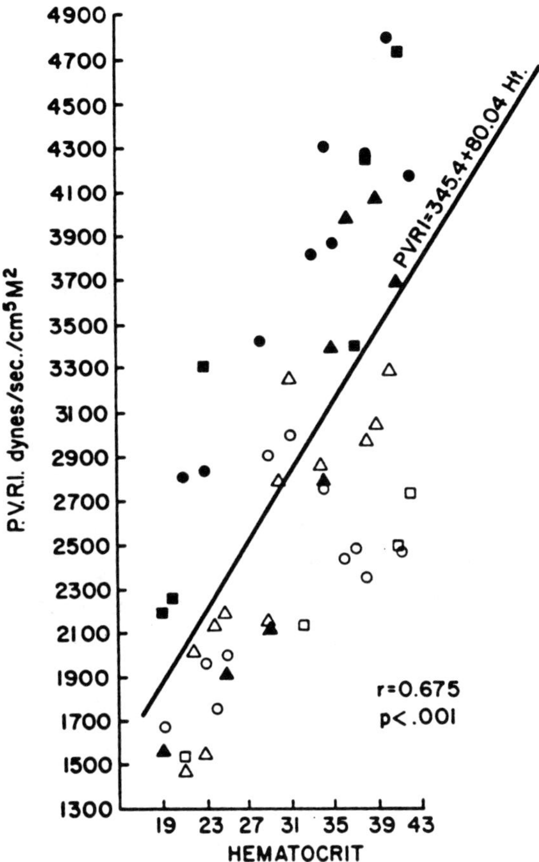

Fig. 2. Change in peripheral vascular resistance index induced by raising the hematocrit. Different symbols represent the different patients (n = 6). [From Ref. 11, with permission.]

10 weeks [14]. Hemoglobin concentration was 146 $\pm$ 10 g/l before venesection (control state) and 110 $\pm$ 7 g/l in the anemic state. Exercise tests were performed in the control state and in the anemic state. Maximal O_2 uptake was 4.55 $\pm$ 0.6 and 3.74 $\pm$ 0.7 l/min, respectively. The adaptive response to submaximal exercise (cycling at 150–175 W) in anemia was mediated to 50% by an increase in cardiac output (mainly on basis of an increased heart rate), and 50% was due to increased O_2 extraction in the peripheral tissue. In conclusion, this study confirmed the strong positive relationship between hemoglobin concentration and max VO_2. Animal experimental research showed that the relationship between max VO_2 and exercise endurance is dependent upon muscle oxidative

Table 1.   Exercise test results [16]

	HD	CAPD	Rtx
Work performed (kg/min)	526 ± 51*	502 ± 51*	899 ± 78
Max VO_2 (ml/kg/min)	19.1 ± 5.8*	21.1 ± 5.4*	31.7 ± 7.0
Max VO_2 (l/min)	1.3 ± 0.4*	1.6 ± 0.6*	2.3 ± 0.6
Max HR (beats/min)	131 ± 23*	153 ± 21*	171 ± 16
Max systolic BP (mm Hg)	194 ± 29	165 ± 44	188 ± 21

HD, hemodialysis; CAPD, chronic ambulatory peritoneal dialysis; Rtx, renal transplantation.
*p < 0.01 when compared to Rtx.

capacities. Anemic trained animals had the same max VO_2 as anemic untrained animals, but trained animals had higher muscle oxidative capacities and greater endurance [15].

Exercise testing has also been performed in hemodialysis patients. Painter et al. studied maximal exercise in 18 hemodialysis, 12 CAPD, and 20 renal transplant patients using a treadmill test [16]. Hematocrit levels were 24.4, 31.6, and 45.1%, respectively. Exercise was continued in all patients until symptoms of excessive fatigue, shortness of breath, or leg fatigue prevented continuation (Table 1).

Max VO_2 compared to average values for normal healthy volunteers proved to be 93% of average in renal transplant patients, 62% in CAPD patients, and 64% in hemodialysis patients. Maximal heart rates were 76% of normal in hemodialysis patients, 84% in CAPD patients, and 93% in renal transplant patients (Fig. 3).

Max VO_2 is an important denominator of maximum exercise capacity. However, an anemic patients' ability to perform endurance exercise could be limited. Endurance exercise capacity can be assessed by determination of the anaerobic threshold during incremental exercise. The cause of a decreased anaerobic threshold could be multifactorial: low hematocrit, decreased left ventricular workload, no optimal increase in heart rate. This was further evaluated by Mayer et al. [17], who studied exhaustive exercise tests in 13 patients on chronic intermittent hemodialysis. The hemoglobin level was 5.1–12.2 g/100 ml O_2 uptake at the anaerobic threshold (r = 0.69) as well as maximum peripheral O_2 uptake (r = 0.63) were severely impaired and were positively correlated with hemoglobin concentration. They concluded that exercise capacity in patients on chronic intermittent hemodialysis is severely impaired and that the impairment of aerobic and anaerobic capacity is significantly correlated with the severity of renal anemia.

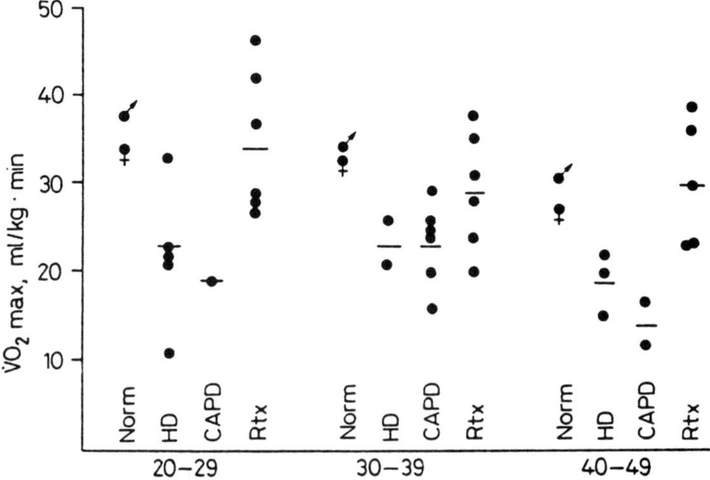

Fig. 3. Maximal VO$_2$ values of hemodialysis (HD), CAPD, and renal transplantation (Rtx) compared to average normal values for age group. ♂ = male norm. ♀ = female norm. [From Ref. 16, with permission.]

Hemodynamic Effects of rhEPO Therapy in Patients with End-Stage Renal Disease

Correction of the anemic state by rhEPO would greatly improve the cardio-vascular state of the patient and his or her quality of life. Hemodynamic studies during rhEPO therapy revealed a decrease of cardiac output and heart rate and an increase of systemic vascular resistance after reaching the target hematocrit level (Fig. 4) [17–23]. The diminished peripheral vasodilation due to improved tissue oxygenation and the increased blood viscosity in combination with structural vessel wall abnormalities at macro- and microcirculatory levels in hemodialysis patients may all contribute to the reported increase in systemic vascular resistance during treatment with rhEPO. While directly studying forearm and calf blood flow a decrease was found during rhEPO therapy, whereas forearm and calf arterial resistances increased. Furthermore, a significant decrease in forearm and calf venous distensibility and an increase in venous tone was found during rhEPO [24]. According to London et al., the increased venous tone helps to maintain an adequate venous return and cardiac filling [24].

The decrease of cardiac output is partly due to a decrease in stroke volume and partly to a decrease in heart rate. The decrease in stroke volume can be explained by a decreased venous return [24]. The increase in peripheral resistance and the decrease in cardiac output usually results in a stable blood

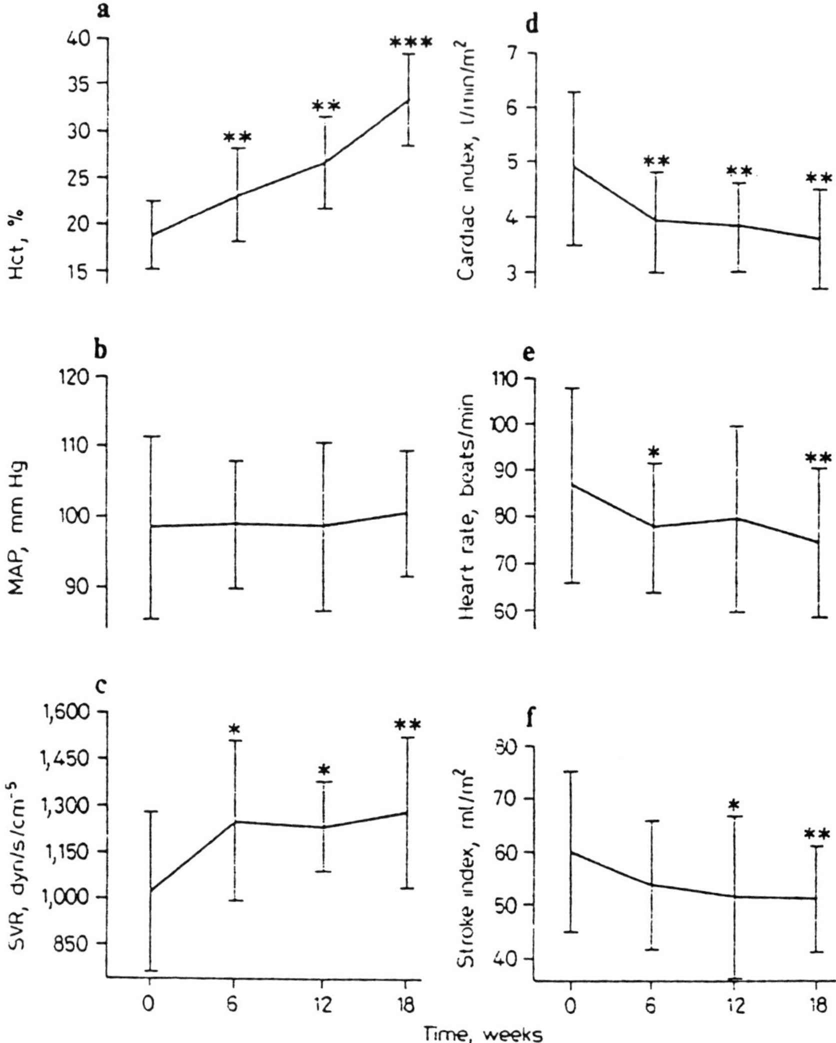

Fig. 4. Effects of rhEPO on (a) hematocrit, (b) mean arterial pressure, (c) systemic vascular resistance, (d) cardiac index, (e) heart rate, and (f) stroke index. *p < 0.05; **p < 0.02; ***p < 0.001, compared to values before (0 weeks) rhEPO treatment. [From Ref. 7, with permission.]

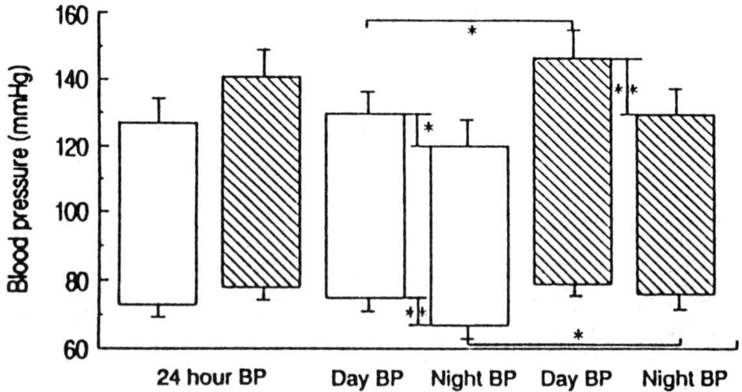

Fig. 5. Twenty-four hour, daytime, nighttime systolic and diastolic blood pressure (BP) before (open bars) and after (hatched bars) correction of renal anemia with rhEPO (n = 13). *p < 0.05; **p < 0.005. [From Ref. 27, with permission.]

pressure. Hypertension has been reported in 20–30% of patients [25, 26]. Patients with preexistent hypertension are prone to a further increase in blood pressure during rhEPO therapy. However, 24-h ambulatory blood pressure measurements in 13 chronic dialysis patients treated with rhEPO revealed a significant increase of systolic/diastolic blood pressure for the whole group (Fig. 5) [27]. The pathophysiological explanation for the increased blood pressure is still a matter of debate. The fact that hypertensive patients were prone to an increase in blood pressure during rhEPO therapy resulted in the hypothesis that the increased blood viscosity in combination with the more severe structural vascular changes of hypertensives resulted in a more exaggerated increase in peripheral vascular resistance, and hence to higher blood pressure [7, 21]. Nonnast-Daniel et al. found an inadequate decrease in cardiac output in patients with increasing blood pressure during rhEPO therapy [18].

Pollok et al. [28] reported an increased number of α_2-receptors (on thrombocytes) and a high blood pressure sensitivity to noradrenaline infusion in anemic dialysis patients. Twelve weeks after correction of the renal anemia by rhEPO, the number of α_2-receptors were still elevated and normalized slowly afterwards. Even 24 weeks after correction of the anemia, blood pressure was still more sensitive to noradrenaline infusion compared to normals. The plasma noradrenaline concentrations decreased but were not related to blood pressure.

Of interest also are the data of Radermacher et al. [29], who found an in vitro enhancement of norepinephrine-induced contraction of rabbit and human arteries via modulation in prostaglandin balance. There was a significant increase in the production of $PGF_{2\alpha}$ and a minor increase of TxB_2 after stimulation of the rabbit aortic rings with rhEPO. Indomethacin and aspirin stopped the increase in prostanoid production. These effects were not dependent on the presence of endothelial cells.

Kokot et al. [30] reported during rhEPO treatment a suppression of baseline plasma renin activity and plasma aldosterone and an increase of plasma α human atrial natriuretic peptide, while plasma concentration of vasopressin remained unchanged. No correlation was found between blood pressure and rhEPO-induced changes of plasma renin activity, aldosterone, plasma atrial natriuretic peptide, and vasopressin.

Whether rhEPO exerts a direct vasoconstrictive effect is still a matter of debate. Bund et al. could find no direct vasoconstrictive effect of rhEPO in subcutaneous resistance arterioles [31]. In conclusion, the only known risk factors for developing hypertension are preexistent hypertension and rapid increase of hematocrit. The cause of the hypertension, however, is not yet fully elucidated.

Despite a decrease in peripheral blood flow [24], tissue oxygenation improved due to increased erythrocyte mass [21, 32]. Transcutaneous oxygen pressure (37 and 44°C) increased significantly (Fig. 6). Nevertheless, maximal

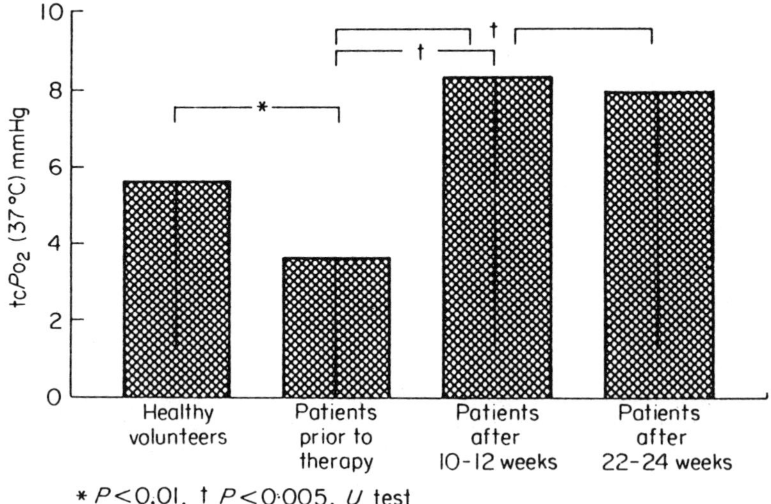

Fig. 6. Forefoot transcutaneous oxygen pressure (tcPo₂) at an electrode core temperature of 37°C in patients with renal anemia before and during rhEPO therapy compared with healthy subjects. (X and SD.) [From Ref. 32, with permission.]

capillary perfusion after prolonged local ischemia decreased during rhEPO therapy, probably due to the increased blood viscosity in combination with the higher degree of tortuous capillaries in the end-stage renal failure patients [7]. These macro- and microcirculatory functional changes were found after 3–4 months of rhEPO therapy [21]. However, longitudinal studies after 14 months of rhEPO therapy did not reveal significant changes compared to the 3-month rhEPO therapy period [21].

To detect structural changes in the cardiovascular system, many studies have been conducted using echography. Except for decreases in left ventricular end-diastolic/systolic and left atrial diameter and left diastolic/systolic volume [33–36], the most important finding was the decrease of left ventricular mass index as reported by Cannella et al. [37] (133.0 ± 30.8 vs. 109.8 ± 13.6 g/m^2, p < 0.05) and others [38]. Wirtz et al. [20] also reported a decrease in left ventricular mass index (Fig. 7) and found a significant correlation between the initial left ventricular mass index and the decrease in left ventricular mass index during rhEPO therapy [20]. The decrease in left ventricular mass index during rhEPO therapy was not related to the change in blood pressure, indicating the possible role of renal anemia in inducing left ventricular hypertrophy in anemic chronic

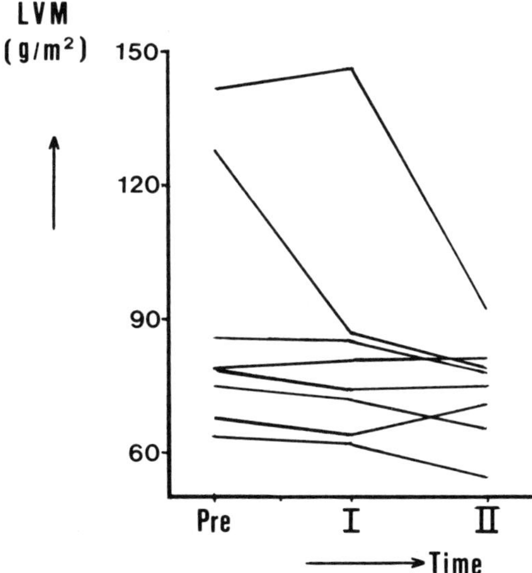

Fig. 7. Left ventricular mass index in normotensive hemodialysis patients treated with rhEPO after 4 months (I) and 14 months (II) of treatment. LVM, left ventricular mass index.

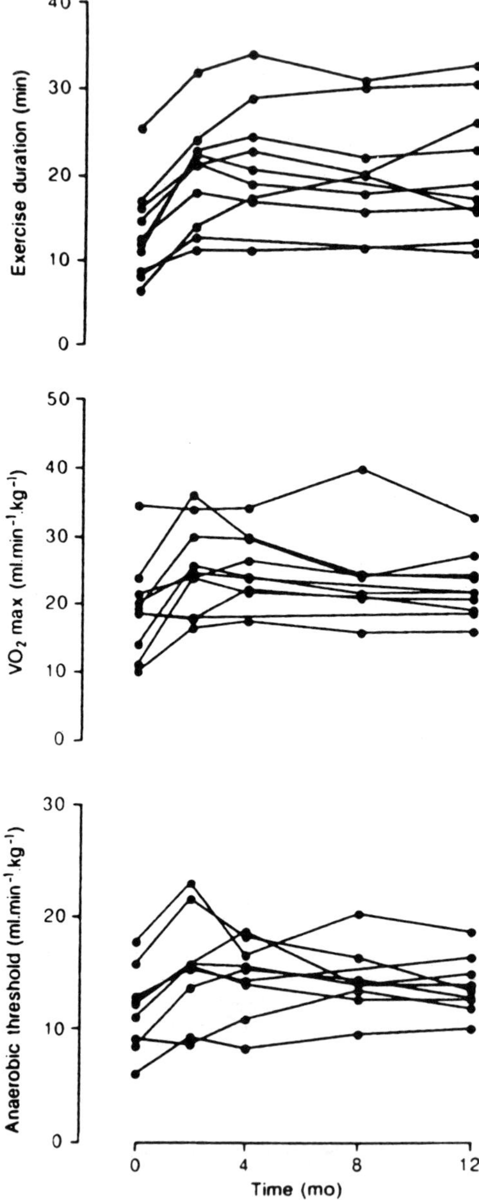

Fig. 8. Changes in exercise duration, maximum oxygen consumption (VO$_2$ max)
and anaerobic threshold during rhEPO treatment. [From Ref. 41, with permission.]

renal failure patients. Cannella et al. [37] found some evidence for a decreased neurosympathetic outflow to the heart during rhEPO therapy from which a decrease in left ventricular mass index can result in the long term. These data on left ventricular mass index also support the importance of early rhEPO treatment of anemic chronic renal failure patients in the predialysis period. Because of these cardiac changes during rhEPO therapy, left ventricular wall stress decreased significantly [19], which results in a decrease in left ventricular oxygen consumption [39].

No structural changes have been reported in the arterial and venous vascular systems. Decreased venous distensibility as found by London et al. is a functional phenomenon, i.e., increased venous tone, [24]. The same is true for increased peripheral vascular resistance, which is not directly related to structural vascular changes. More important, Wirtz et al. found a decreasing number of tortuous capillaries in the finger nailfold studied by intravital microscopy [20], as has also been found after a successful renal transplantation. The percentage of tortuous capillaries after 3 and 14 months decreased from 34.7% to 10.2% and 7.1%, respectively. Knowing the light microscopic structure of the capillaries in hemodialysis patients, the effect of rhEPO on pruritus as shown by De Marchi et al. is very interesting [40]. They found a decrease in plasma histamine concentration, which could indicate a decrease in mast cells, known to be a part of the inflammatory substrate around the capillaries of hemodialysis patients.

rhEPO Therapy and Exercise Capacity

A significant correlation has been described in chronic end-stage renal failure patients between hemoglobin and impairment of exercise capacity. We may therefore conclude that correction of anemia with rhEPO would greatly improve exercise capacity. Macdougall et al. [41] investigated exercise capacity in 10 hemodialysis patients after 12 months of rhEPO therapy. Apart from maximum exercise testing according to the Weber treadmill protocol, duration of exercise, maximum oxygen consumption, and anaerobic threshold were determined 2, 4, 8, and 12 months after starting rhEPO therapy. There were significant increases in exercise time (13.2 $\pm$ 5.5 to 20.0 $\pm$ 6.2 min), maximum oxygen consumption (19.1 $\pm$ 7.0 to 25 $\pm$ 6.7 ml/min/kg), and anaerobic threshold (11.7 $\pm$ 3.6 to 15.4 $\pm$ 4.8 ml/min/kg) after 2 months of rhEPO therapy. These improvements were maintained but did not increase further after 4, 8, and 12 months of therapy (Fig. 8).

These results were also reported by Grunze et al. [42], who found a 20% increase in oxygen uptake, exercise capacity, and anaerobic threshold (Table 2).

Table 2. Physical work capacity and oxygen uptake [42]

	Before treatment		After treatment
PWC AT (W)	43.7 ± 11.5	*	62.5 ± 13.3
VO_2 AT (l/min)	0.83 ± 0.16	*	1.04 ± 0.15
PWC max (W)	87.5 ± 18	*	96.8 ± 20
VO_2 max (l/min)	1.19 ± 0.25	*	1.37 ± 0.3

Mean values ± SD.
PWC, physical work capacity; AT, anaerobic threshold; VO_2, oxygen uptake.
*p < 0.05.

Analysis of the underlying mechanisms by pulmonary function tests and ergospirometry demonstrated that improved oxygen transport in the blood and its concomitant changes of the anaerobic threshold and heart rate appeared to be main causes of improvement. Parameters of respiratory mechanics and gas exchange remained unaltered [42]. The oxygen uptake at anaerobic threshold per heart beat (O_2 pulse) increased from 7.48 to 10.0 ml/beat, while the respiratory equivalent for oxygen (i.e., ventilation necessary for the uptake of 1 liter of oxygen) remained constant. Similar changes occurred at maximal exercise. Correction of anemia by rhEPO provides more relief for the heart than for the respiratory system. The increased oxygen transport capacity, on the basis of the rise in hemoglobin concentration and right shift of the ODC as compared with healthy controls [43], leads to a decrease in heart rate and improved oxygenation of working muscle. Thus, the onset of anaerobic metabolism occurs later during exercise. However, Thompson et al. [44] pointed out that exercise training is still of importance to increase the ability to utilize delivered O_2.

The effect of rhEPO on muscle energy metabolism, i.e., the rate of recovery of phosphocreatinine, has been studied using ^{31}P magnetic resonance spectroscopy. Since the rate of recovery of phosphocreatinine is a function of oxidative phosphorylation, slow recovery reflects either inadequate oxygen delivery or defective oxygen utilization. The studies of Park et al. [45] and Szerlip et al. [46] showed an improvement of exercise capacity either objectively or subjectively assessed. However, Park et al. found normalized values for phosphocreatinine–to–inorganic phosphate ratios at rest and at the maximum recovery point after all-out handgrip exercise, while Szerlip et al., testing the plantar flexors of the foot, could not demonstrate any improvement in the same parameters under rhEPO therapy. From these conflicting results it seems impossible to conclude whether the slow rate of recovery of muscular phosphocreatinine in anemic hemodialysis patients is related to the effects of uremia per se on energy utilization or to inadequate oxygen delivery, which would be improved by normalization of hematocrit as suggested by Park et al. Also of interest is the study of Bárány et al. [47], who used a bioluminescence method to measure ATP production in isolated muscle mitochondria obtained from a biopsy of the quadriceps femoris muscle. Their anemic hemodialysis patients had higher ATP production rates before rhEPO treatment than the normal controls. During rhEPO therapy ATP production rates decreased and reached normal levels. This suggests that correction of the anemia reversed enhanced mitochondrial metabolism, which is a metabolic adaptation to decreased oxygen transport.

Because of the improvement in exercise capacity and exercise endurance as discussed above, rhEPO therapy has an important impact on quality of life. Some well-organized multicenter questionnaires have been developed and will be discussed in the last part of this article.

Subjective Improvements of Exercise Capacity during rhEPO Therapy

The correction of renal anemia by rhEPO will also improve the subjective quality of life in dialysis patients. Lundin [48] found that 32 of 35 patients in whom the hematocrit rose from 20.4 to 34.3% reported improved well-being and exercise capacity. In a multicenter study of the Canadian Erythropoietin Study Group [49, 50], 118 patients treated with rhEPO reported significant clinical improvement in their response to questions on fatigue and physical symptoms like strength. On the sickness impact profile, there were significant improvements in the response of patients to questions on body care and movement, home maintenance, ambulation, communication, and work among those treated with rhEPO. The difference in the time walked in the exercise stress test between patients given rhEPO and those given placebo was significant, but no significant improvement was found in results of the 6-min walk test. A significant correlation was found between the change in hemoglobin concentration and the change in physical scores on the sickness impact profile. Generally, dialysis patients receiving rhEPO were much less fatigued, complained of less severe physical symptoms, and had greater exercise tolerance than patients given placebo.

Conclusion

Correcting anemia in hemodialysis patients by rhEPO results in a decrease of cardiac output towards normal and an increase of peripheral vascular resistance. There is a clinically significant blood pressure rise in 20–30% of the patients. Patients with preexistent hypertension and patients in whom there was a rapid rise in hematocrit were prone to an exaggerated rise in blood pressure. The pathophysiological cause of the hypertension is not yet fully elucidated.

Left ventricular dimensions, especially left ventricular end-diastolic dimension, decreased as was left ventricular mass, leading to a decreased left ventricular workload. Tissue oxygenation improved despite the decrease in tissue perfusion on basis of increased O_2 transport capacity.

These changes resulted in an increase in exercise capacity (max VO_2) and exercise endurance (anaerobic threshold). Subjective parameters of quality of life also improved considerably.

rhEPO therapy has a great impact on the quality of life. Whether the induced hemodynamic changes related to rhEPO will improve the cardiovascular prognosis of dialysis patients in the long term is still unknown. Predialysis patients treated with rhEPO could be an interesting group to study in this regard.

References

1   Duke M, Abelmann WH: The hemodynamic response to chronic anemia. Circulation 1969;39:503–515.
2   Murray JF, Escobar E, Rapaport E: Effects of blood viscosity on hemodynamic responses in acute normovolaemic anemia. Am J Physiol 1969;216(3):638–642.
3   Capelli JP, Kasparian H: Cardiac work demands and left ventricular function in end-stage renal disease. Ann Int Med 1977;86:261–267.
4   Grossman W: Cardiac hypertrophy: Useful adaptation or pathologic process? Am J Med 1980;69:576–584.
5   Silberberg JS, Rahal DP, Patton DR, Sniderman AD: Role of anemia in the pathogenesis of left ventricular hypertrophy in end-stage renal disease. Am J Cardiol 1989;64:222–224.
6   Florenzano F, Diaz G, Regonesi C, Escobar E: Left ventricular function in chronic anemia: Evidence of noncatecholamine positive inotropic factor in the serum. Am J Cardiol 1984;54:638–645.
7   Wirtz JJJM, Leunissen KML, van Esser JWJ, Cheriex EC, Slaaf DW, Reneman RS, van Hooff JP: Recombinant human erythropoietin and its effect on macro- and microcirculation during normovolaemia. Blood Purif 1990;8:285–294.
8   Matsumoto M, Ichimaru K, Horie A: Pruritus and mast cell proliferation of the skin in end-stage renal failure. Clin Nephrol 1985;23:285–288.
9   Ichimaru K, Horie A: Microangiopathic changes of subepidermal capillaries in end-stage renal failure. Nephron 1987;46:144–149.
10 Gilchrest B, Rowe JW, Mihm MC: Clinical and histological skin changes in chronic renal failure: evidence for a dialysis-resistant transplant responsive microangiopathy. Lancet 1980;2:1271–1275.
11 Neff MS, Kim KE, Persoff M, Onesti J, Swartz Ch: Hemodynamics of uremic anemia. Circulation 1970;43:876–883.

12   Wirtz JJJM, van Esser JWJ, Hamulyak K, Leunissen KML, van Hooff JP: The effects of recombinant human erythropoietin on hemostasis and fibrinolysis in hemodialysis patients. Clin Nephrol 1992;38:277–282.

13   Steffen HM, Brunner R, Müller R, Degenhardt S, Pallok M, Lang R, Baldamus CA: Peripheral hemodynamics, blood viscosity and the renin-angiotensin system in hemodialysis patients under therapy with recombinant human erythropoietin. Contrib Nephrol 1989;76:292–298.

14   Celsing F, Nyström J, Pihlstedt P, Werner B, Ekblom B: Effects of long-term anemia and retransfusion of central circulation during exercise. J Appl Physiol 1986;61(4):1358–1362.

15   Gregg SG, Willis WI, Brooks GA: Interactive effects of anemia and muscle oxidative capacity on exercise endurance. J Appl Physiol 1989;67(2):765–770.

16   Painter P, Messer-Rehak D, Hanson P, Zimmerman SW, Glass NR: Exercise capacity in hemodialysis, CAPD, and renal transplant patients. Nephron 1986;42:47–51.

17   Mayer G, Thum J, Graf H: Anaemia and reduced exercise capacity in patients on chronic haemodialysis. Clin Science 1989;76:265–268.

18   Nonnast-Daniel B, Schäffer J, Frei U: Hemodynamics in hemodialysis patients treated with recombinant human erythropoietin. Contrib Nephrol 1989;76:283–291.

19   Satoh K, Masuda T, Ikeda Y, Kurokawa S, Kamata K, Hikawada R, Tahamoto T, Marumo F: Hemodynamic changes by recombinant erythropoietin therapy in hemodialyzed patients. Hypertension 1990;15:262–266.

20   Wirtz JJJM, Leunissen KML, van Kuijk W, van Hooff JP: The long-term effects of recombinant human erythropoietin on macro- and microcirculation in chronic hemodialysis patients. Blood Purif 1991;9:41.

21   Nonnast-Daniel B, Deschodt G, Brunkhorst R, Crentzig A, Bahlmann J, Shaldon S, Koch KM: Long-term effects of treatment with recombinant human erythropoietin on hemodynamics and tissue oxygenation in patients with renal anaemia. Nephrol Dial Transplant 1990;5:444–448.

22   Hori K, Onoyama K, Iseki K, Fujimi S, Fujishima M: Hemodynamic and volume changes by recombinant human erythropoietin in the treatment of anemic hemodialysis patients. Clin Nephrol 1990;33:293–298.

23   Teruel JC, Pascual J, Jimenez M, Liano F, Rivera M, Martinez J, Moya JL, Ortimo J: Hemodynamic changes in hemodialyzed patients during treatment with recombinant human erythropoietin. Nephron 1991;58:135–137.

24   London GM, Zins B, Pammic B, Naret C, Berthelot J-M, Jacquot C, Safar M, Drueke T: Vascular changes in hemodialysis patients in response to recombinant human erythropoietin. Kidney Int 1989;36:878–882.

25   Brunkhorst R, Nonnast-Daniel B, Koch KM, Frei U: Hypertension as a possible complication of recombinant human erythropoietin therapy. Contrib Nephrol 1991;88:118–125.

26   Eschbach JW, Egrie JC, Douring MR, Browne JK: Correction of the anemia of end-stage renal disease with recombinant human erythropoietin: Results of a combined phase I and II clinical trial. N Engl J Med 1987;316:73–78.

27   Van de Borne P, Tielemans C, Vanherweghem J-L, Degaute J-P: Effect of recombinant human erythropoietin therapy on ambulatory blood pressure and heart rate in chronic haemodialysis patients. Nephrol Dial Transplant 1992;7:45–49.

28 Pollok M, Behrenbeck HP, Steffen HM, Mueller R, Scigalla P, Baldamus CA: The effect of erythropoietin corrected anemia on the sympathetic system JASN 1991;2:385.

29 Radermacher J, Bodebäger SM, Böger RH, Frölich JC, Koch KM: Erythropoietin enhances norepinephrine induced contractions via modulation in prostaglandin balance in rabbit and human arteries. Blood Purif 1992;10:79–80.

30 Kokot F, Wiçcek A, Grzeszczak W, Klepacha J, Klin M, Lao M: Influence of erythropoietin treatment on endocrine abnormalities in haemodialyzed patients. Contrib Nephrol 1989;76:257–272.

31 Bund SJ, Heagerty A, Edmunds M, Walls J: Erythropoietin does not induce vasoconstriction directly in human subcutaneous resistance arterioles. Nephron 1989;53:173.

32 Creutzig A, Caspary L, Nonnast-Daniel B, Bahlmann J, Kühn K, Brunkhorst R, Reimers E, Koch KM, Alexander K: Skin microcirculation and regional peripheral resistance in patients with chronic renal anaemia treated with recombinant human erythropoietin. Eur J Clin Invest 1990;20:219–223.

33 Löw I, Grützmacher P, Bergmann M, Schoeppe W: Echocardiographic findings in patients on maintenance hemodialysis substituted with recombinant human erythropoietin. Clin Nephrol 1989;31:26–30.

34 Cannella G, la Canna G, Sandrini M, Gaggiotti M, Nordio G, Movilli E, Maiorca R: Renormalization of high cardiac output and of left ventricular size following long-term recombinant human erythropoietin treatment of anemic dialyzed uremic patients. Clin Nephrol 1990;34:272–278.

35 Löw-Friedrich I, Grützmacher P, März W, Bergmann M, Schoeppe W: Therapy with recombinant human erythropoietin reduces cardiac size and improves heart function in chronic haemodialysis patients. Am J Nephrol 1991;11:54–60.

36 Grützmacher P, Scheuermann E, Löw I, Baum R, Heuzer J, Schoeppe W: Correction of renal anaemia by recombinant human erythropoietin: Effects on myocardial function. Contrib Nephrol 1988;66:176–184.

37 Cannella G, La Canna G, Sandrini M, Gaggiotti M, Nordio G, Movilli E, Momebelloni S, Visioli O, Maiorca R: Reversal of left ventricular hypertrophy following recombinant human erythropoietin treatment of anaemic dialysed uraemic patients. Nephrol Dial Transplant 1991;6:31–37.

38 Colan S, Jabs K, Harmon W: Treatment with epoetin alfa is associated with a reduction in ventricular mass and an increase in exercise tolerance in young hemodialysis patients. JASN 1991;2:374.

39 Strauer BE: Myocardial oxygen consumption in chronic heart disease: role of wall stress, hypertrophy and coronary reserve. Am J Cardiol 1979;44:730–740.

40 De Marchi S, Cecchin E, Villalta D, Sepiacci G, Santini G, Bartoli E: Relief of pruritus and decreases in plasma histamine concentrations during erythropoietin therapy in patients with uremia. N Engl J Med 1992;326:969–974.

41 Macdougall IC, Lewis NP, Saunders MJ, Cochlin DL, Davies ME, Hutton RD, Fox KAA, Coles GA, Williams JD: Long-term cardiorespiratory effects of amelioration of renal anaemia by erythropoietin. Lancet 1990;335:489–493.

42 Grunze M, Kohlmann M, Mulligan M, Grüner I, Koeppel M, Bommer J: Mechanisms of improved physical performance of chronic haemodialysis patients after erythropoietin treatment. Am J Nephrol 1990;10(Suppl. 2):15–23.

43 Böcker A, Reimers E, Noumast-Daniel B, Kühn K, Koch KM, Scigalla P, Braumann K-M, Brunkhorst R, Böning D: Effect of erythropoietin treatment on D2 affinity and performance in patients with renal anaemia. Contr Nephrol 1988;66:165–175.

44 Thompson JR, Stray-Gunderson J: Cardiovascular adaptation in maximal exercise among patients with end-stage renal disease after graded increases in hemoglobin. JASN 1991;2:389.

45 Park JS, Park SK, Kim SB, Lim TW, Lee DK, Hong CD: Effect of recombinant human erythropoietin on muscle energy metabolism measured by 31p-NMR spectroscopy in patients with end-stage renal disease. JASN 1991;2:384.

46 Szerlip H, Noyszewski E, Leigh J: Correction of anemia by erythropoietin in hemodialysis patients: effect on muscle metabolism. JASN 1991;2:389.

47 Bárány P, Wibom R, Hultman E, Bergström J: ATP production in isolated muscle mitochondria from hemodialysis patients: Effects of anemia correction with erythropoietin. JASN 1991;2:371.

48 Lundin AP: Quality of life: Subjective and objective improvements with recombinant human erythropoietin therapy. Semin Nephrol 1989;9(Suppl. 1):22–29.

49 Canadian Erythropoietin Study Group: Association between recombinant human erythropoietin and quality of life and exercise capacity of patients receiving haemodialysis. Br Med J 1990;300:573–578.

50 Laupacis A (for the Canadian Erythropoietin Study Group): Changes in quality of life and functional capacity in hemodialysis patients treated with recombinant human erythropoietin. Semin Nephrol 1990;10(Suppl. 1):11–19.

K. M. L. Leunissen, MD, PhD, Department of Nephrology, University Hospital Maastricht, P. O. Box 5800, NL/6202 AZ Maastricht, The Netherlands

Discussion

to the Paper by K. M. L. Leunissen et al.

Erslev (*Philadelphia*): Many peoples' concern has been the acceptance by professional athletes that erythropoietin, like blood doping, could do something for their performance. Obviously if it is given without being monitored, and the hematocrit goes up dramatically because of EPO and excessive dehydration, the athletes may risk their lives. My question to you and the previous speaker is: Is there a benefit in physical performance for a highly trained professional athlete to have a hematocrit of 51 instead of 47 by taking erythropoietin?

Leunissen: As we look at the slide of the previous speaker which showed the relation between increased viscosity, hematocrit, and oxygen-transport capacity, I think that a small increase in hematocrit when you are still on the climbing limb of the curve of the O_2 transport capacity would improve physical performance. But when you are over the top of the O_2-transport-capacity curve, I think the effects would be negative due to the negative effects of increasing viscosity.

Eschbach (*Seattle*): The Swedish psychologist Dr. Ekblom has studied athletes and has shown that exercise performance improves with modest increases in hematocrit.

Wardrop (*Cardiff*): I am surprised that Dr. Erslev does not invoke the diagram in his chapter in *Hematology*, edited by Williams, in 1977. It is a diagram which showed that the impact of total circulating blood volume influenced the optimal hematocrit for maximal oxygen transport. And if the subject is hypervolemic, a higher hematocrit is associated with better oxygen transport.

Erslev: In some way, I have hoped that that would not be the case and that erythropoietin, like steroids, did not need to be outlawed for Olympic games.

Shaldon (*Nimes*): Is that why athletes train at high altitude to make it physiological rather than doping?

Koch (*Hannover*): Dr. Winearls asked a similar question before: Presently nephrologists in general are only partially correcting renal anemia with erythropoietin. The desired level of hematocrit is 30–35 vol.%. Would you advise to go above this level—what is your opinion?

Leunissen: No, I would not advise to go above this, because when you look at our microcirculatory studies in the skin showing a decreased perfusion at maximal ischemic vasodilation, I agree these are studies in physiologically not so important tissue. Inducing maximal vasodilation by longstanding local ischemia there is still a disturbance of the microcirculation, according to the increased time to peak, as compared to normals with an even higher hematocrit. So I think that, increasing the hematocrit, the effect on perfusion is dependent on structural abnormalities in the micro- and macrocirculation. And I think when there are structural abnormalities also in other tissues, except from the skin, increasing hematocrit very high would have an important impact on the microcirculatory flow through these tissues. So I would not advise to go higher than 30 vol.%.

Erythropoietin and Hypertension

Jörg Radermacher, Karl M. Koch

Department of Nephrology, Hannover Medical School, Hannover, Germany

Introduction

Recombinant human erythropoietin (rhEPO) has been successfully used for the treatment of the anemia of end-stage renal disease for more than 5 years. Development or aggravation of hypertension has been reported as the most relevant side effect and may, in the long term, counteract the beneficial cardial effects of r-HuEPO treatment. Hypertension is considered the most important risk factor for cardiac and cerebrovascular complications in end-stage renal failure patients [1, 2]. It has been shown that left ventricular hypertrophy, which is frequently associated with hypertension, appears to be an important, independent determinant of survival in patients on hemodialysis treatment [3, 4].

This review will show incidence rates of rhEPO induced hypertension as well as the associated hemodynamic changes and will discuss the pathophysiological mechanisms possibly involved.

Incidence of rhEPO-Induced Hypertension

The aggravation of pre-existing hypertension or the development of hypertension in normotensive hemodialysis patients was recognized and reported as a major side effect soon after the introduction of rhEPO into clinical therapy [5–11]. Hypertension develops after a lag time of 2–12 weeks [5]; some studies report a reduction of the hypertensinogenic effect with time [12–14], although reports to the contrary exist [15–17]. An immediate rise of blood pressure after intravenous application of rhEPO has never been reported. Incidence rates vary according to the definition of hypertension chosen. Summing up the results of uncontrolled studies, hyptertension according to WHO criteria developed in 21% of patients [18–23]; hypertension defined as the start or increase in antihypertensive treatment developed in 26% [5, 8, 11, 18, 24–42] and hypertension defined as an increase in MAP of 10 mm Hg or more developed in 29% [11, 19, 20, 25, 27, 28, 36, 37, 42–46]. If hypertension was defined as either the start or increase in antihypertensive treatment and/or an increase in MAP of 10 mm Hg or more (so-called blood pressure responders), an incidence rate of 33% was reported [25, 47–50]. Incidence rates are lower if placebo-controlled studies only are evaluated (Table 1). Abraham and Macres [51] reported an increase in MAP of $\geq$10 mm Hg in 30% of placebo-treated and 45% of erythropoietin-treated patients, resulting in a net increase of 15% due to erythropoietin. Thirty-seven percent of placebo treated, as compared to 58% of rhEPO-treated patients had to be started on antihypertensives or placed on higher doses of antihypertensive medication and/or experienced a rise in blood pressure of 10 mm Hg or more resulting in a net increase of the incidence of hypertension due to rhEPO of 21%. When hypertension was defined according to WHO criteria, the net increase of the incidence of hypertension due to erythropoietin was 13% (13% placebo versus 26% rhEPO). Suzuki et al. [12], also defining hypertension according to WHO criteria but using lower doses of erythropoietin and correcting hematocrit to 26% only, found considerably lower incidence rates of 0% in placebo and 2.5% in rhEPO-treated patients. Most studies used start or increase in antihypertensive treatment as a marker of the hypertensinogenic effect of rhEPO and reported increases of the incidence of hypertension ranging from 6 to 18% [12, 51–54]. (Table 1).

These values may underestimate the development of hypertension, since it has been shown that rhEPO therapy in regular dialysis treatment (RDT) patients increased the percentage of abnormal 24-hour ambulatory blood pressure measurements (defined as systolic blood pressure greater than 140 mm Hg and/or diastolic blood pressure greater than 90 mm Hg) from 33% to 52% ($p < 0.05$), while in contrast, mean pre- and posthemodialytic blood pressure values remained unchanged [28]. With 24-hour ambulatory blood pressure monitoring it could be shown that especially nocturnal diastolic and systolic blood pressure is elevated with rhEPO treatment [30], resulting in a decrease in diurnal blood pressure variation.

Central neurological symptoms possibly related to rhEPO-induced hypertension, such as seizures, have been frequently reported in uncontrolled studies [7–9, 55–58]. In placebo-controlled studies [12, 52–54, 59–61] there also seem to be more cases of CNS complications in the erythropoietin-treated groups (rhEPO:4/643 vs. placebo:0/320). These usually hypertension-associated complications are rarely accompanied by fundoscopic evidence of accelerated phase hypertension such as retinal hemorrhage, soft exudates, and papilloedema [55].

Table 1. Placebo-controlled studies with rhEPO in hemodialysis patients

Ref.	Number of patients, placebo/EPO	Hct/Hb increase, mean values	r-HuEPO dose (U/kg BW/week), range or mean $\pm$ SD	Duration of rhEPO treatment (weeks)	% of patients with start and/or increase in antihypertensive treatment, Placebo/EPO
51	78/151	70 $\rightarrow$ 108 g/l	900 – 1350	12	13/20
52	40/82	21,5 $\rightarrow$ 34,2 %	150 – 450	12	5.0/11.3
53	40/78	70 $\rightarrow$ 109 g/l	204 $\pm$ 167 – 248 $\pm$ 146	26	9/27
12	58/118	19 $\rightarrow$ 26 %	85 – 170	8	1.7/7.6
54	46/53	23 $\rightarrow$ 31 %	120 – 240	24	10.9/28.3

Severe hypertension, defined as an increase in diastolic blood pressure >110 mm Hg, has not been shown to be more frequent in patients treated with erythropoietin as compared to placebo controls [53].

Effect of rhEPO on Nonuremic Patients

As new indications for the use of rhEPO emerge, the question arises whether rhEPO also causes hypertension in nonuremic patients. Up to now the development of hypertension in nonuremics has rarely been reported [62–72] and, if so, only in non–placebo-controlled studies. Even with extremely high doses of rhEPO (100.000 IU 2 times/week), Casadevall et al. [69] did not see hypertension in patients with anemia of myelodysplastic syndrome (Table 2). Berglund and Ekblom [65] reported small but significant increases in systolic blood pressure after 6 weeks of rhEPO treatment during submaximal exercise at 200 watts in 15 healthy male subjects, the initial and final values for systolic blood pressure being 177 ± 14.2 vs. 191 ± 19.5 mm Hg (p < 0,01; mean ± SD). The hematocrit increased from 44.5% to 49.7%. With the possible exception of this study, rhEPO-induced hypertension has been shown to occur exclusively in uremic patients.

Pathogenesis of Hypertension in Uremics

The restriction of rhEPO-induced hypertension to uremic patients suggests that the general disposition of these patients towards hypertension must play a role in the hypertensinogenic response to rhEPO treatment. Hypertension occurs in up to 75% of patients with end-stage renal disease [73] before the initiation of renal replacement therapy. The underlying causes for this high incidence of hypertension are not fully understood [74]. There is little doubt, however, that sodium-volume excess is the basic derangement that induces hypertension in advanced renal failure [73]. Renin-angiotensin system hyperactivity [75–79], autonomic nervous system hyperactivity [80–85], and deficits in antihypertensive systems such as prostaglandins [86, 87] and nitric oxide/EDRF [88, 89] may play a complementary role, although findings with these systems are controversial.

In response to the hypertensive state, structural adaptation of the vasculature in the form of medial hypertrophy and an increased wall-to-lumen ratio will occur. These adaptive changes have been studied extensively [90–92] and may

Table 2. Effect of rhEPO on blood pressure (BP) in nonuremic patients

	n	Placebo/EPO	Dose (IU/kg/week)	Duration of treatment (weeks)	BP response ↑ ↔ ↓
Autologous blood donation [64]	10	5/5	400	3	↔
Autologous blood donation [68]	26	13/13	1200	12	↔
Myelodysplastic syndrome [69]	14	—	2900	12	↔
AIDS-related anemia [62]	63	39/29	300	12	↔
Autologous blood donation [63]	47	24/23	1200	3	↔
Anemia in collagenoses [66]	11	11/11	300	6	↔
Anemia of prematurity [71]	20	10/10	210	6	↔
Anemia of prematurity [72]	93	50/43	75	4	↔
Anemia of collagenoses [70]	17	4/13	150–450	32	↔
Bone marrow transplant at [67]	21	13/8	900	4	↔
Healthy male subjects [65]	15	—	60–120	6	↔ resting BP ↑ Systolic BP at exercise (200 W)
		self-control			

be involved in maintenance of hypertension, even if the underlying cause has been resolved [93].

The pathogenesis of the hypertension of end-stage renal disease obviously is based on multiple factors, and a participation of some of these factors in rhEPO-induced hypertension cannot be excluded. Most studies report on increased hypertensinogenic effects to rhEPO in uremic patients with preexisting hypertension [9, 33, 34, 53, 56, 59, 94], however, studies to the contrary exist [36, 50, 51, 95]. How is the rhEPO-induced increase in blood pressure in uremic patients characterized hemodynamically?

Hemodynamics of Erythropoietin-Induced Hypertension

Blood pressure is determined by cardiac output and systemic vascular resistance. An increase of both under rhEPO treatment would lead to hypertension. In the majority of studies, decreased cardiac output and increased peripheral vascular resistance have been observed [13, 19–21, 25, 46, 58, 95–100]. This is in agreement with transfusion studies in uremics showing the same hemodynamic effects of correction of anemia [101, 102]. Is the erythropoietin-induced hypertension due to inadequately decreased cardiac output, or is it due to inadequately increased vascular resistance? Inadequately decreased cardiac output can occur in individual patients [21, 103, 104] and is sometimes observed in blood pressure responders [20, 21]. However, if one evaluates all the studies [20, 21, 95, 97, 100, 104] that compare so-called blood pressure responders to nonresponders, systemic vascular resistance seems to be inadequately increased in blood pressure responders, while there is no significant difference in the degree of reduction of cardiac output between the two groups (Table 3 and Fig. 1).

Is an Increase in Total or Effective Blood Volume Causative for rhEPO-Induced Hypertension?

Since erythropoietin increases total red cell mass, an increase in total blood volume leading to volume expansion seems likely. However, a number of studies have shown that total blood volume remains unchanged after correction of renal anemia with rhEPO due to a reduction in plasma volume [21, 30, 98, 105]. It has been shown that rhEPO treatment leads to an increase in venous tone in the lower limb in RDT patients [25]. If venous capacitance were generally reduced following rhEPO treatment an increase in the effective blood volume [106] might be

Table 3. Studies comparing hemodynamic effects of blood pressure responding[a] (R) and nonresponding (Non-R) hemodialysis patients

Ref.	n R/Non-R	% Hct increase	Dose range (IU/kg BW/week)	Duration of treatment (weeks)	Method for determination of cardiac output
100	6/6	20 → 30	75–150	12	ECHO
95	4/13	21 → 34	150–4500	24	ECHO
21	10/2	19 → 30	90–300	15	dye dilution
20	9/9	20 → 31	90–360	12	ECHO
97	6/6	24 → 31	120–360	12	ECHO
104	4/3	21 → 37	120	12	thermodilution

[a]Blood pressure responder = Start of increase in antihypertensive treatment and/or increase in MAP ≥ 10 mmHg

expected to occur. This assumption could be supported by the finding that ANP levels are significantly correlated with blood pressure in rhEPO-treated hemodialysis patients [38]. An increased venous filling pressure would result in an increase in cardiac stroke volume. If cardiac output were increased, an increase in blood pressure could result. However, as just stated above, an increase in cardiac output under rhEPO treatment has been observed very rarely. Furthermore, an increase in stroke volume has not been shown to occur in clinical studies investigating the hemodynamic effects of rhEPO therapy. The average stroke volume decreased after rhEPO treatment by about 8% (54 ± 8.7 vs. 49.5 ± 11.8 ml/m^2, mean ± SD) [15, 20, 21, 38, 96–98]. Thus increased venous tone, possibly resulting in increased effective blood volume, does not seem to be involved in the increase in blood pressure observed after treatment.

Pathophysiology of rhEPO-Induced Hypertension

What mechanisms can cause an inadequate increase in systemic vascular resistance? Poiseuille's law predicts that vascular resistance varies directly with blood viscosity and inversely with the fourth power of vessel radius [107]. Therefore, either increased whole blood viscosity or changes in vessel diameter due to so-called reversal of hypoxic vasodilatation have been frequently named as the major causes of increased peripheral vascular resistance in rhEPO-induced hypertension. Reversal of hypoxic vasodilatation in this context can only be considered as a hypothetical concept to explain vasoconstriction after rhEPO treatment, since the precise mechanisms leading to hypoxia-induced vasodilata-

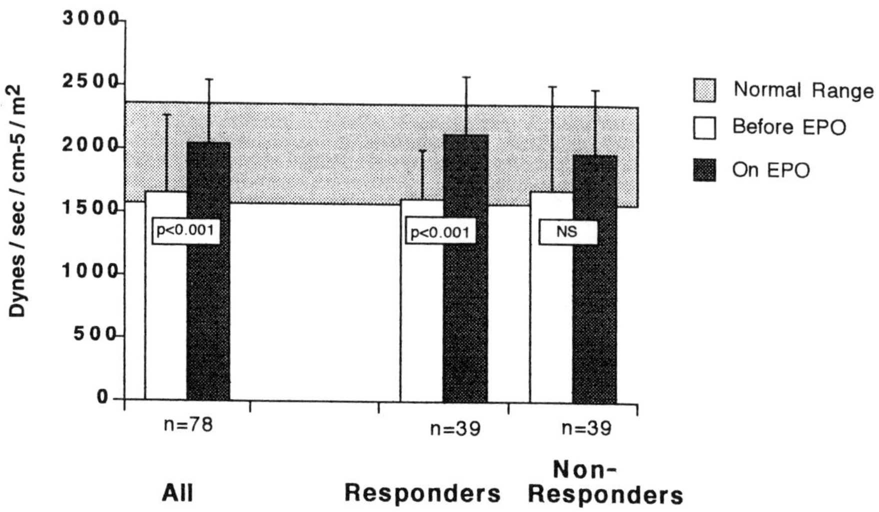

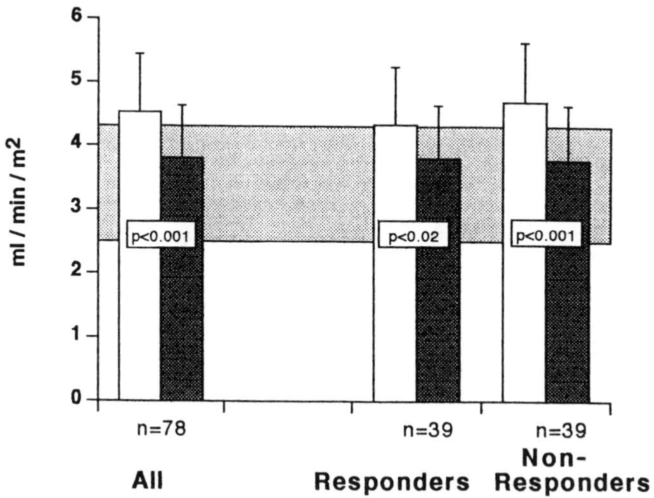

Fig. 1. Changes in (top) total peripheral resistance index and (bottom) cardiac index in patients on hemodialysis at the start of erythropoietin treatment and when target hematocrit was reached. The results are combined from 6 studies [20, 21, 95, 97, 100, 104] with a total of 78 patients. Data are expressed as mean $\pm$ S.D. Responder = Start or increase in antihypertensive treatment and/or an increase in MAP $\geq$ 10 mm Hg.

tion are not known. In the following section we will discuss whether viscosity changes and/or vasoconstrictor effects induced by rhEPO may explain the inadequate increase in vascular resistance.

Relation Between Hematocrit, Viscosity, and Vascular Resistance

Whole blood viscosity is a complex variable, depending on hematocrit, vessel radius, plasma viscosity, and cell aggregation and deformability [108], hematocrit being the most important single determinant of whole blood viscosity [35, 109]. However, there is no linear relationship between whole blood viscosity and hematocrit. In the anemic range up to a hematocrit of 30%, viscosity increases only slowly with increasing hematocrit [107, 110]. Furthermore, erythropoietin leads to increased red cell deformability and reduced red cell aggregation [111–113], at least in the first weeks of rhEPO treatment, probably due to the production of young erythrocytes. This effect may be less pronounced after long-term rhEPO treatment [111, 114]. Therefore, viscosity does not increase as much in the first weeks of rhEPO therapy as would be predicted by the rise in hematocrit. Due to these complex interactions, valid predictions on the effect of an increase in hematocrit on in vivo whole blood viscosity cannot be easily made. Ex vivo, however, an increase in whole blood viscosity with erythropoietin treatment at both high and low shear stress of 14–40% can be found [18, 19, 26, 103, 113, 115, 116] correlating with the increase in hematocrit. Plasma viscosity is generally reported as unchanged [115]. Since vascular resistance and whole blood viscosity are directly related [107], a similar increase in the former can therefore be expected.

Is an Increase in Hematocrit a Cause of the Hypertensinogenic Effect of rhEPO?

A direct though weak correlation between blood pressure and viscosity has been found in normo- and hypertensive nonuremic patients [117]. In uremic patients with preexisting hypertension, Neff et al. [101] found an increase in diastolic blood pressure of 20 mm Hg and an inappropriate rise of peripheral vascular resistance when these patients were transfused up to a hematocrit around 40%. Thus, an increase in blood pressure accompanies increases in hematocrit if target hematocrits of about 40% are achieved. However, presently target hematocrits in rhEPO treatment of renal anemia are about 30%. In the majority of placebo-controlled and uncontrolled studies aiming at target hematocrits in this range, neither final levels [51, 53, 95] of hematocrit nor the rate of hematocrit increase [5, 36, 51, 53, 94, 95] were found to be correlated with increases in blood pressure. In contrast to these findings, Polok et al. [33] and Samtleben et al. [34], in a large multicenter study of 95 patients (separated in three groups with different doses of erythropoietin) reported a higher incidence of hypertension with faster rises in hematocrit. However, since the incidence of hypertension also correlated with the erythropoietin dose, it cannot be stated with certainty whether the increased incidence of hypertension was due to more rapid changes of hematocrit or to a dose effect of erythropoietin independent of changes in hematocrit.

A retrospective study of 100 hemodialysis patients [118], all of whom received 2 units of blood to increase their mean hemoglobin rapidly from 6.7 to 9.3 g/dl, failed to demonstrate any increase in blood pressure. Actually there was a small decrease in mean arterial pressure, while antihypertensive treatment remained unchanged. Thus rapid correction of hemoglobin levels does not necessarily cause hypertension in hemodialysis patients. Pascual et al. [119] corrected hematocrit in anemic hemodialysis patients up to 30% with either rhEPO or iron or androgens. The amount of antihypertensive drugs had to be increased in rhEPO-treated patients only, whereas blood pressure remained constant and hematocrit increased to comparable levels in all groups.

From all these findings one can conclude that other factors, in addition to increases in viscosity, must be responsible for the development of rhEPO-induced hypertension at a target hematocrit of about 30% in uremic patients.

*Possible Mediators of Vasoconstrictor Effects Induced
by rhEPO*

Data on the effect of rhEPO treatment on effectors of the neurohumoral system are contradictory. Most studies have reported no change or a decrease in plasma levels of renin [21, 35, 38, 61, 120, 121], angiotensin II [35], and catecholamines [19, 21, 38, 46, 120, 122]. However, increased angiotensin II [21, 120] and norepinephrine [61, 123] concentrations have also been reported. One study [103] reports increased plasma renin activity before the start of rhEPO treatment in those patients in whom blood pressure increased under rhEPO treatment. In these patients the response to exogenous angiotensin II after, as compared to before, rhEPO treatment was enhanced. Alpha 2 receptor density is reported to decrease with rhEPO treatment [19, 61] with improved receptor function [19]. Probably due to variations in the study populations, controversial findings regarding the blood pressure response to exogenous norepinephrine were reported. A placebo-controlled study not separating blood pressure responders from nonresponders found a decrease of blood pressure response to norepinephrine after treatment [61]. Another study reported enhanced responses in patients in whom blood pressure increased under rhEPO treatment [103].

A direct relation between platelet intracellular free calcium and blood pressure in essential hypertension has been described [124, 125], and there is some evidence that rhEPO may affect intracellular calcium homeostasis. Studies in platelets of uremic children on hemodialysis treated with rhEPO have shown significant increases in thrombin-stimulated platelet cytosolic free calcium over control [126]. Schiffl reported a close correlation between increases in platelet free calcium concentration and mean arterial pressure in uremic patients developing hypertension after 12 weeks of treatment with rhEPO [123]. Furthermore, high doses of erythropoietin (250 IU/ml) increased cytosolic free calcium concentrations in platelets from hypertensive, but not in platelets from normotensive rats [127]. rhEPO-induced constriction of rat isolated resistance vessels could be abolished by the removal of calcium from the incubation medium [128]. Thus, rhEPO-induced hypertension may be mediated by increased intracellular calcium levels.

Vasoconstrictor effects of rhEPO either by direct actions on smooth muscle cells or secondary to effects on other cells, leading to the release of vasomodulator substances, appeared unlikely in the past, since receptors for rhEPO were only known to be present on erythroid precursor cells. Early experimental studies performed seemed to support this assumption. Vascular resistance of the isolated perfused rat kidney was not affected by rhEPO perfusate concentrations ranging from 0.01 to 1 IU/ml [129], and the same concentration range did not cause changes in the tone of isolated human resistance vessels in vitro [130]. However, it has been shown that endothelial cells may possess erythropoietin receptors [131]. Erythropoietin could therefore cause vasoconstrictor effects by modulating the release of vasoactive substances from endothelial cells. Indeed, high concentrations of erythropoietin (10–200 IU/ml) have been reported to cause contraction of rat isolated resistance arteries of the renal and mesenteric bed [128]. With the same high doses, we have reported enhanced norepinephrine vasoconstrictor effects in rabbit aorta and renal artery with and without endothelium [123, 133]. How erythropoietin evokes responses in an endothelium-denuded vessel preparation remains unclear; it could be hypothesized that erythropoietin also acts directly on smooth muscle cells. In our model the enhancement could be partially blocked with cyclooxygenase inhibitors. When we measured prostaglandins we found a vasopressor shift in prostaglandin release in various vessels and cells: In human renal artery rings thromboxane B_2 production was stimulated 10-fold by 200 IU/ml of rhEPO from 84 $\pm$ 36 to 878 $\pm$ 34 pg/ring/15 min (mean $\pm$ SD). In human umbilical vein endothelial cells, prostacyclin production was inhibited significantly by the same dose of rhEPO (4399 $\pm$ 503 vs. 1375 $\pm$ 854 pg/10^6 cells). Thus, erythropoietin might lead to an increase in vasopressor or a decrease in vasorelaxant prostaglandins, resulting in enhanced responses to exogenous norepinephrine or angiotensin II in vivo. Large doses of erythropoietin had to be used in order to observe the above-mentioned in vitro effects. This may have been due either to a loss of functional integrity of the in vitro vessel preparation or to the choice of insensitive vessel preparations.

rhEPO-induced hypertension has only been observed in uremic patients. Studies in different vessels or organs from uremic animals are needed to determine whether these vessels are more sensitive to rhEPO-induced vasoconstriction. Regarding the finding of a vasopressor shift of prostaglandins, a 36% decrease in serum levels of 6-keto-PG-1α (a stable metabolite of prostacyclin) after treatment was actually reported in hemodialysis patients treated with rhEPO [38], however, no relation to blood pressure response could be found. Thromboxane levels have been reported as unchanged or reduced [115,134] although no correlation was performed regarding blood pressure response.

We also found a significant increase in endothelin production of almost 100% with 200 IU/ml of rhEPO in human umbilical vein endothelial cells. Elevated plasma endothelin concentrations after rhEPO treatment have also been observed in hemodialysis patients [43], and endothelin levels could be weakly correlated with mean arterial pressure, hypertensive patients having higher levels.

Since free hemoglobin inhibits the action of NO/EDRF in vitro [38, 135], it has been speculated that increasing hemoglobin concentrations may trap the vasorelaxant nitric oxide/EDRF—which is continuously released from endothelial cells—thereby causing increases in blood pressure. However, there is no evidence that intrinsic modulation of vascular tone by NO/EDRF is affected significantly in vivo by increases in hematocrit [136]. In in vivo experiments in nonuremic rats NO/EDRF release seemed to be increased in response to rhEPO treatment in spontaneously hypertensive rats [137] and normotensive rats made polycytemic by rhEPO [138].

As has been shown in the above-mentioned experimental and clinical studies, a variety of changes possibly causing vasoconstriction may be induced by rhEPO treatment. However, presently none of these mechanisms has been definitively shown to be causative in the hypertensinogenic response to rhEPO treatment in uremic, anemic patients.

Treatment

Frequent blood pressure measurement during the first 1–4 months of therapy are mandatory, and 24-hour ambulatory blood pressure measurements could be useful to reveal nighttime hypertension, which has been described with rhEPO therapy. If hypertension develops when the target hematocrit has been reached or surpassed, the dose of erythropoietin needs to be reduced or, if necessary, discontinued until blood pressure has normalized before reintroduction at a lower dose. Treatment of malignant hypertension with phlebotomy has been reported [139, 140]. If hypertension occurs at lower hematocrit levels, fluid and sodium removal during dialysis and the use of conventional antihypertensive treatment (β-adrenergic antagonists, calcium entry blockers, converting enzyme inhibitors) usually controls increased blood pressure with erythropoietin treatment.

Summary

1. Hypertension is the major side effect of rhEPO treatment of end-stage renal failure patients (incidence rates: 10–24%).
2. In the majority of patients, rhEPO-induced hypertension is due to inadequately increased systemic vascular resistance.
3. The exact mechanism leading to the inadequately increased systemic vascular resistance is unknown. At target hematocrits around 30% other rhEPO-induced mechanisms in addition to viscosity changes must be involved in the induction of hypertension.
4. In experimental and clinical studies, multiple vasoconstrictor mechanisms have been shown to be activated by rhEPO treatment. However, at the present time no single factor has been clearly shown to be causative involved in the pathogenesis of rhEPO-induced hypertension in uremic patients.
5. rhEPO-induced hypertension occurring in uremic patients only could be due to a further derangement of the already disturbed vasoregulating mechanism in these patients, which cannot be compensated, as obviously is the case in anemic, nonuremic patients.

References

1 Charra B, Colemard E, Cuche M, Laurent G: Control of hypertension and prolonged survival on maintenance hemodialysis. Nephron 1983;33:96–99.
2 Vincenti F, Amend WJ, Abele J, Feduska NJ, Salvatierra O: The role of hypertension in hemodialysis-associated atherosclerosis. Am J Med 1980;68:363–369.
3 Silberberg JS, Barre PE, Prichard SS, Sniderman AD: Impact of left ventricular hypertrophy on survival in end-stage renal disease. Kidney Int 1989;36:286–290.
4 Sniderman AD, Silberberg J, Prichard S, Barré PE: Anemia and left ventricular function in end-stage renal disease; in Parfrey PS, Harnett JD (ed): Cardiac Dysfunction in Chronic Uremia. Kluwer Academic Publishers, 1992, pp 161–170.
5 Samtleben W, Baldamus CA, Bommer J, Fassbinder W, Nonnast-Daniel B, Gurland HJ: Blood pressure changes during treatment with recombinant human erythropoietin. Contr Nephrol 1988;66:114–122.
6 Bommer J, Alexiou C, Müller-Bühl U, Eifert J, Ritz E: Recombinant human erythropoietin therapy in hemodialysis patients—dose determination and clinical experience. Nephrol Dial Transplant 1987;2:238–242.
7 Casati S, Passerini P, Campise MR, Graziani G, Cesana B, Perisic M, Ponticelli C: Benefits and risks of protracted treatment with human recombinant erythropoietin in patients having haemodialysis. Br Med J Clin Res Ed 1987;295:1017–1020.
8 Eschbach JW, Egrie JC, Downing MR, Browne JK, Adamson JW: Correction of the anemia of end stage renal disease with recombinant human erythropoietin. N Engl J Med 1987;316:73–78.
9 Winearls CG, Oliver DO, Pippard MJ, Reid C, Downing MR, Cotes PM: Effect of human erythropoietin derived from recombinant DNA on the anaemia of patients maintained by chronic haemodialysis. Lancet 1986;2:1175–1178.
10 Jacquot CH, Feragu-Haguet M, Lefebvre A, Berthelot J-M, Peterlongo F, Castaigne JP: Recombinant erythropoietin and blood pressure. Lancet 1987;2:1083.
11 Schaefer RM, Kurner B, Zech M, Krahn R, Heidland A: Therapy of renal anemia with recombinant human erythropoietin. Dtsch Med Wochenschr 1988;113: 125–129.
12 Suzuki M, Hirasawa Y, Hirashima K, Arakawa M, Odaka M, Ogura Y, Yoshikawa Y, Sanaka T, Shinoda A, Morii H: Dose-finding, double-blind, clinical trial of recombinant human erythropoietin (Chugai) in Japanese patients with end-stage renal disease. Research Group for Clinical Assessment of rhEPO. Contrib Nephrol 1989;76:179–192.
13 Nonnast-Daniel B, Deschodt G, Brunkhorst R: Long-term effects of treatment with recombinant human erythropoietin on haemodynamics and tissue oxygenation in patients with renal anemia. Nephrol Dial Transplant 1990;5:444–448.
14 Berkley V, Fouad F, Currie P, Thomas T, Paganini EP: Serial echocardiographic evaluation of chronic haemodialysis pts during long term correction of anemia with recombinant human erythropoietin. Kidney Int 1989;35:240.
15 Abdulhadi MH, Fouad TF, Thomas T, Bravo EL, Paganini EP: The haemodynamic effects of correction of anaemia in haemodialysis patients using recombinant human erythropoietin. Nephrol Dial Transplant 1990;5:102–108.
16 MacDougall IC, Lewis NP, Saunders MJ, Cochlin DL, Davies ME, Hutton RD,

Fox KAA, Coles GA, Williams JD: Long term cardiorespiratory effects of amelioration of renal anemia by erythropoietin. Lancet 1990;335:489–493.

17 Tagawa H, Nagano M, Saito H, Umezu M, Yamakado M: Echocardiographic findings in hemodialysis patients treated with recombinant human erythropoietin: proposal for a hematocrit most beneficial to hemodynamics. Clin Nephrol 1991;35:35–38.

18 Schaefer RM, Leschke M, Strauer BE, Heidland A: Blood rheology and hypertension in hemodialysis patients treated with erythropoietin. Am J Nephrol 1988;8:449–453.

19 Müller R, Steffen HM, Brunner R, Pollok M, Baldamus CA, Kaufmann W: Disturbed function of alpha-2-adrenoceptors in renal anemia: a possible reason for increase in blood pressure after recombinant human erythropoietin? Klin Wochenschr 1991;69:742–748.

20 Kamata K, Marumo F, Onoyama K: Hemodynamic mechanism of the elevation in blood pressure following the improvement of anemia with recombinant human erythropoietin. Jpn Circ J 1991;55:649–656.

21 Hori K, Onoyama K, Iseki K, Fujimi S, Fujishima M: Hemodynamic and volume changes by recombinant human erythropoietin (rHuEPO) in the treatment of anemic hemodialysis patients. Clin Nephrol 1990;33:293–298.

22 Burghard R, Gordjani N, Leititis JU: Treatment of renal anemia with recombinant human erythropoietin. Monatsschr Kinderheilkd 1989;137:174–177.

23 Zehnder C, Blumberg A: Treatment of anemia in hemodialysis patients using recombinant human erythropoietin: advantages and disadvantages. Schweiz Med Wochenschr 1989;119:269–275.

24 Nonnast-Daniel B, Creutzig A, Kühn K, Bahlmann J, Reimers E, Brunkhorst R, Caspary L, Koch KM: Effect of treatment with recombinant human Erythropoietin on peripheral hemodynamics and oxygenation. Contr Nephrol 1988;66:185–194.

25 London GM, Zins B, Pannier B, Naret C, Berthelot J-M, Jacquot C, Safar M, Drueke T: Vascular changes in hemodialysis patients in response to recombinant human erythropoietin. Kidney Int 1989;36:878–892.

26 Canaud B, Donadieu P, Polito C, Rivory JP, Mathieu DJ, Peterlongo F, Mion C: Erythropoietin-associated hypertension: what role for blood viscosity changes? Nephron 1989;51:430–431.

27 Duff DR, Golper TA, Sloan RS, Brier ME, Aronoff GR: Low-dose recombinant human erythropoietin therapy in chronic hemodialysis patients. Am J Kidney Dis 1991;18:60–64.

28 van de Borne P, Tielemans C, Vanherweghem J-L, Degaute J-P: Effect of recombinant human erythropoietin therapy on ambulatory blood pressure and heart rate in chronic haemodialysis patients. Nephrol Dial Transplant 1992;7:45–49.

29 Bianchetti MG, Hammerli I, Roduit C, Neuhaus TJ, Leumann EP, Oetliker OH: Epoetin alfa in anaemic children or adolescents on regular dialysis. Eur J Pediatr 1991;150:509–512.

30 Abraham PA, Opsahl JA, Keshaviah PR, Collins AJ, Whalen JJ, Asinger RW, McLain LA, Hanson G, Davis MG, Halstenson CE: Body fluid spaces and blood pressure in hemodialysis patients during amelioration of anemia with erythropoietin. Am J Kidney Dis 1990;16:438–446.

31 Stenver D, Nielsen B: On the need for erythropoietin treatment in dialysis patients. A Copenhagen City Dialysis Unit study. Int J Artif Organs 1990;13:474–476.

32 Acchiardo SR, Quinn BP, Burk LB, Moore LW: Are high flux dialysis and erythropoietin treatment in a collision course? Asaio Trans 1989;35:308–310.

33 Pollok M, Bommer J, Gurland HJ, Koch KM, Schoeppe W, Scigalla P, Baldamus CA: Effects of recombinant human erythropoietin treatment in end-stage renal failure patients. Results of a multicenter phase II/III study. Contrib Nephrol 1989;76:201–211.

34 Samtleben W, Baldamus CA, Bommer J, Grutzmacher P, Nonnast DB, Scigalla P, Gurland HJ: Indications and contraindications for recombinant human erythropoietin treatment. Results in hemodialysis patients. Contrib Nephrol 1989;76:193–200.

35 Steffen HM, Brunner R, Muller R, Degenhardt S, Pollok M, Lang R, Baldamus CA: Peripheral hemodynamics, blood viscosity, and the renin-angiotensin system in hemodialysis patients under therapy with recombinant human erythropoietin. Contrib Nephrol 1989;76:292–298.

36 Akizawa T, Koshikawa S, Takaku F, Urabe A, Akiyama N, Mimura N, Otsubo O, Nihei H, Suzuki Y, Kawaguchi Y, Ota K, Kubo K, Marumo F, Maeda T: Clinical effect of recombinant human erythropoietin on anemia associated with chronic renal failure. A multi-institutional study in Japan. Int J Artif Organs 1988;11:343–350.

37 Schaefer RM, Kuerner B, Zech M, Denninger G, Borneff C, Heidland A: Treatment of the anemia of hemodialysis patients with recombinant human erythropoietin. Int J Artif Organs 1988;11:249–254.

38 Verbeelen D, Bossuyt A, Smitz J, Herman A, Dratwa M, Jonckheer MH: Hemodynamics of patients with renal failure treated with recombinant human erythropoietin. Clinical Nephrol 1989;31:6–11.

39 Creutzig A, Caspary L, Nonnast-Daniuel B, Bahlmann J, Kühn K, R.B, Reimers E, Koch KM, Alexander K: Skin microcirculation and regional peripheral resistance in patients with chronic renal anemia treated with recombinant human erythropoietin. Eur J Clin Invest 1990;20:219–223.

40 Pascual J, Teruel JL, Liano F, Ortuno J: Evidence for two different blood pressure responses after long term erythropoietin treatment in hemodialysis patients. JASN 1991;2:385.

41 Frenken LAM, Verberckmoes R, Michielsen P, Koene RAP: Efficacy and tolerance of treatment with recombinant-human erythropoietin in chronic renal failure (pre-dialysis) patients. Nephrol Dial Transplant 1989;4:782–786.

42 Löw-Friedrich I, Grützmacher P, März W, Bergmann M, Schoeppe W: Long-term echocardiographic examinations in chronic hemodialysis patients substituted with recombinant human erythropoietin. Blood Purif 1990;8:272–278.

43 Takahashi K, Totsune K, Sone M, Nozuki M, Murakami O, Sekino H, Saito T, Yoshinaga K, Mouri T: Elevated plasma endothelin-1 concentrations in hemodialysis patients with recombinant human erythropoietin therapy-induced blood pressure elevation. JASN 1991;2:418.

44 Epstein D, Valeri A, Neusy A-J, Lowenstein J: Endalin activity in Epogen® recipients. JASN 1991;2:376.

45 Roger SD, Baker LRI, Raine AEG: Erythropoietin induced hypertension is not related to autonomic dysfunction. JASN 1991;2:386.

46 Onoyama K, Hori K, Osato S, Fujishima M: Haemodynamic effect of recombinant human erythropoietin on hypotensive haemodialysis patients. Nephrol Dial Transplant 1991;6:562–565.

47 Eschbach JW, Downing MR, Egrie JG, Browne JK, Adams JW: USA multicenter clinical trial with recombinant human erythropoietin (AMGEN): results in hemodialysis patients. Contr Nephrol 1989;76:160–165.

48 Di Paolo B, Di LL, Summa R, Catucci G, Del RG, Muscianese P, Albertazzi A: Clinical effects of recombinant human erythropoietin in hemodialysis patients. Results of the "Abruzzo" Multicenter Trial. Asaio Trans 1991;37:M380–M381.

49 Lim VS, Flanigan MJ: Blood pressure and r HuEPO therapy. JASN 1991;2:381.

50 Eschbach JW, Abdulhadi MH, Browne JK, Delano MD, Downing M, Egrie JC, Evans RW, Friedman EA, Graber SE, Haley R, Korbet S, Krantz SB, Lundin P, Nissenson AR, et al.: Recombinant human erythropoietin in anemic patients with end stage renal disease: results of a phase III, multicenter clinical trial. Ann Intern Med 1989;111:992–1000.

51 Abraham PA, Macres MG: Blood pressure in hemodialysis patients during amelioration of anemia with erythropoietin. J Am Soc Nephrol 1991;2:927–936.

52 Bennett WM: A multicenter clinical trial of epoetin beta for anemia of end-stage renal disease. J Am Soc Nephrol 1991;1:990–998.

53 Canadian Erythropoietin Study Group: Effect of recombinant human erythropoietin therapy on blood pressure in hemodialysis patients. Am J Nephrol 1991;11:23–26.

54 Bahlmann J, Schoter KH, Scigalla P, Gurland HJ, Hilfenhaus M, Koch KM, Muthny FA, Neumayer HH, Pommer W, Quelhorst E, Sieberth HG, Weber U: Morbidity and mortality in hemodialysis patients with and without erythropoietin treatment: a controlled study. Contrib Nephrol 1991;88:90–106.

55 Edmunds ME, Walls J, Tucker B, Baker LR, Tomson CR, Ward M, Cunningham J, Moore R, Winearls CG: Seizures in haemodialysis patients treated with recombinant human erythropoietin. Nephrol Dial Transplant 1989;4:1065–1069.

56 Sundal E, Businger J, Kappeler A: Treatment of transfusion-dependent anaemia of chronic renal failure with recombinant human erythropoietin. A European multicentre study in 142 patients to define dose regimen and safety profile. Nephrol Dial Transplant 1991;6:955–965.

57 Edmunds ME, Walls J: Blood pressure and erythropoietin. Lancet 1988;2:351.

58 Mayer G, Cada EM, Watzinger U, Barnas U, Graf H: Hemodynamic effects of partial correction of chronic anemia by recombinant human erythropoietin in patients on dialysis. Am J Kidney Dis 1991;17:286–289.

59 Sobota JT: Recombinant human erythropoietin in patients with anemia due to end stage renal disease. US multicenter trials. Contrib. Nephrology 1989;76:166–178.

60 Canadian Erythropoietin Study Group: Association between recombinant human erythropoietin and quality of life and exercise capacity of patients receiving haemodialysis. Canadian Erythropoietin Study Group. Br Med J 1990;300:573–578.

61 Fritschka E, Neumayer HH, Seddighi S, Thiede HM, Distler A, Philipp Th: Effect of erythropoietin on parameters of sympathetic nervous activity in patients undergoing chronic haemodialysis. Br J Clin Pharmacol 1990;30:135S–138S.

62 Fischl M, Galpin JE, Levine JD: Recombinant human erythropoietin for patients with AIDS treated with Zidovudine. N Engl J Med 1990;322:1488–1493.

63 Goodnough LT, Rudnick S, Price TH: Increased preoperative collection of autol-

ogous blood with recombinant human erythropoietin therapy. N Engl J Med 1989;321:1163–1168.

64 Bormann B, Weidler B, Friedrich M, Andrian-Werburg HV: Recombinant erythropoietin in autologous blood donation. Anaesthesist 1991;40:386–390.

65 Berglund B, Ekblom B: Effect of recombinant human erythropoietin treatment on blood pressure and some haematological parameters in healthy men. J Intern Med 1991;229:125–130.

66 Kaltwasser JP, Praeve F, Wigand R, Brune T: The use of recombinant human erythropoietin in the treatment of the anemia of chronic disorders; in Pagel H, Weiss C, Jelkmann W (ed): Pathophysiology and Pharmacology of Erythropoietin. Berlin, Springer, 1992, pp 271–278.

67 Vannucchi AM, Grossi A, Bosi A, Rafanelli D, Guidi S, R.S, Longo G, Miele AR, Rossi-Ferrini P: Erythropoietin in bone marrow transplantation: Pathophysiology and clinical use; in Pagel H, Weiss C, Jelkmann W (ed): Pathophysiology and Pharmacology of Erythropoietin. Berlin, Springer, 1992, pp 311–314.

68 Busch ORC, Hoynck MAWvP, Marquet RL, Jeekel J: Experimental and clinical results of perioperative treatment with recombinant human erythropoietin; in Pagel H, Weiss C, Jelkmann W (ed): Pathophysiology and Pharmacology of Erythropoietin. Berlin, Springer, 1992, pp 315–320.

69 Casadevall N, Belanger C, Goy A, Varet B, Lang J, Poisson D: High-dose recombinant human erythropoietin administered intravenously for the treatment of anaemia in myelodysplastic syndromes. Acta Haematol 1992;1:25–27.

70 Pincus T, Olsen NJ, Russel IJ, Wolfe F, Harris ER, Schnitzer TJ, Boccagno JA, Krantz SB: Multicenter study of recombinant human erythropoietin in correction of anemia in rheumatoid arthritis. Am J Med 1990;89:161–168.

71 Mentzer WC, Shannon KM, Abels RI, Freeman P, Newton N, Thompson D, Phibbs R: A randomized, placebo-controlled clinical trial of recombinant human erythropoietin in the anemia of prematurity. Contrib Nephrol 1991;88:306–312.

72 Obladen M, Maier R, Segerer R, Grauel EL, Holland BM, Stewart G, Jorch G, Rabe H, Linderkamp O, Hoffmann HG, Houghton F, Herrmann Z, Scigalla P, Wardrop C: Efficacy and safety of recombinant human erythropoietin to prevent the anemia of prematurity. Contrib Nephrol 1991;88:314–326.

73 Wilkinson R: Clinical approach to hypertension; in Cameron S, Davison AM, Grünfeld JP, Kerr D, Ritz E (ed): Oxford Textbook of Clinical Nephrology. Oxford, England, Oxford University Press, 1992, pp 2047–2058.

74 Zuchelli P, Santoro P, Zuccala A: Genesis and control of hypertension in hemodialysis patients. Semin Nephrol 1988;8:163–168.

75 Weidemann P, Beretta-Piccoli C, Steffen F, Blumberg A, Reubi FC: Hypertension in terminal renal failure. Kidney Int 1976;9:294–301.

76 Wilkinson R, Scott DF, Uldall PR, Kerr DNS, Swinney J: Plasma renin and exchangeable sodium in the hypertension of chronic renal failure. The effect of bilateral nephrectomy. Quar J Med 1970;39:377–394.

77 Brass H, Ocks HG, Armbruster H, Heintz R: Plasma renin activity and aldosterone in patients with chronic renal glomerulonephritis and hypertension. Clin Nephrol 1976;5:57–60.

78 Boer P, Dorhout Mees EJ, Ross JC, Koomons HA, Geyskes GG: Renin and body fluid volumes in chronic renal disease. Acta Med Scand 1981;210:207–212.

79 Cangiano JL, Ramirez-Muno O, Ramirez-Gonzales K, Trevino A, Campos JA: Normal renin uremic hypertension; study of cardiac hemodynamics, plasma volume, extracellular fluid volume, and the renin angiotensin system. Arch Intern Med 1976;136:17–26.

80 Zucchelli P, Zuccala A: Control of blood pressure in patients on haemodialysis; in Cameron S, Davison AM, Grünfeld JP, Kerr D and Ritz E (ed): Oxford Textbook of Clinical Nephrology. Oxford, England, Oxford University Press, 1992, pp 1458–1467.

81 Beretta-Piccoli C, Weidmann P, Schiffl H, Cottier C, Reubi FC: Enhanced cardiovascular pressor reactivity to norepinephrine in mild renal parenchimal desease. Kidney Int 1982;22:297–303.

82 Campese VN, Romoff MS, Levitian D, Kenneth L, Massry SG: Mechanisms of autonomic nervous dysfunction in uremia. Kidney Int 1981;20:246–253.

83 Converse RL, Jacobsen TN, Toto RD, Jost CMT, Cosentino F, Fouad-Tarazi F, and Victor RG: Sympathetic overactivity in patients with chronic renal failure. N Engl J Med 1992;327:1912–1918.

84 Daul AE, Wang XL, Michel MC, Brodde OE: Arterial hypotension in chronic hemodialyzed patients. Kidney Int 1987;32:728–735.

85 Muller R, Steffen HM, Brunner R, Saric J, Pollok M, Baldamus CA, Kaufmann W: Changes in the alpha adrenergic system and increase in blood pressure with recombinant human erythropoietin (rHuEpo) therapy for renal anemia. Clin Invest Med 1991;14:614–22.

86 Kishimoto T, Terada T, Okohara T, Abe Y, Yamagami S, Mackacoa M: Correlation between blood prostaglandins and blood pressure in chronic renal failure. Nephron 1987;47:49–55.

87 Ylikorkala O, Huttunen K, Jarvi J, Viunikka L: Prostacyclin and thromboxane in chronic uremia, effect of hemodialysis. Clin Nephrol 1982;18:83–87.

88 Gordge MP, Neild GH: Platelets from patients on hemodialysis show impaired responses to nitroc oxide. Clin Sci 1992;83:313–318.

89 Vallance, P, A.L, Calver A, Collier J, Moncada S: Accumulation of an endogenous inhibitor of nitric oxide synthesis in chronic renal failure. Lancet 1992;339:572–575.

90 Folkow B, Grimby G, Thulesius O: Adaptive structural changes of the vascular walls in hypertension and their relation to the control of peripheral resistance. Acta Physiol Scand 1958;44:255–272.

91 Folkow B: The hemodynamic consequence of adaptive structural changes of the resistance vessels in hypertension. Clin Sci 1971;41:1–12.

92 Folkow B: Structural factor in primary and secondary hypertension. Hypertension 1990;16:89–101.

93 Helmchen U, Kneissler U, Bohle RM, Reher A, Groene HJ: Adaptation and decompensation of intrarenal small arteries in experimental hypertension. J Cardiovasc Pharmacol 1984;6:S696–S705.

94 Sundal E, Kaeser U: Correction of anaemia of chronic renal failure with recombi-

nant human erythropoietin: safety and efficacy of one year's treatment in a European multicentre study of 150 haemodialysis-dependent patients. Nephrol Dial Transplant 1989;4:979–987.

95   Buckner FS, Eschbach JW, Haley NR, Davidson RC, Adamson JW: Hypertension following erythropoietin therapy in anemic hemodialysis patients. Am J Hypertens 1990;3:947–955.

96   Pascual J, Teruel JL, Moya JL, Liano F, Jimenez MM, Ortuno J: Regression of left ventricular hypertrophy after partial correction of anemia with erythropoietin in patients on hemodialysis: a prospective study. Clin Nephrol 1991;35:280–287.

97   Löw-Friedrich I, Grutzmacher P, Marz W, Bergmann M, Schoeppe W: Therapy with recombinant human erythropoietin reduces cardiac size and improves heart function in chronic hemodialysis patients. Am J Nephrol 1991; 11:54–60.

98   Wirtz JJJM, Leunissen KML, Esser JWJV, Cheriex EC, Slaaf DW, Reneman RS, Hooff JPV: Recombinant human erythropoietin and its effect on macro- and microcirculation during normovolemia. Blood Purif 1990;8:285–294.

99   Nonmast DB, Deschodt G, Brunkhorst R, Creutzig A, Bahlmann J, Shaldon S, Koch KM: Long-term effects of treatment with recombinant human erythropoietin on haemodynamics and tissue oxygenation in patients with renal anaemia. Nephrol Dial Transplant 1990;5:444–448.

100 Akiba T, Kurihara S, Katoh H, Yoneshima H, Marumo F: Hemodynamic changes of hemodialyzed patients by recombinant human erythropoietin treatment. Kidney Int 1989;35:237.

101 Neff MS, Kim KE, Persoff M: Hemodynamics of uremic anemia. Circulation 1971;43:876–883.

102 Kim KE, Onesti G, Schwarz AB, Chinitz JL, Swartz C: Hemodynamics of hypertension in chronic end-stage renal disease. Circulation 1972;46:456–464.

103 Yamakado M, Umezu M, Nagano M, Tagawa H: Mechanisms of hypertension induced by erythropoietin in patients on hemodialysis. Clin Invest Med 1991;14:623–629.

104 Nonnast-Daniel B, Daniel WG, Brabant EG, Talartschik J, Frei U, Koch K-M: Personal communication, 1992.

105 Satoh K. Masuda T, Ikeda Y, Kurokawa S, Kamata K, Kikawada R, Takamoto T, Marumo F: Hemodynamic changes by recombinant erythropoietin therapy in hemodialyzed patients. Hypertension 1990;15:262–266.

106 Dorhout Mees EJ: Fluid retention in renal disease: the genesis of renal oedema, in Cameron S, Davison AM, Grünfeld JP, Kerr D, Ritz E (ed): Oxford Textbook of Clinical Nephrology. Oxford, England, Oxford University Press, 1992, pp 262–275.

107 Pirofsky B: The determination of blood viscosity in man by a method based on Poiseuille's law. J Clin Invest 1953;32:292–298.

108 Schmidt-Schönbein H, Rieger HFT: Blood fluidity as a consequence of red cell fluidity. Flow properties of blood and flow behaviour of blood in vascular diseases. Angiology 1980;31:301–319.

109 Stuart J, Kenny MW: Blood rheology. J Clin Path 1980;33:417–429.

110 Whittaker S, Winton FR: Apparent viscosity of blood flowing in isolated hind limb of dog and variation with corpuscular concentration. J Physiol 1933;78:339–369.

111 Brunner R, Steffen HM, Pollok M, Heidel M, Muller R, Degenhardt S, Baldamus

CA: Blood rheology in hemodialysis patients treated with recombinant human erythropoietin. Contrib Nephrol 1989;76:306–312.

112 Delamaire M, Durand F, Hamel D, Joyeux V, Lepogamp P, Genetet B: Improvement of hemorheological parameters in patients on hemodialysis, treated with recombinant human erythropoietin. J Mal Vasc 1991;16:289–294.

113 Lerche D, Schmidt R, Zoellner K: Rheology in whole blood and in red blood cells under recombinant human erythropoietin therapy. Contrib Nephrol 1989; 76: 299–305.

114 Jacquot C, Berthelot JM, Chiappini JD, Ferragu HM, Lefebvre A, Masselot JP, Moynot A, Frydman MO, Peterlongo F: Treatment of anemia in chronic hemodialysis patients with recombinant human erythropoietin: long-term results in 15 patients. Nephrologie 1990;11:11–16.

115 Gordge MP, Leaker B, Patel A, Oviasu E, Cameron JS, Neild GH: Recombinant human erythropoietin shortens the uremic bleeding time without causing intravascular haemostatic activation. Thromb Res 1990;57:171–182.

116 Canaud B, Polito-Bouloux C, Garred LJ, Rivory J-P, Donnadieu, P, Taib J, Florence P, Mion C: Recombinant human erythropoietin: 18 months' experience in hemodialysis patients. Am J Kidney Dis 1990;15:169–175.

117 Letcher RL, Chien S, Pickering TG, Sealey JE, Laragh JH: Direct relationship between blood pressure and blood viscosity in normal and hypertensive subjects. Am J Med 1981;70:1195–1202.

118 Williams B, Edmunds ME, Thompson JP, Burton PR, Feehally J, Walls J: Does increasing haemoglobin concentration and haematocrit have a pressor effect in dialysis patients? Nephrol Dial Transplant 1989;4:878–891.

119 Pascual J, Teruel JL, Marcen R, Gamez C, Liano F, Ortuno J: Blood pressure after three different forms of correction of anemia in hemodialysis. Int J Artif Organs 1992;15:393–396.

120 Ono K, Hisasue Y: The rate of increase in hematocrit, humoral vasoactive substances and blood pressure changes in hemodialysis patients treated with recombinant human erythropoietin or blood transfusion. Clin Nephrol 1992;37:23–27.

121 Arik N, Demirkan F, Erbas B, Arinsoy T, Sungur C, Yasavul U, Turgan C, Koray Z, Caglar S: Acute effect of erythropoietin on plasma renin activity and aldosterone levels in endstage renal disease. Nephron 1992;60:111.

122 Canella G, G.L, Sandrini M, Gaggiotti M, Nordio G, Movilli E, Mombelloni S, Visioli O, Maiorca R: Reversal of left ventricular hypertrophy following recombinant human erythropoietin treatment of anaemic dialysed uraemic patients. Nephrol Dial Transplant 1991;6:31–37.

123 Schiffl H: Correlation of blood pressure in end-stage renal disease with platelet cytosolic free calcium concentration during treatment of renal anemia with recombinant human erythropoietin. Int J Artif Organs 1992; 15:343–348.

124 Pritchard K, Raine AEG, Ashley CC, Castell LM, Somers V, Osborn C, Ledingham JGG, Conway J: Correlation of blood pressure in normotensive and hypertensive individuals with platelet but not lymphocyte intracellular free calcium concentrations. Clin Sci 1989;76:631–635.

125 Erne P, Bolli P, Bürgisser E, Bühler FR: Correlation of platelet calcium with blood pressure. N Engl J Med 1984; 310: 1084–1088.

126 VanGeet C, Damme-Lombaerts Rv, Vanrusselt M, Mol Ad, Proesmans W, Ver-

mylen J: Recombinant human erythropoietin increases blood pressure, platelet aggregability and platelet free calcium mobilization in uremic children: a possible link? Thromb Haemost 1990;64:7–10.

127 Tepel M, Wischniowski H, Zidek W: Erythropoietin increases cytosolic free calcium concentration and thrombin induced changes in cytosolic free calcium in platelets from spontaneously hypertensive rats. Biochem Biophys Res Commun 1991;177:991–997.

128 Heidenreich S, Rahn KH, Zidek W: Direct vasopressor effect of recombinant human erythropoietin on renal vascular resistance. Kidney Int 1991;39:259–265.

129 Pagel H, Jelkmann W, Weiss C: Erythropoietin and blood pressure. Hormone Metabol Res 1989;21:224.

130 Bund SJ, Heagarty A, Edmunds ME, Walls J: Erythropoietin does not induce vasoconstriction directly in human subcutaneous resistance vessels. Nephron 1989;53:173.

131 Anagnostou A, Lee ES, Kessimian N, Levinson R, Steiner M: Erythropoietin has a mitogenic and positive chomtactic effect on endothelial cells. Proc Natl Acad Sci USA 1990;87:5978–5982.

132 Radermacher J, Bode-Böger SM, Böger R, Frölich JC, Koch K-M: Erythropoietin enhances norepinephrine induced contractions via modulation in prostaglandin balance in rabbit and human arteries. Blood Purification 1992; 10:79–80.

133 Bode-Böger SM, Böger RH, Kuhn M, Radermacher J, Frölich JC: Endothelin release and shift in prostaglandin balance are involved in the modulation of vascular tone by recombinant erythropoietin. J Cardiovasc Pharmacol 1992;20:S25–S28.

134 Vigano G, Benigni A, Mendogni D, Mingardi G, Mecca G, Remuzzi G: Recombinant human erythropoietin to correct uremic bleeding. Am J Kidney Dis 1991;18:44–49.

135 Martin J, Moncada S: Blood pressure, erythropoietin, and nitric oxide [letter]. Lancet 1988;1:644.

136 Vallance P, Benjamin N, Collier J: Erythropoietin, haemoglobin, and hypertensive crises [letter]. Lancet 1988;1:1107.

137 Muntzel M, Hannedouche T, Lacour B, Drücke T: Erythropoetin therapy and endogenous nitric oxide in normotensive and hypertensive rats. JASN 1991;2:383.

138 Doll Ha, Welch WJ, Wilcox CS: Role of Nitric Oxide in the renal and circulatory adjustement to erythropoetin induced polycythemia in the rat. JASN 1991;2:375.

139 Fahal IH, Yaqoob M, Ahmad R: Phlebotomy for erythropoietin-associated malignant hypertension. Lancet 1991;337:1227.

140 Roger SD, Macdougall IC, Raine AE: Phlebotomy for erythropoietin-associated malignant hypertension. Lancet 1991;337:1606.

Jörg Radermacher, Abt. Nephrologie, Zentrum Innere Medizin, Konstanty-Gutschow-Str.8, D-W-3000 Hannover, Germany

Discussion

to the paper by J. Radermacher and K.M. Koch

Shaldon (Nimes): Do you think erythropoietin was developed too late for the dialysis patients? Twenty years ago, one controlled blood pressure by salt and water depletion very effectively and one had long hours of dialysis and one had occasional patients who had normal hematocrits and I think when one added testosterone one had several. I don't recollect there being any problem with hypertension in that population. Do you think the volume effect is one of the determinant factors in today's anxiety concerning the association of hypertension with erythropoietin therapy?

Koch: I think that the background of dialysis we provide in these patients of course plays a role, and you are quite right—the spontaneous incidence of hypertension in the dialysis population today and in the '70s, at least in our country, was different. There was rarely a need to use antihypertensives in the '70s, and when EPO was introduced about 60 or 50% of the dialysis population were on antihypertensive drugs. So the background of dialysis changed, and this may also affect the incidence of hypertension under erythropoietin treatment.

Wardrop (Cardiff): I support what I think Dr. Shaldon has just said. It is likely to be important. Remember that the hematocrit is but a ratio of plasma to red cells. If total plasma volume is considered—i.e., blood volume parameters are considered, as well as hematocrit—you might get a clue as to the basis of hypertension in some of the EPO-treated patients. Secondly, and perhaps related to that, there are whole new systems of vasomotor tone control of neurogenic origin being described, mediated by nitric oxide. Perhaps somebody here has data on deficiencies in these systems in hypertensive renal-failure patients?

Koch: Regarding your first comment, I think Neff in his very early studies, where he was acutely correcting the anemic state of hemodialysis patients by transfusion, showed an increase of blood pressure with normal plasma volumes. In some of our patients who became hypertensive after erythropoietin, we also performed volume measurements and we found normal plasma volumes.

Klinkmann (Rostock): Are there any reliable data available showing that there is a difference in the incidence rate of hypertension between the different routes of administration, subcutaneously or intravenously?

Koch: No, I don't think there is data demonstrating that subcutaneous application is accompanied by less hypertension than intravenous administration.

Gaehtgens (Berlin): I would like to come back to the question of nitric oxide, and this comment is also related to the previous presentations, discussing the occurrence of vasodilation during anemia. It was mentioned several times that this dilation is due to hypoxia. However, I know of no data to demonstrate that that is actually true. In fact, there are data showing that there is no tissue hypoxia during hemodilution. Therefore, an alternative explanation of the dilation would be the release of EDRF or nitric oxide from the endothelium in response to elevated flow: If you have anemia, you have reduced viscosity; therefore you have increased flow, and as a result you have vasodilation due to NO release. In uremic patients or in patients subjected to dialysis, this flow-dependent release of EDRF is somehow disturbed. This will lead to increased vascular hindrance which goes unnoticed as long as viscosity is reduced. As soon as you treat with erythropoietin, increase hematocrit, and thereby increase viscosity, you may actually unmask the vasoconstrictor effect that results from the absence of an adequate response to flow or an adequate NO release from endothelial cells. I'm wondering whether this could be a mechanism explaining at least in part the elevated peripheral resistance and hypertension observed.

Koch: Referring to your first comment, there are data from experimental studies in hamsters showing that there is a relation between PO_2 of the bath and the vasoconstriction of resistance vessels, so I think there is at least experimental proof for the existence of hypoxic vasodilatation. Concerning your question regarding the EDRF system in the uremic, this is an interesting question but there are no data yet available.

Kokot (Katowice): What is the importance of volume-related hormones in the pathogenesis of EPO-induced hypertension?

Koch: There are many studies where investigators tried to correlate plasma levels of many hormones with the occurrence of hypertension, but I don't think there are any conclusive data; there is a lot of controversy. I can't answer your question.

Wardrop: May I just come back to Dr. Koch, that the methods used for measurement of plasma volume may have given false high values and that a reliable method of measuring plasma volume is most important. I can't tell you what that is, but perhaps we can discuss this later.

Koch: You are asking what method I used?

Wardrop: I wonder if the methods that you report where plasma volume was measured depend on the volume of distribution of albumin, as in Evans blue?

Koch: We measured plasma volume indirectly by use of chromium-labeled red cells and hematocrit.

Long-Term Changes of α_2 Receptors in Recombinant Human Erythropoietin–Corrected Anemia

M. Pollok, H. M. Steffen,[a] R. Müller,[a] H. P. Behrenbeck, C. A. Baldamus

Medical Clinic II[a] and V, University Hospital Cologne, Cologne, Germany

The increased incidence of hypertension in erythropoietin (rhEPO)-treated dialysis patients stimulated research in blood pressure regulation in patients undergoing rhEPO therapy. This so far has not led to a definite explanation of the pathogenesis of hypertension. It seems to be multifactorial. Among other factors [1–3] the dysregulation of the sympathetic nervous system [4] has been discussed as a possible mechanism for hypertension following erythropoietin therapy.

The aim of this study was to investigate the time course of blood pressure, the pressure response to catecholamines, and the sympathetic status in erythropoietin-corrected renal anemia in otherwise stable hemodialysis patients.

Methods

Ten stable hemodialysis patients—6 females, 4 males—between 26 to 80 years of age with a mean age of 55 were studied. They had been on regular dialysis treatment for 10 months to 6 years and were dialyzed 3 times weekly for 4–5 hours with bicarbonate dialysate. Erythropoietin treatment was started with 3 times 120 U/kg BW/week i.v. until the target hematocrit of 30–35 vol% was reached. Then individual dosage adaptation was started to maintain this hematocrit. Patients were controlled over a period of 24 weeks.

In addition, nine stable additional hemodialysis patients with the highest hemoglobin concentration but not on rhEPO treatment were selected from a population of about 150 patients to correlate hemoglobin concentration with α_2 receptor concentration. For this group only, a hematocrit value >30 vol% was a selection criterion.

None of the patients in the two patient groups was on antihypertensive drugs or on any medication known to interfere with sympathic regulation.

The following outcome parameters were measured: hematocrit in vol%, arterial blood pressure in mm Hg, heart rate in beats/min, noradrenaline dosage to increase systolic blood pressure for 20 mm Hg, given as ng/kg/min, resting noradrenaline plasma levels in pmol/ml, measured by the COMT method [5], and α_2 receptor concentration on thrombocytes, given in fmol/mg protein, analyzed by the yohimbin ligand assay [6].

Results

Figure 1 gives the mean values (± SD) for blood pressure, heart rate, and hematocrit response. Hematocrit started at 24 vol% and met the target value at 8 weeks after beginning rhEPO therapy with 34%, and this value was maintained above 30 vol% throughout (24 weeks). Blood pressure did not change over the entire observation period. Between the 14th and the 24th week, the systolic blood pressure dropped slightly from 130 to 125 mm Hg. Heart rate did not change and remained at 76 beats/min throughout. Therefore, in the patient population studied, no one developed erythropoietin-associated hypertension.

Table 1 shows data about the noradrenaline dosage necessary to increase systolic blood pressure 20 mm Hg. 88 ng/kg/min in the anemic state were needed before treatment with erythropoietin. This value then increased with correction of renal anemia to 118 ng/kg/min. Although the hematocrit did not change further, the noradrenaline dosage increased to 136 ng/kg/min at week 24.

Compared to normal healthy controls, noradrenaline plasma levels in hemodialysis patients [7] are increased. With correction of renal anemia plasma, noradrenaline concentration (Table 1) decreased, and even in patients with a stable corrected renal anemia (24 weeks) plasma noradrenaline tended to drop even further.

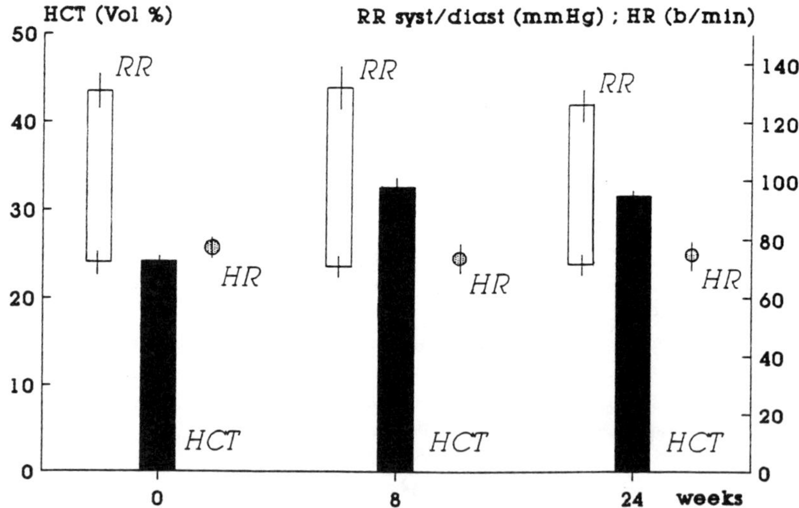

Fig. 1.   Time course of blood pressure (RR), heart rate (HR), and hematocrit (HCT) during correction of renal anemia by rhEPO.

Table 1. Noradrenaline dosage (NAD) to increase systolic arterial blood pressure by 20 mm Hg, resting noradrenaline plasma level and α_2 receptor concentration (A2R) on thrombocytes before and under long-term rhEPO treatment of hemodialysis patients at 8 and 24 weeks

	NAD (ng/kg/min)	NA (pmol/ml)	A2R (fmol/mg)
pre-EPO	88 ± 17	492 ± 88	587 ± 117
EPO, 8 weeks	117 ± 22*	368 ± 76*	392 ± 67*
EPO, 24 weeks	136 ± 29*	244 ± 57*	206 ± 34*

*p < 0.05, paired t-test.

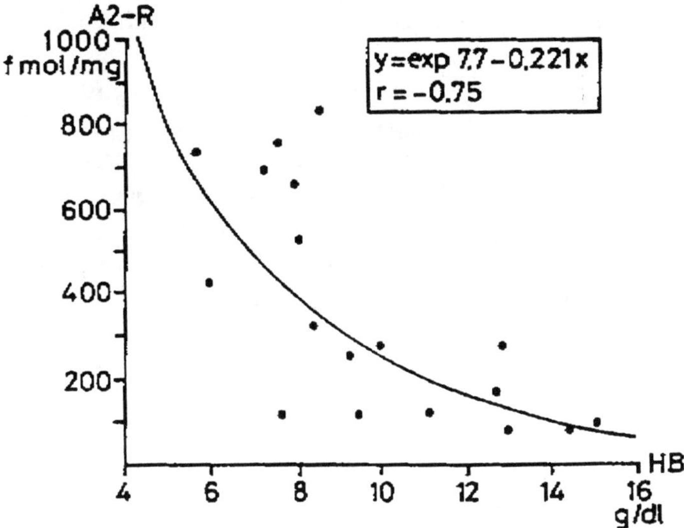

Fig. 2. Correlation between thrombocyte α_2 receptor (A2-R) concentration and blood hemoglobin concentration. In renal anemia A2-R concentration increases exponentially.

With correction of renal anemia the α_2 receptor concentration on thrombocytes (Table 1) decreases. Although hematocrit remains stable between 8 and 24 weeks, α_2 receptors seem not to have reached a new steady state.

In Figure 2 the α_2 receptor concentration is correlated against the hemoglobin concentration in hemodialysis patients not on rhEPO therapy with varying degrees of anemia. With decreasing hemoglobin concentration, the α_2 receptor concentration on thrombocytes increases exponentially.

Discussion

Due to the fact that none of the patients tested developed hypertension as described for the dialysis population treated with rhEPO [1–4], little can be contributed to the pathogenesis of hypertension in rhEPO treated patients. Regardless of the development of hypertension, however, correction of anemia in hemodialysis patients is associated with several changes in hemodynamic regulation.

The vascular responsiveness to an intravenous noradranaline infusion decreased with correction of anemia. Although hematocrit remained stable from the 8th to the 24th week, the noradrenaline dosage increased further (Table 1). From these results it cannot be determined whether a new steady state is already reached at 24 weeks or whether it takes even longer to establish. Little data are published on this issue yet. In a similar study Fritschka et al. [9, 10] also observed a blunted vascular response to noradrenaline with correction of anemia at half a year. They also described a decrease in α_2 receptor concentration. In contrast to our results, however, they observed an increase in resting plasma noradrenaline concentrations. To explain this discrepancy, the different experimental conditions must be considered. Fritschka et al. studied their patients one hour after dialysis, whereas we investigated our patients on the day between two dialyses. Their data might be influenced by the dialysis procedure with reequilibration of solutes and water, whereas a steady-state situation is reached the day after dialysis.

As can be seen from Figure 2, together with the data in Table 1, the change in α_2 receptors after correction of renal anemia reaches the regression line at only 24 weeks, but values are relatively too high early (8 weeks) after correction of renal anemia.

It remains difficult to explain a decrease in resting catecholamine level associated with a decrease of α_2 receptor concentration. The opposite was expected [8], as was found by Fritschka [9, 10]. No data are available for anemic patients with normal renal function to compare the described dialysis data with hemodynamic regulation in nonrenal patients. It might be that the steady state between the α_2 receptor and catecholamine concentration is hemoglobin dependent. Our data in dialysis patients suggest this.

Nothing is known about α_2 receptors in states of stable severe anemia. The data established here in dialysis patients suggest an inverse logarithmic correlation with hemoglobin concentration. Patients with high hematocrit values reach the range of normal volunteers (8).

In hemodialysis patients, plasma noradrenaline concentrations were found elevated [11], but so far no clear explanation has been given. A multifactorial pathogenesis [12, 13] was favored. The data from this study add another possible interpretation: the plasma noradreanaline elevation might be partly due to the anemic state of the patient.

References

1 Brunkhorst R, Nonnast-Daniel B, Koch KM, Frei U: Hypertension as a possible complication of recombinant human erythropoietin therapy. Contrib Nephrol 1991;88:118–125.
2 Akiba T, Kurhara S, Kotoh H, Yoneshima H, Marumo F: Hemodynamic changes of hemodialyzed patients by erythropoietin treatment. Kidney Int 1989;35:237.
3 Buckner FS, Eschbach JW, Haley NR, Davidson RR, Adamson JW: Correction of anemia in hemodialysis patients with recombinant erythropoietin: hemodynamic changes and risk for hypertension. Kidney Int 1989;35:237.
4 Frei U, Nonnast-Daniel B, Koch KM: Erythropoietin and Hypertonie. Klin Wschr 1988;66:914–919.
5 Passon PG, Peuler JD: A simplified radiometric assay for plasma norepinephrine and epinephrine. Anal Biochem 1973;51:618–631.
6 Brodde OE, Engel G, Hoyer D, Bock KD, Weber F: The beta-adrenergic receptor in human lymphocytes: subclassification by use of a new radioligand, $(-)^{-125}$ iodo-cyanopindolol. Life Sci 1981;29:2189–2189.
7 Baldamus CA, Ernst W, Frei U, Koch KM: Sympathetic and hemodynamic response to volume removal during different forms of renal replacement therapy. Nephron 1982;31:324.
8 Brodde OE: Die Rolle adrenerger alpha- und beta-Rezeptoren in der Pathogenese von Hypertonie und Herzerkrankungen. Internist 1988;29:397–413.
9 Fritschka E, Neumayer HH, Seddighi S, Distler A, Philipp T: Einfluß einer Erythro-poietintherapie auf die alpha-Adrenozeptoren-Dichte bei chronischen Dialysepa-tienten. Med Klinik 1991;86:353–359.
10 Fritschka E, Neumayer HH, Seddighi S, Thiede HM, Distler A, Philipp T: Effect of erythropoietin on parameters of sympathetic nervous activity in patients undergoing chronic hemodialysis. Br J Clin Pharm 1990;30:135S–138S.
11 Zucchelli P, Catizone L, Esposti ED, Fusaroli M, Ligabue A, Zuccala A: Influence of ultrafiltration on plasma renin activity and adrenergic system. Nephron 1978;21:317.
12 Brecht HM, Ernst W, Koch KM: Plasma noradrenaline levels in regular hemo-dialysis patients. Proc Eur Dial Transpl Ass 1976;12:281–289.
13 Lilley JJ, Golden J, Stone RA: Adrenergic regulation of blood pressure in chronic renal failure. J Clin Invest 1976;57:1190–1200.

M. Pollak, Medical Clinic, University of Cologne, Joseph-Stelzmann-Str. 9, 50931 Cologne, Germany

Discussion

to the paper by M. Pollok et al.

Kokot (Katowice): I am very happy to see that during EPO therapy there was a decrease of plasma noradrenalin level. We also found similar results; e.g., both noradrenalin and adrenalin plasma levels declined significantly at the beginning of EPO therapy. If we checked these parameters after 1 year of EPO treatment, there was a rising tendency of plasma noradrenalin levels. Therefore, my question is: Did you estimate the alpha-2 receptors after 1 year of EPO treatment?

Baldamus: No, the longest period we tested it was 24 weeks. After that, I really cannot tell you whether they increase or whether they decrease. Concerning adrenalin plasma levels, we did not find any change during the course of treatment. Usually there is a negative relationship between the number of alpha-2 receptors and noradrenalin plasma levels; that is, the higher the noradrenalin levels are, the lower the alpha-2 receptors become, and vice versa. This is not true in the cases we studied: Here we find a drop in alpha-2 receptors and a drop in noradrenalin concentrations.

Shaldon (Nimes): I was rather unimpressed by your exponential correlation. If I took your patients who had anemia without erythropoietin you had a scatter of 6 to 7 grams of hemoglobin, but you went through the whole range of concentration of the alpha-2 receptors. My question really is: What is the reproducibility of measurement to the alpha-2 receptor on a diurnal basis in this population, and what is the error of measurement?

Baldamus: It has not been studied. Measurements have not been repeatedly performed in the same patients under comparable conditions.

Shaldon: But I mean they are presumably varying depending on whatever signal is causing them to be expressed.

Baldamus: But this certainly would be true for all patients regardless of their degree of anemia. The scatter which bothers you is, however, only in the very-low-hematocrit patients, not in those with high hematocrit.

Shaldon: Well, then I will ask you the question: Did you in fact plot the data on a log scale and get significant correlation, or was your slide just art?

Baldamus: We did not plot the data on a logarithmic scale, but if we had I am sure we would have found a significant correlation.

Horina (Graz): What would be your explanation for the improvement of sympathic dysfunction; I mean, is that a matter of a feedback mechanism or better oxygenation, or would there be any other explanation?

Baldamus: I really cannot tell you. We were astonished when we found a drop in alpha-2 receptors with increasing hemoglobin in hemodialysis patients. We are in the process of following this and finding out whether this is true also for patients who are anemic for different reasons but have normal renal function.

Kaltwasser (Frankfurt): Do you have an explanation for this enormous time gap in the down-regulation of alpha-2 receptors between 4 and 24 weeks after EPO treatment shown in one of your slides, in respect to normal hematocrit in that population?

Baldamus: First of all, the hematocrit is not normal; the state of anemia is only partially corrected. I can't give you an explanation why it takes so long; usually the adaptation of the sympathetic system is a fast change. So I really cannot explain why this happened with such a time delay.

Eschbach (Seattle): Do you have any data for normal controls?

Baldamus: The control values for alpha-2 receptors in normal controls with normal renal function?

Eschbach: Yes.

Baldamus: It is about the same as that of patients with high hematocrit.

Gaehtgens (Berlin): Regarding the mechanism, you showed alpha-2 receptor density as a function of hemoglobin, thereby implying that there is a cause-and-effect relationship. I would like to stimulate you to speculate about this explanation: Is it possible that the general level of sympathetic activity simply decreases because these patients are better off after treatment?

Baldamus: Why the sympathetic system tends to normalize after correction of renal anemia I cannot tell you. Whether or not there is a cause–effect relationship, it is too early to say. At the moment I would interpret it as only an association.

Goldwasser (Chicago): I ask this question out of absolute ignorance: Are all alpha-2 receptors the same? You measure them on platelets, but it seems to me there might be different target cells.

Baldamus: That is a good question. It is the only way we can attack this question, but there is solid data in the literature that the number of alpha-2 receptors on thrombocytes represents the number of alpha-2 receptors in the periphery. These data are gained from analyzing tissue samples and correlating them to alpha-2 receptor measurements on thrombocytes.

Erslev (Philadelphia): Another question of ignorance: Does the number of receptors depend on the number of platelets?

Baldamus: No.

Iron and Erythropoiesis

J. W. Adamson

New York Blood Center, New York, N.Y., USA

This review will focus on the path of iron through the body as it relates to erythropoiesis. It will also examine the effects of erythropoietin (EPO) therapy on some aspects of iron metabolism and will analyze the effect of iron deficiency, at the progenitor cell level, to provide information as to where iron deficiency becomes manifest in erythroid cellular proliferation. And, finally, we will discuss an aspect of iron metabolism that may prove to be useful in predicting effective responses to EPO therapy in certain groups of patients.

Iron Metabolism

Figure 1 provides an overview of the internal cycle of iron metabolism in humans. Iron enters the body in human beings by two routes: through gastrointestinal absorption, which is the normal route, and through blood transfusions, as is true for many patients with chronic anemia. The iron molecule is transported in the plasma by the iron-binding protein, transferrin. Transferrin delivers its iron through specific cell surface receptors to developing erythroid cells; there, the iron is incorporated into hemoglobin. At the end of the erythroid maturation process, which takes approximately 5 days, the cells are released from the marrow. Under normal conditions, the bulk of iron in the body is in the form of circulating hemoglobin, which remains in the circulation for an average of 120 days, unless there is blood loss or premature red cell destruction.

The scavenging system for senescent red cells involves the reticuloendothelial (RE) cell. This is an extremely efficient internal metabolism pathway, with only a very small fraction of the body's iron being lost on a day-to-day basis. In males, that loss is on the order of 0.5–1 mg per day, but the average loss is 2 mg/day in menstruating females. In nonmenstruating females or adult males, the source of iron loss is largely the sloughing of epithelial cells from the gastrointestinal tract and skin.

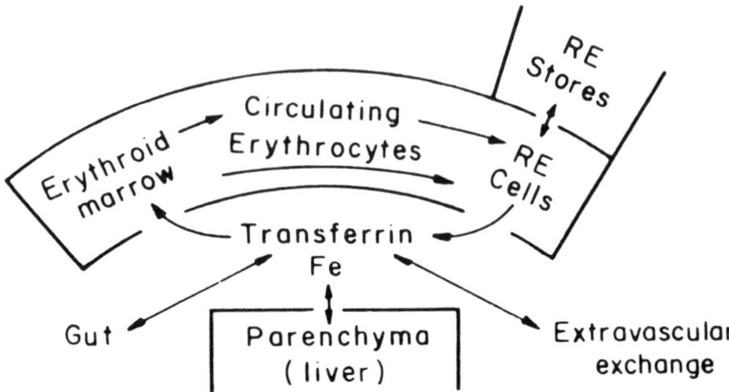

Fig. 1. The pathway of internal iron metabolism in humans. (From Hillman and Finch, 1974. Reprinted with permission.)

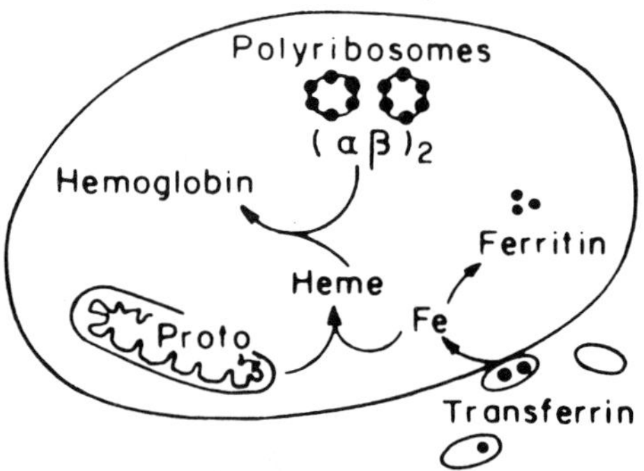

Fig. 2. The pathways of iron metabolism within the developing erythroid cell. (From Hillman and Finch, 1974. Reprinted with permission.)

Internally, there is a small amount of exchange of transferrin-bound iron with extravascular pools, as well as parenchymal cells such as those in the liver. The degree of parenchymal iron loading depends directly on the transferrin saturation; individuals with a persistently high transferrin saturation will have some degree of parenchymal iron overload.

Iron is presented to the erythroid cell in the form of the transferrin-iron complex (Fig. 2). The transferrin molecule has two iron-binding sites and thus can exist as diferric, monoferric, or aferric transferrin. The iron-loaded transferrin interacts with specific transferrin receptors on the surface of the developing erythroid cell. While all cells in the body require iron for survival, erythroid cells are unique in the amount of iron that is required in order for them to carry out the function for which they were designed. One of the characteristics that sets the erythroid cell apart from other cells in the body is the number of transferrin receptors, which may be as high as 750,000 per cell at certain stages of erythroid development. There is evidence for preferential recognition by the transferrin receptor for the diferric form of transferrin. Following binding of transferrin to its receptor, there is internalization of the complex—iron, transferrin, and receptor—into the cytoplasm of the cell. Within the endosome, at low pH, there is a release of iron from the complex, making the iron available for binding to protoporphyrin to form heme; heme and globin then combine to form hemoglobin. Any iron in excess of that needed for hemoglobin synthesis is shunted into a storage pathway and bound to apoferritin to form ferritin. Microscopically, ferritin granules appear within the cytoplasm of the developing erythroid cell and are recognized by specific iron stains; such a cell is called a sideroblast. In the absence of an adequate iron supply, a number of changes are seen in the developing erythroid cell which signal iron deficiency: the inadequate hemoglobinization of the cell; an increase in free erythrocyte protoporphyrin; the absence of stainable ferritin; an increase in transferrin receptor numbers on the cells.

The majority of iron turned over internally per day is made available as a result of the senescence of red cells. The signals or changes that allow a red cell to be recognized as being at the end of its life span are largely unknown. However, once the red cell is taken up by reticuloendothelial cells, globin is broken down, its components returned to the amino acid pool, and iron is released. At this point, iron can be bound to apoferritin for storage purposes, or the iron can be shuttled back to the surface of the reticuloendothelial cell and made available to transferrin to form, once again, the transferrin-iron complex. This is an extremely efficient step in the pathway of iron metabolism. In fact, if one radiolabels the iron in red cells, heat damages the cells, and reinfuses them into the body, radioactive iron, now bound to transferrin, appears in the circulation within minutes.

The size and distribution of iron pools within the body is summarized in Table 1. On average, adult males have about 1 g of elemental iron stored

Table 1. Body iron content

	Adult male	Adult female
Erythron iron (erythroid marrow and circulating red cells)	2400 mg	1700 mg
Iron stores	1000 mg	300 mg
Myoglobin/Tissue iron	160 mg	120 mg
Transferrin iron	6 mg	4 mg

From Hillman and Finch, 1974. Reprinted with permission.

throughout the body, generally in reticuloendothelial cells; there are about 3 mg of elemental iron bound to transferrin in the circulation. The average adult male has a red cell mass of slightly over 2000 ml, which is equivalent to 2000 to 2300 mg of elemental iron. There is a smaller component of tissue iron throughout the body.

One can assess the size of the body's iron stores clinically through a reasonably simple laboratory test that quantitates the level of ferritin in the plasma. As shown in Figure 3, there is a relationship between the plasma ferritin

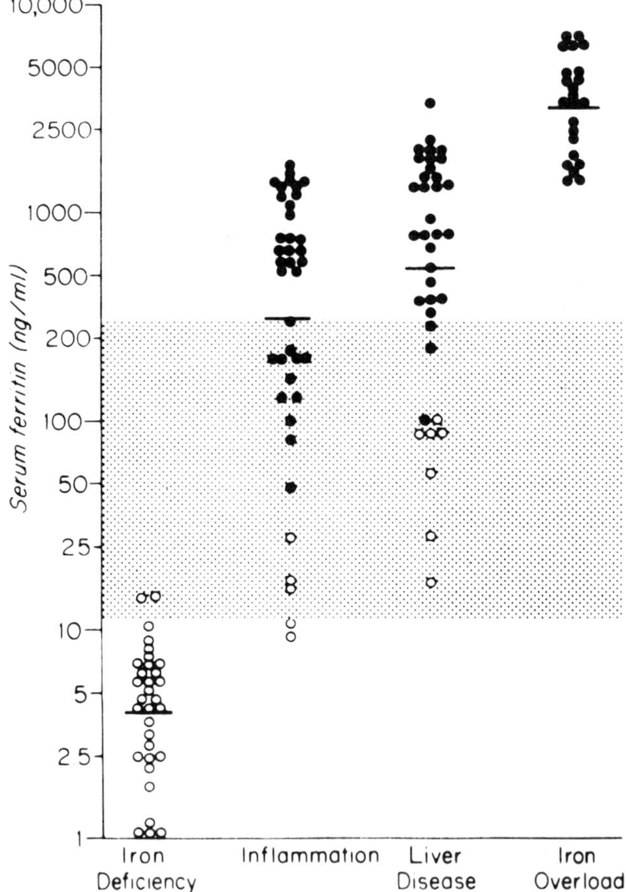

Fig. 3. Serum ferritin levels in normal individuals (shaded area) and in groups of patients with iron-deficiency anemia, inflammation, active liver disease, or iron overload. Because ferritin is an acute phase reactant, inflammation results in a false elevation of the ferritin value and can bring ferritin values for patients with true iron deficiency into the normal range. (From Lipschitz et al., N Engl J Med 1974;290:1213–1216. Reprinted with permission.)

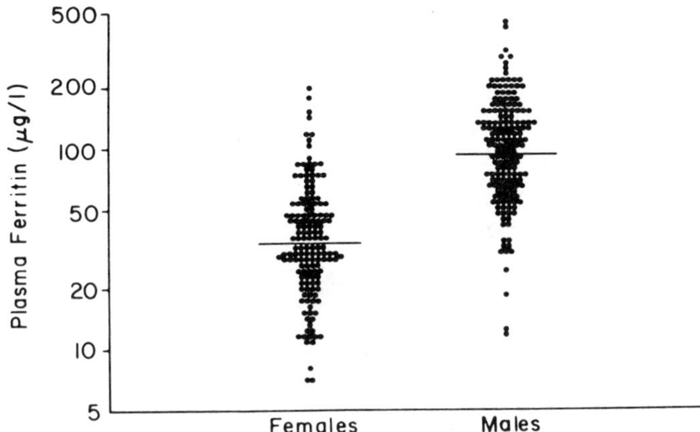

Fig. 4.   Plasma ferritin concentrations in 152 normal females and 174 normal male subjects. The geometric means are 34 µg/l in females and 94 µg/l in males. (From Cook JD, Am J Clin Nutr 1974;27:681–687 © American Society for Clinical Nutrition.)

level and storage iron in a given individual. Figure 4 demonstrates the difference in plasma ferritin levels between female and male adults. The normal value for adult males is approximately 100 µg of ferritin per liter of plasma. The lower value for females reflects the lower iron stores that result from menstrual blood loss. With iron deficiency, plasma ferritin levels are low. The converse is true in patients with iron overload, where serum ferritin levels are elevated. It is important to note, however, that while ferritin is a form of storage protein for iron, it is also an acute phase reactant. Thus, with active inflammation, plasma levels of ferritin can rise sharply in the absence of any change in total body iron stores.

In the overall scheme of iron metabolism, iron absorption is regulated by total body iron stores. Figure 5 demonstrates the changes in the absorption of labeled food iron in normal subjects and in patients with chronic renal failure who were on dialysis. The data indicate that with iron deficiency (as reflected by a plasma ferritin of 5–15 µg/l), dietary iron absorption is increased. In subjects with normal or increased iron stores, as reflected by the plasma ferritin, iron absorption is reduced. The results also indicate that, beginning at a plasma ferritin level of 50–100 µg/l, there is an inverse correlation between the amount of iron that is absorbed from dietary sources and the plasma ferritin level. Finally, patients with renal failure who are iron deficient have the same relationship of dietary iron absorption to plasma ferritin as do normal subjects.

Figure 6 relates total erythropoiesis in humans to the plasma iron level. The relationship indicates that if one is to see sustained rates of red cell production of

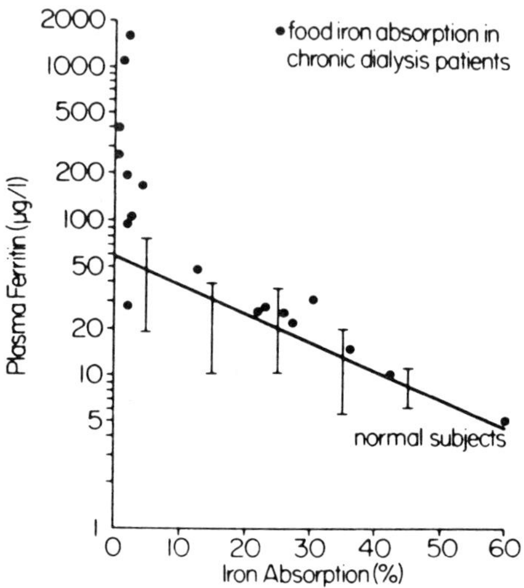

Fig. 5.   Food iron absorption in 19 chronic dialysis patients is indicated by closed circles. The absorption in 83 normal subjects (± 2 SD) is plotted as a solid line. It can be seen that absorption in the patients with chronic renal failure is appropriate to the iron status. (From Eschbach et al., Ann Intern Med 1977;87:710–713.)

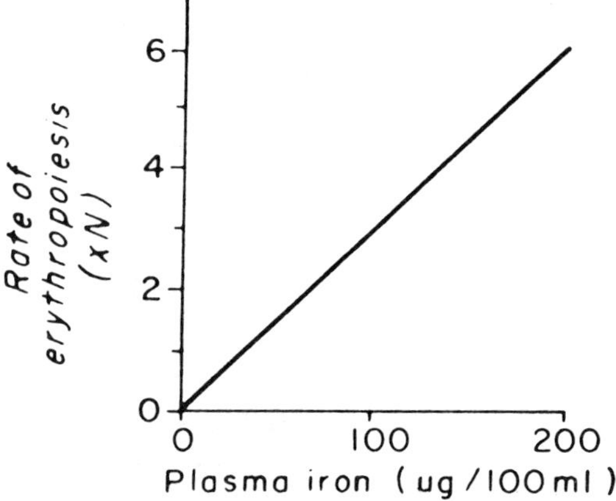

Fig. 6.   Sustainable rates of erythropoiesis (times the normal value) as related to the plasma iron concentration. (From Hillman and Finch, 1974. Reprinted with permission.)

three or four times normal, the plasma iron level has to be above 100 µg/dl. It should be emphasized that the test that reflects the iron immediately available for hemoglobin synthesis is the serum iron concentration in conjunction with the total iron-binding capacity. This is true despite the size of the body's iron stores as reflected by the plasma ferritin level.

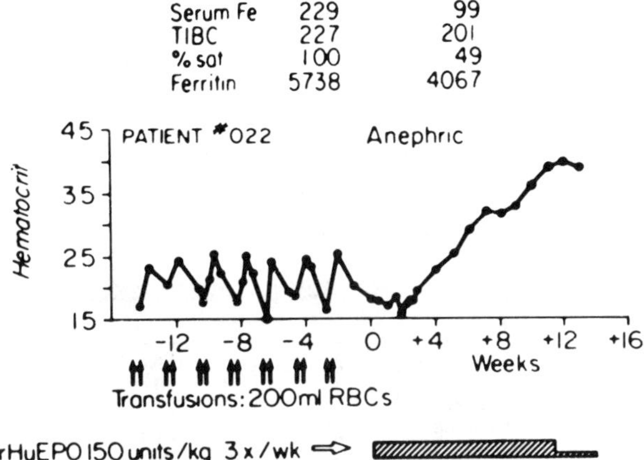

Fig. 7. The effect of the administration of rhEPO on the iron stores and the serum iron of a patient with chronic renal failure on dialysis. (From Eschbach et al., N Engl J Med 1987;316:73–78. Reprinted with permission.)

EPO Treatment and Changes in Iron Metabolism

Figure 7 illustrates some of the changes in storage iron and in serum iron as a result of administering recombinant human EPO (rhEPO) to a patient with renal failure. This patient was transfusion-dependent and had iron overload, as indicated by a plasma ferritin of nearly 6000 ng/ml and a transferrin saturation of 100%. With the initiation of EPO therapy, there was a reticulocytosis and gradual correction of the anemia. In addition, there was a fall in the serum iron due to the fact that iron was being removed from the circulation at a more rapid rate than it could be mobilized from storage sites. The utilization of iron stores to support the increasing circulating hemoglobin mass was reflected by a fall in the plasma ferritin level. In such patients, the iron overload state was reversed by EPO therapy.

However, EPO treatment can also result in functional iron deficiency, as shown in Figure 8. This patient had a moderate amount of iron overload with a plasma ferritin of nearly 900 ng/ml and a 50% transferrin saturation. After a period of rhEPO therapy—even though the plasma ferritin level was nearly 600 ng/ml—the percent transferrin saturation fell to 13%. This is a state of functional iron deficiency in terms of the iron immediately deliverable to the developing erythroid marrow. Under these circumstances, rhEPO becomes less effective.

Figure 9 demonstrates some of the changes in iron metabolism that are associated with EPO therapy in patients with renal failure. As is shown, the change in serum iron is relatively modest. In this study, most of the patients had high serum iron levels at the outset, averaging about 120 ng/ml. After 4 doses

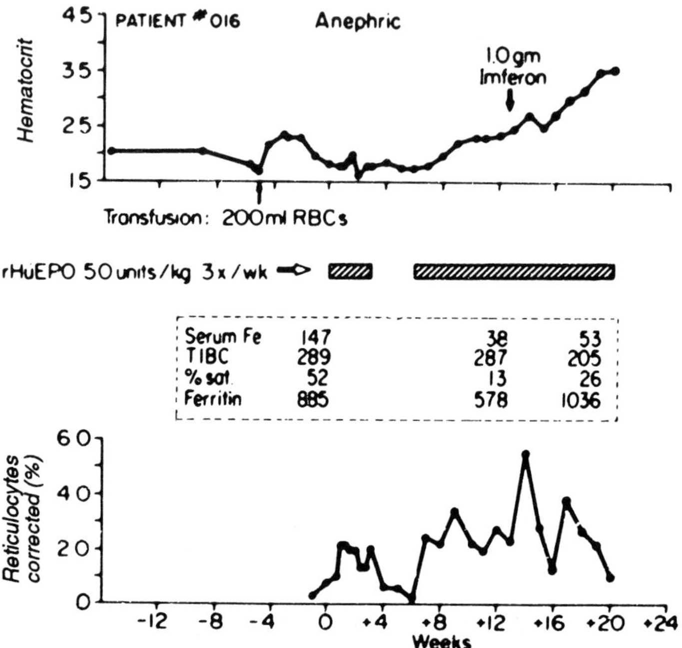

Fig. 8. The effect of rhEPO on iron metabolism in a patient on dialysis with chronic renal failure. As can be seen, after 4–8 weeks of EPO therapy, the patient became relatively iron deficient despite the fact that the serum ferritin remained well above normal. (From Eschbach et al., N Engl J Med 1987;316:73–78. Reprinted with permission.)

(given every other day) of EPO therapy (and at a time the hematocrit clearly would not have changed) the serum iron had fallen to about 80 μg/ml. The plasma iron turnover and erythron transferrin uptake, which reflect total erythropoiesis in humans, increased substantially, reflecting the effective response of the erythroid marrow to EPO administration.

The response to rhEPO administration of 5 normal subjects is shown in Figure 10. The dose of EPO was 150 units/kg given every other day i.v. for a total of 4 doses. Again, while there was no change in the hematocrit, the average serum iron, which was 100 ng/ml at the initiation of EPO dosing, fell to 40. At this point, the percent transferrin saturation is 15–17%. Thus, these doses of EPO in individuals with a fully functional erythroid marrow may induce a state of relative iron deficiency. As expected, there were appropriate changes in plasma iron turnover and erythron transferrin uptake.

Iron metabolism is also disturbed in normal individuals who experience inflammation or tissue injury. Simple examples of inflammation are viral infections or surgery. Figure 11 demonstrates the change in total iron-binding capacity

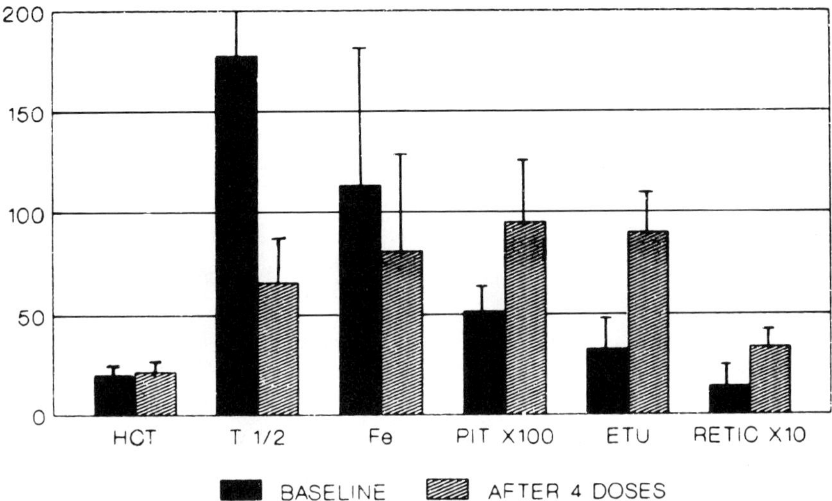

Fig. 9. The changes in a variety of hematopoietic parameters in 15 hemodialysis patients treated with 4 doses of 150 units rhEPO/kg. The parameters include the $T_{1/2}$ clearance time of radioactive iron, the serum iron (Fe), the plasma iron turnover (PIT), the erythron transferrin uptake (ETU), and the reticulocyte count.

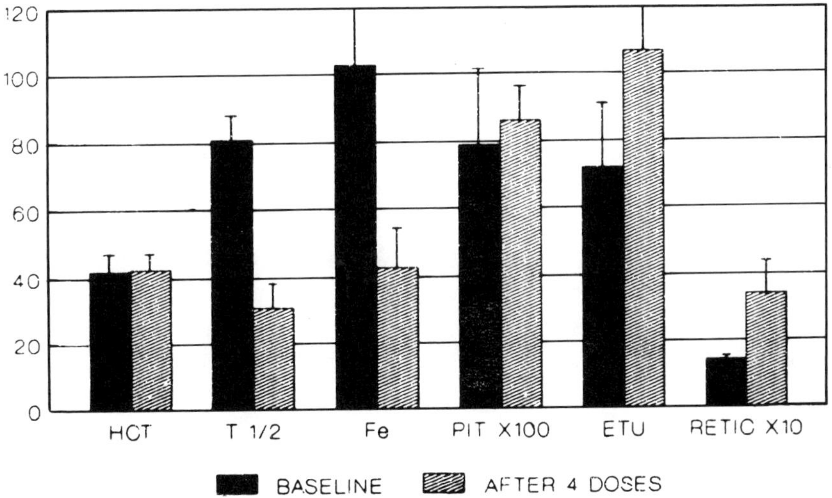

Fig. 10. The erythropoietic response of 5 normal subjects to the administration of 4 doses of rhEPO given in an identical fashion as that shown in Figure 9.

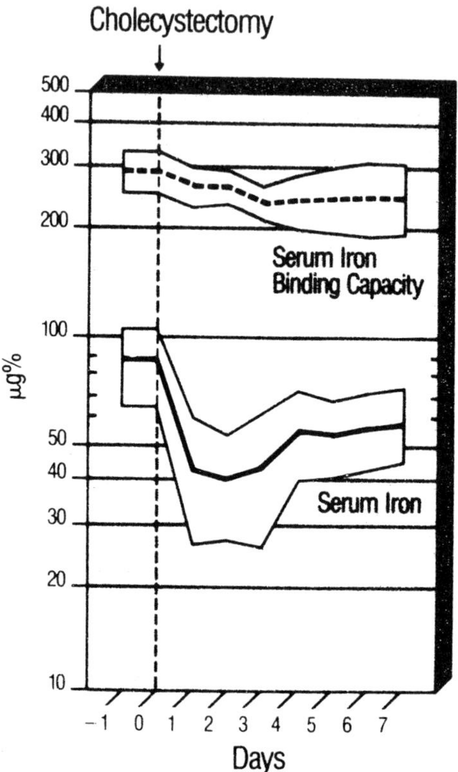

Fig. 11. The effect of tissue injury induced by a surgical procedure on the serum iron and iron-binding capacity in otherwise normal individuals. (From Erslev AJ, Curr Issues Anemia 1987;2:1–14. Reprinted with permission.)

and serum iron in a group of patients undergoing cholecystectomy. The serum iron averages about 90 ng/ml and then, over a period of a few days after surgery, falls to 40. The total iron-binding capacity over this period of time does not change appreciably, but at this time the patient has relative iron deficiency.

This point is emphasized in Figure 12, which presents a patient on dialysis who is chronically receiving rhEPO. The patient undergoes hip surgery. EPO treatment had allowed this patient—who had previously required transfusion support—to donate blood for autologous use at the time of the surgery. The percent transferrin saturation progressively fell over several days post-operatively, despite the fact that the ferritin level remained high. In fact, in response to the tissue injury induced by the surgical procedure, the plasma ferritin nearly tripled.

In this clinical setting, we have a percent transferrin saturation and a serum iron consistent with relative or functional iron deficiency. It was not until the

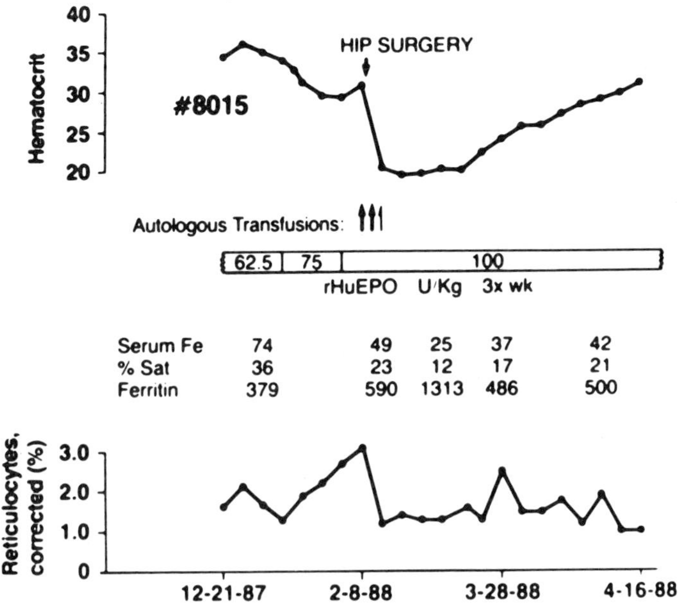

Fig. 12. The effect of surgery on iron metabolism and the response to rhEPO in a patient with chronic renal failure on dialysis. (From Adamson and Eschbach, Ann Rev Med 1990;41:357. Reprinted with permission.)

inflammation abated, as reflected by a return of the plasma ferritin level to presurgical values and a rise in the serum iron, that the hematocrit began to respond.

In this and other clinical situations, one could question the value of maintaining EPO therapy during a period of relative iron deficiency. Experimental evidence bearing on this question is provided by studies that examined the effect of iron deficiency on erythroid and nonerythroid progenitor cell compartments. The earliest erythroid progenitor that can be assayed in culture is the erythroid burst-forming cell (BFU-E). BFU-E give rise to erythroid colony-forming cells (CFU-E). In individuals or animals with an intact erythroid marrow, the ratio of CFU-E to BFU-E can rise severalfold in response to anemia or EPO administration. The study employed a model of chronic severe iron deficiency in the rat. The total body numbers of BFU-E and CFU-E were compared between normal animals and anemic, iron-deficient animals. Granulocyte/macrophage colony-forming cells (CFU-GM) were also monitored as a control for the lineage-specific effects of anemia and iron deficiency on erythropoiesis. In this model of chronic iron deficiency and severe anemia, there was a 3.5-fold increase in the numbers of CFU-E over normal animals (Fig. 13). This was not increased further by acutely replacing iron in individual animals while maintaining the anemia

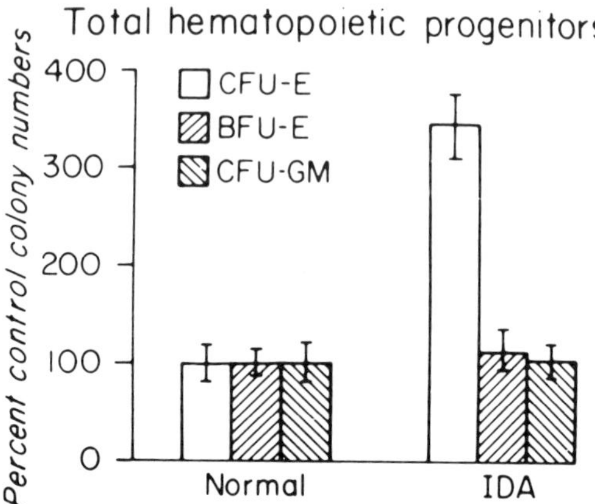

Fig. 13. Relative changes in progenitor cell compartments in rats made severely iron deficient and anemic (IDA) compared to normal. A selective and specific increase in erythroid colony-forming cells (CFU-E) was observed.

through phlebotomy. There were no differences seen in the total body numbers of BFU-E or CFU-GM. Under these circumstances, it would appear that the expansion of the CFU-E compartment—driven by high endogenous EPO levels—still occurs even in the face of iron deficiency. Consequently, to the extent that priming of the marrow with exogenous EPO is deemed clinically important, EPO should work.

Finally, can changes in iron metabolism be used to predict effective responses to EPO administration in certain patients? Recently, several investigators have demonstrated a close correlation between the erythron transferrin uptake (ETU)—a classic ferrokinetic measurement of iron turnover—and plasma levels of transferrin receptor protein (TFRP). As is true for many cell surface receptors, there is a soluble form of TFRP, which can be measured in plasma by sensitive immunological assays. Table 2 shows the correlation between the ETU and plasma levels of TFRP in normal subjects and patients with a variety of red cell production disorders. Chronic renal failure patients are anemic and have suppressed erythroid marrow function, as reflected by below-normal values for the ETU and TFRP. In cases of expanded erythropoiesis, there is a markedly increased ETU and increased plasma levels of TFRP. Figure 14 shows the correlation between these measurements in over 80 patients and normal subjects. The correlation indicates that plasma levels of TFRP are a good approximation of total erythropoiesis in humans.

Table 2. Plasma transferrin receptors in subjects with a variety of hematological disorders

	N	Age (yrs)	Hct (%)	Receptors[a] (μg/L)	Range	P Value
Normal subjects	56	37 ± 16	43 ± 6	8,279 ± 1,261	5,307-11,063	—
Hypoplastic erythropoiesis						
Aplastic anemia	16	35 ± 16	16 ± 5	3,871 ± 1,145	2,175-5,930	.0000
Marrow transplantation	14	30 ± 10	32 ± 5	3,842 ± 1,348	2,073-6,017	.0000
Chronic renal failure	43	45 ± 14	21 ± 3	4,973 ± 2,276	1,044-10,205	.0000
Hyperplastic erythropoiesis						
Immune hemolytic anemia	9	50 ± 13	35 ± 5	23,258 ± 5,640	14,558-31,117	.0000
Hereditary spherocytosis	7	31 ± 19	33 ± 4	37,076 ± 12,847	16,457-51,794	.0001
β-thalassemia/Hb E	72	26 ± 8	22 ± 4	70,049 ± 22,417	29,710-142,941	.0000
Hemoglobin H disease	11	40 ± 13	35 ± 3	32,900 ± 8,352	22,083-48,386	.0000
Altered iron status						
Iron deficiency	13	47 ± 16	32 ± 15	360,325 ± 23,490	11,237-80,707	.0000
Idiopathic hemochromatosis	7	61 ± 9	41 ± 5	9,497 ± 3,712	5,321-16,617	NS
Malignancies						
Polycythemia vera	13	57 ± 16	54 ± 8	22,011 ± 11,846	10,715-51,794	.0000
Myelofibrosis	10	70 ± 9	29 ± 6	12,615 ± 3,103	8,076-18,067	.0000
Myelodysplastic syndrome	10	57 ± 19	31 ± 10	12,310 ± 5,582	4,814-22,083	NS
Acute myelogenous leukemia	3	53 ± 8	35 ± 4	8,352 ± 3,364	5,495-12,035	NS
Chronic myelogenous leukemia	4	64 ± 9	38 ± 3	8,192 ± 2,131	5,307-10,382	NS
Essential thrombocythemia	5	47 ± 6	41 ± 2	7,525 ± 957	6,278-8,830	NS
Lymphoid malignancies	14	67 ± 10	41 ± 7	9,497 ± 3,190	6,343-17,425	NS
Solid tumors	9	63 ± 7	44 ± 2	7,859 ± 1,450	5,858-10,034	NS

Values as mean ± SD.
[a]Values refer to the transferrin receptor molecule complexed with transferrin.
From Huebers et al., Blood 1990;75:102–107.

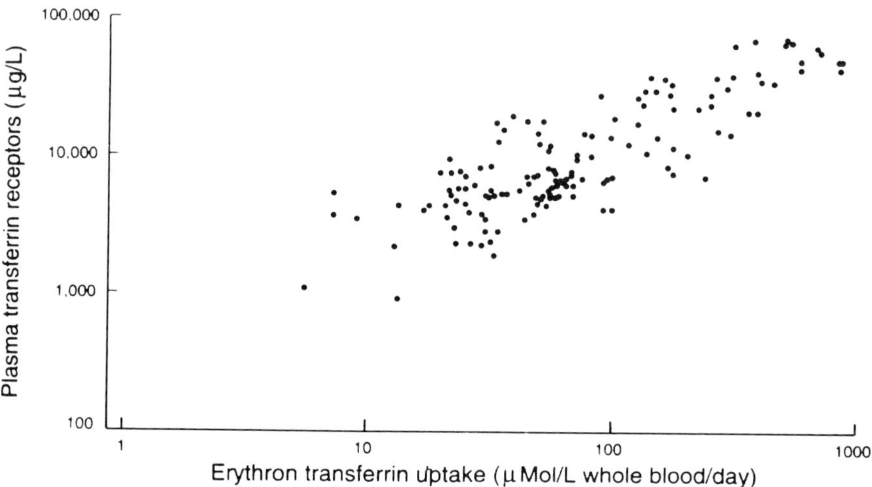

Fig. 14. The correlation between plasma levels of transferrin receptor protein and the erythron transferrin uptake in normal individuals and patients with a variety of hematological disorders. (From Huebers et al., Blood 1990;75:102–107. Reprinted with permission.)

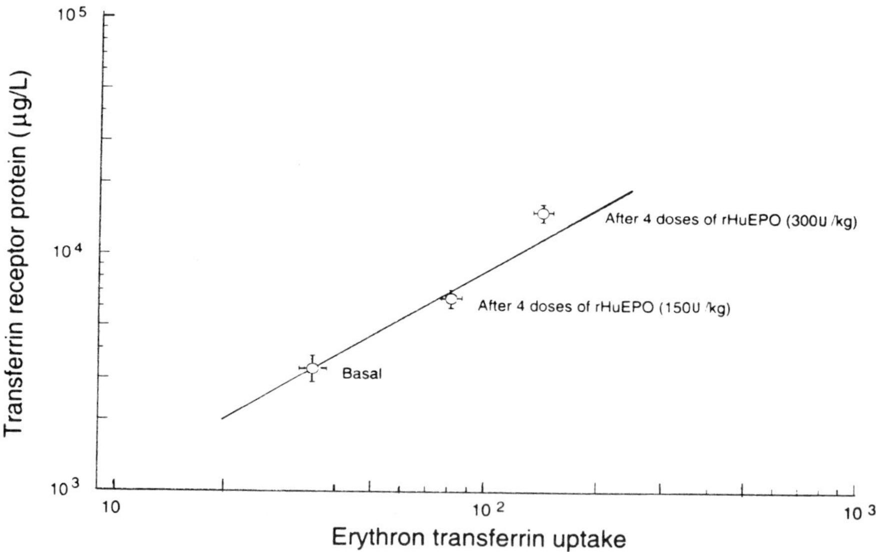

Fig. 15. The correlation between quantitative ferrokinetics as reflected by the erythron transferrin uptake and plasma concentrations of transferrin receptor protein in patients with renal failure at baseline and then after 4 subcutaneous doses of either 150 or 300 U/kg rhEPO. (From Adamson et al., Acta Haematologica 1992;87(suppl 1):20–24. Reprinted with permission.)

We then looked at changes in plasma levels of TFRP and measured the ETU in groups of dialysis patients who were treated with different doses of recombinant human EPO. Figure 15 shows the results of these studies in patients at baseline and then after 4 doses of either 150 U/kg or 300 U/kg of rhEPO. The correlation that was derived based on acute changes in TFRP follows the same regression that characterizes the patient groups shown in Figure 14.

Based on these observations, we and others have proposed that by monitoring acute changes in plasma levels of TFRP following a limited number of EPO doses, one might identify those patients who would have an effective response to EPO with increases in hemoglobin and hematocrit.

In early studies of patients with a variety of anemias, both success and failure have been reported. These results are early, however, and it is likely that some combination of laboratory tests will allow an accurate prediction of the eventual clinical response to EPO therapy. Such a development would assist early decisions concerning continuing therapy or altering EPO dosing in patient groups known to have a less than uniform response to this important therapeutic.

Source Materials

The principles of iron metabolism summarized in this review can be found in the 4th edition of the *Red Cell Manual*, by Robert S. Hillman and Clement A. Finch (F.A. Davis Company, Philadelphia, 1974), and *Iron Metabolism in Man*, edited by Thomas H. Bothwell, Robert W. Charlton, James D. Cook, and Clement A. Finch (Blackwell Scientific Publications, Oxford, England, 1979.

J. W. Adamson, New York Blood Center, 310 East 67th Street, New York, NY 10021-6295 (USA)

Discussion

to the paper by J. W. Adamson

Breymann (Zurich): You said you can increase the erythropoiesis if you have higher iron plasma levels. Do you think with parenteral iron it is possible to enhance EPO effectiveness on the red blood cell production due to high plasma levels?

Adamson: Certainly you can enhance the response to erythropoietin by having higher rather than lower serum iron levels. Where the break comes I am not sure, but I draw on the experience of hematologists to reflect on the fact that patients with idiopathic hemachromatosis who have very high serum iron levels tend to run slightly high hemoglobin levels, and they also have larger than normal red cells. Consequently, iron availability will influence the amount of hemoglobin being made both on a per-cell basis and by the erythroid marrow. We have seen patients with marginal iron availability increase their response to erythropoietin therapy as a result of administration of parenteral iron. So, I think, exogenous iron can enhance the response to either erythropoiesis too or the response to erythropoietin therapy. There probably is a limit in patients, depending upon the serum iron levels and the dose of EPO.

Horina (Graz): I would like to come back to that patient with the hip surgery. You showed that shortly after the hip surgery he developed "falsely" high ferritin levels and at the same time serum iron levels and the iron saturation went down. Would intravenous iron improve erythropoiesis in this case?

Adamson: It may depend on the form of iron. The commercially available parenteral form of iron in the U.S. would not be effective because—and I do not want to steal Professor Kaltwasser's thunder here—the release of iron from the complex requires processing by the reticuloendothelial cell. With inflammation, reticuloendothelial cell processing of iron is suppressed.

Influence of Recombinant Human Erythropoietin on Iron Metabolism in Healthy Subjects

Barry S. Skikne, James D. Cook

Division of Hematology, Department of Medicine, Kansas University Medical Center, Kansas City, Kans., USA

Introduction

Erythropoiesis is closely linked to iron metabolism because it is highly dependent on a continuous supply of iron from the circulation. The process of iron uptake by red cell precursors has been defined more clearly in recent years. The uptake of circulating transferrin iron is accomplished by the presence of a specific receptor for transferrin on the external surface of normoblasts [1]. The binding affinity of the transferrin receptor is greater for diferric transferrin than for monoferric transferrin [2, 3]. When the supply of circulating iron is diminished, there is an up-regulation of the transferrin receptor to permit more effective competition for the limited supply of transferrin iron. A deficiency in iron supply for hemoglobin synthesis, referred to as iron-deficient erythropoiesis, has previously been defined only on the basis of a diminished saturation of circulating transferrin below 20%. A more appropriate definition of iron-deficient erythropoiesis is based on the disparity between circulating transferrin iron and the total mass of erythroid transferrin receptor. Thus, iron-deficient erythropoiesis could occur with a normal transferrin saturation but markedly expanded erythroid requirement for iron. In support of this concept, increased free erythrocyte protoporphyrin in circulating red cells, an established laboratory index of iron-deficient erythropoiesis, has been reported in patients with thalassemia major who have normal or increased transferrin saturation but a massive expansion in erythroid precursor mass [4]. There is also evidence that the enhanced erythropoiesis resulting from erythropoietin (EPO) administration can also induce at least a temporary state of iron-deficient erythropoiesis in iron-replete patients.

The iron requirements for erythropoiesis are normally met by a combination of iron derived from the breakdown of senescent red blood cells in the reticuloendothelial system, from absorption, and from iron stores. Under conditions of basal erythropoiesis, iron recovered from red cell catabolism remains the major source of iron supply to circulating transferrin. However, when erythropoiesis is accelerated following the administration of EPO, iron supply from body stores and from the gastrointestinal tract becomes increasingly important. This is particularly true in anemic patients who have a more limited contribution from senescent red cells than normal subjects. When iron stores are ample, much of the heightened marrow iron requirements following EPO administration can be supplied from the storage compartment. However, when iron stores are diminished, the erythroid response to EPO administration becomes highly dependent on the amount of iron that can be assimilated by the gastrointestinal tract. The extent to which absorption can compensate for heightened iron demands is an important determinant of the severity of iron-deficient erythropoiesis following EPO administration.

Much information has been gained from examining the changes in iron metabolism in patients treated with EPO. However, this population of patients is heterogeneous and contains many variables that could influence iron metabolism independently. In order to eliminate these variables, we undertook a study of the erythroid response to EPO in healthy subjects. A group of 20 normal volunteer subjects were given a daily dose of 100 µg/kg recombinant human erythropoietin (Ortho Biotech, Inc. and R.W. Johnson Pharmaceutical Research Institute, Raritan, N.J.). EPO was injected subcutaneously on 10 days over a 2-week period [5]. The following is a summary of the induced changes in hematopoiesis, iron status, and gastrointestinal iron absorption.

Effect on Hematopoiesis

The effect on hematopoiesis of EPO administration in our normal volunteer subjects was similar to that described in previous studies [6]. Over the 2-week period of administration, the circulating hemoglobin concentration increased from 142 ± 13 g/l to 150 ± 16 g/l (mean $\pm$ 1 SD), a rise of approximately 6%. This was accompanied with a similar increase in circulating red blood cells from $4.58 \pm 0.42 \times 10^{12}$/l to $5.01 \pm 0.5 \times 10^{12}$/l, an increase of 9.1%. The increase in circulating hemoglobin concentration can be used to estimate the additional amount of iron required for the expansion of the circulating red cell mass. Based on individual changes in the hemoglobin concentration, the blood volume of each subject, and the assumption that 1 g hemoglobin contains 3.38 mg iron, it

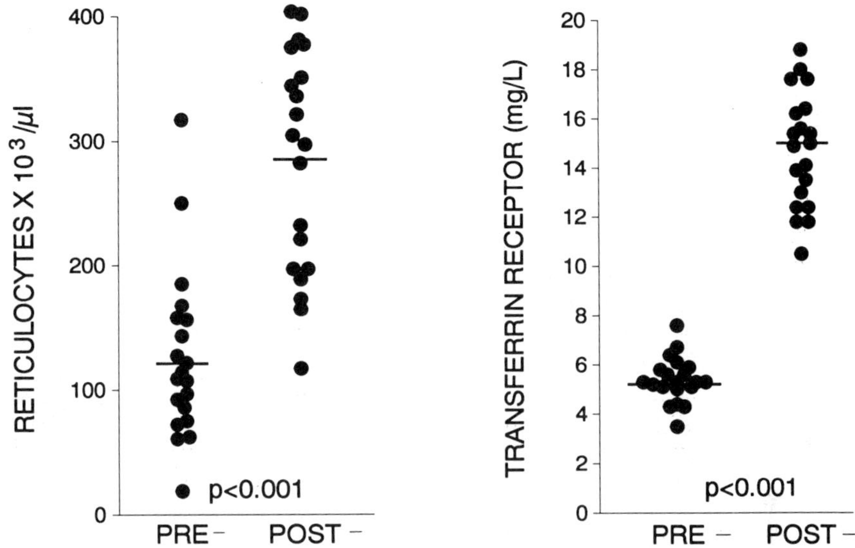

Fig. 1. Measurements of erythroid marrow response reflected as absolute reticulocytes and serum transferrin receptor levels, pre– and post–erythropoietin administration.

was estimated that an average of 120 mg iron was required for the increase in the circulating hemoglobin.

The effects of EPO could be more accurately monitored by specific measurements of erythroid marrow response (Fig. 1). As a measure of effective erythropoiesis, there was an increase in absolute reticulocyte count from $119 \times 10^3/\mu l$ to $285 \times 10^3/\mu l$, a 2.5-fold increase. It was also possible in this study to measure the effect on total erythropoiesis or total erythroid precursor mass, a parameter that previously required the intravenous administration of radioactive iron to measure various ferrokinetic indices. Recent studies have shown that total erythropoiesis can be measured more efficiently by determining the concentration of serum transferrin receptor. The serum transferrin receptor is a truncated, soluble form of intact cellular receptor present in all body cells and in highest concentration in early normoblasts. Comparison with the erythron transferrin uptake, a ferrokinetic measure of total erythropoiesis, has shown a high correlation with serum receptor in a wide variety of hematological disorders [7]. Recent evidence shows that the serum transferrin receptor level increases prior to an increase in circulating reticulocyte count, indicating that it monitors an earlier stage of erythropoietic activity [8]. In the present study, the serum transferrin receptor level increased in normal subjects from a baseline level of 5.4 ± 0.8

mg/l to 14.8 ± 2.4 mg/l following EPO administration. The 2.7-fold rise in serum transferrin receptor paralleled, very closely, the similar increase in reticulocyte production.

Effects on Iron Status

The increased rate of erythropoiesis induced by EPO administration resulted in a sharp increase in iron requirements by the erythroid marrow. In our subjects, this was reflected in a significant fall in serum iron from a baseline of 720 ± 160 µg/l to 380 ± 130 µg/l at the end of the 2-week administration period (p < 0.001) Although there was also an increase in total iron binding capacity (TIBC) from 3780 ± 740 µg/l at baseline to 4090 ± 970 µg/l following rhEPO, the increase was not statistically significant. Due predominantly to the reduction in serum iron concentration, there was a pronounced fall in transferrin saturation from 20 ± 7% at baseline to 10 ± 5% at the end of the 2-week course of EPO (p < 0.01).

The increased iron demand resulting from EPO administration was met by a combination of mobilization of iron stores and increased gastrointestinal absorption of iron. The contribution of iron from the storage compartment could be calculated from changes in the serum ferritin level. Phlebotomy studies in normal subjects have demonstrated that the serum ferritin level provides a reliable quantitative index of storage iron levels [9, 10]. The mean serum ferritin in our normal subjects was 43 µg/l at baseline, which corresponds to average iron stores of approximately 510 mg [11] (Table 1). One subject had absent iron stores based on a baseline serum ferritin <12 µg/l. Following rhEPO administration, there was a marked reduction in iron stores as reflected by a fall in serum ferritin to a mean of 13 µg/l, only slightly above the level of 12 µg/l commonly accepted as denoting absent iron stores. Based on this definition, iron stores became exhausted in 9 of the 20 subjects at the end of the 2-week course of EPO. A calculation of residual iron stores in each individual subject gave a mean level of 135 mg iron. Only 9 subjects had iron stores greater than 100 mg. It was noteworthy that of the 12 individuals with a baseline serum ferritin of 50 µg/L or less, 9, or 75%, had absent iron stores following EPO administration (Table 1).

These calculations indicated that iron stores decreased by an average of 375 mg during the 2-week period of EPO administration. Of this amount, 120 mg could be accounted for by the increase in circulating hemoglobin. The remaining 255 mg represents the iron incorporated into the expanded erythroid marrow compartment. It has been previously estimated that approximately 6.5% of iron in the erythron is contained in bone marrow erythroid precursors, or an average

Table 1. Mobilized iron stores based on change in serum ferritin[a]

Subject	Serum ferritin (ug/l)		Iron stores (mg)		Δ Stores (mg)
	Initial	Post	Initial	Post	
1	151	65	1013	676	337
2	126	39	941	471	470
3	83	24	774	277	497
4	76	23	738	260	478
5	72	20	717	204	513
6	54	23	602	260	342
7	54	16	602	115	487
8	53	19	594	184	410
9	50	9	571	0	571
10	48	13	676	32	523
11	40	8	482	0	482
12	36	8	439	0	439
13	35	8	428	0	428
14	34	13	419	32	385
15	27	11	324	0	324
16	27	6	324	0	324
17	26	19	309	184	125
18	22	5	242	0	242
19	16	4	115	0	115
20	10	5	0	0	0
Mean	43[b]	13[b]	515	135	375

[a]Iron store (mg) = 400 (log SF - log 12).
[b]Geometric mean.

of 130 mg iron in an individual weighing 70 kg. Measurements of the increase in circulating reticulocytes and serum transferrin receptor indicated a 2.5-fold expansion in erythroid mass corresponding to an increase of 325 mg iron in erythroid precursors in our subjects. This is in reasonable agreement with the calculated increase of 255 mg iron in this compartment from stores.

Effect on Iron Absorption

The only other source of iron for the expanded red cell compartment following EPO, apart from iron stores, is newly absorbed iron from the gastrointestinal tract. It is known that iron absorption is controlled by the level of body iron reserves and the rate of erythropoiesis. Of these, iron stores appear to be far more important. The quantitative relationship between iron stores and iron absorption has been well defined [12, 13]. Evidence in support of the effect of erythropoiesis on iron absorption is largely circumstantial. A dramatic increase in iron absorption and iron overload is known to occur in hematological disorders associated with ineffective erythropoiesis such as in patients with thalassemia major or sideroblastic anemia [14, 15]. However, it is the effectiveness rather than total erythropoiesis that is important because patients with compensated hemolytic anemia, such as hereditary spherocytosis, do not develop significant iron overload. By obtaining precise measurements of gastrointestinal iron absorption using radioisotopes, it was possible to evaluate the precise quantitative effect of EPO administration on iron absorption and assess the contribution of oral iron to meet the expanding marrow needs.

The absorption of dietary iron in our subjects was measured by extrinsically tagging the heme and nonheme iron compartment in a standard hamburger meal containing 820 kcal and 4.8 mg iron, of which 1.4 mg was in the form of heme. The methodology for extrinsic radioiron labeling of these two major dietary compartments is well established [16]. There was a dramatic increase in nonheme iron absorption in these subjects, which increased from 5.9 to 31.8% following EPO administration (Fig. 2). This increase corresponded to an increase in absolute iron absorption from 0.3 to 1.5 mg. Because of the dominant effect of iron stores on iron absorption, some of this increase in iron absorption could be attributed to the decrease in iron stores as reflected by the serum ferritin level. In order to independently assess the effect of enhanced erythropoiesis and iron status on iron absorption, nonheme iron absorption before and following EPO administration was corrected to a constant serum ferritin level of 40 μg/l. This correction is based on the known close inverse relationship between log serum ferritin and log nonheme iron absorption from food [17]. There was little change in corrected absorption values prior to EPO but a reduction in nonheme absorption following EPO to 13.1%. Because this corrected value is independent of iron stores, it is estimated that the increase in nonheme iron absorption due to enhanced erythropoiesis was 6.0 to 13.1%, or slightly more than 2-fold.

Because heme iron absorption is less responsive to changes in iron stores, these corrections were not applied to this dietary compartment. Nevertheless, there was a modest, but significant, increase in heme iron absorption from 47.0% prior to EPO to 58.6% following EPO administration. Although this rise is statistically significant, the absolute amount of iron contributed by the increased absorption of heme iron was <0.2 mg/day as compared to a contribution of 1.2 mg from nonheme iron.

The second study was designed to measure the contribution of oral iron tablets to the enhanced marrow iron requirement following EPO administration.

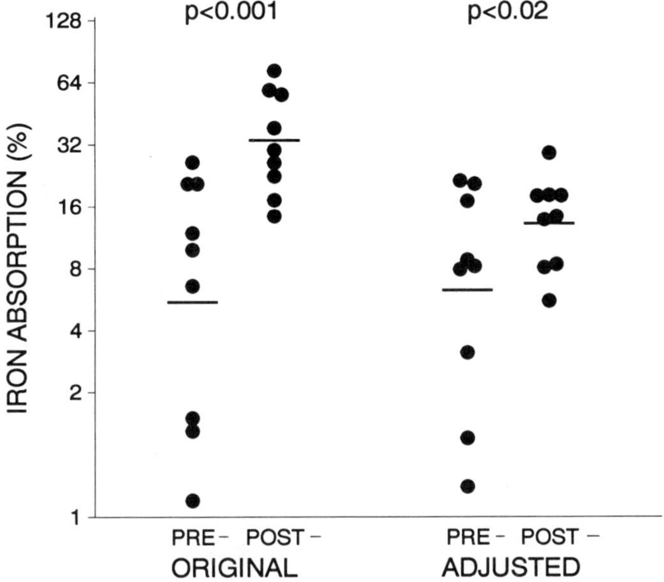

Fig. 2.   Nonheme iron absorption from the standard meal pre– and post–erythropoietin administration. The corrected absorption after adjustment for the change in iron stores due to erythropoietin is also shown.

Absorption from inorganic iron was measured when given with and without food. In the former study, 50 mg iron as ferrous sulfate was given with a standard meal in which the hamburger patty had been removed. Because of the absence of the enhancing effect of meat and the higher iron content of the meal, baseline absorption of nonheme iron was appreciably lower than in the first study, averaging 2.0%. There was a dramatic 8-fold increase in iron absorption to an average of 17.9% following EPO administration (Fig. 3). This corresponded to an increase of from 1.1 to 9.5 mg iron. After correcting for the effect of iron stores as previously described, the values for nonheme iron absorption before and following EPO were 2.5 and 7.6%, respectively. These observations again indicated that enhanced erythropoiesis is associated with a 2- to 3-fold increase in nonheme iron absorption.

Because of the significant inhibiting effect of food on the absorption of therapeutic iron, it was also of interest to study the effect of EPO administration on the absorption of ferrous sulfate given without food. The baseline absorption of 7.0% increased sharply to 24.6%, corresponding to an increase in absorbed iron from 3.5 mg to 12.3 mg (Fig. 3).

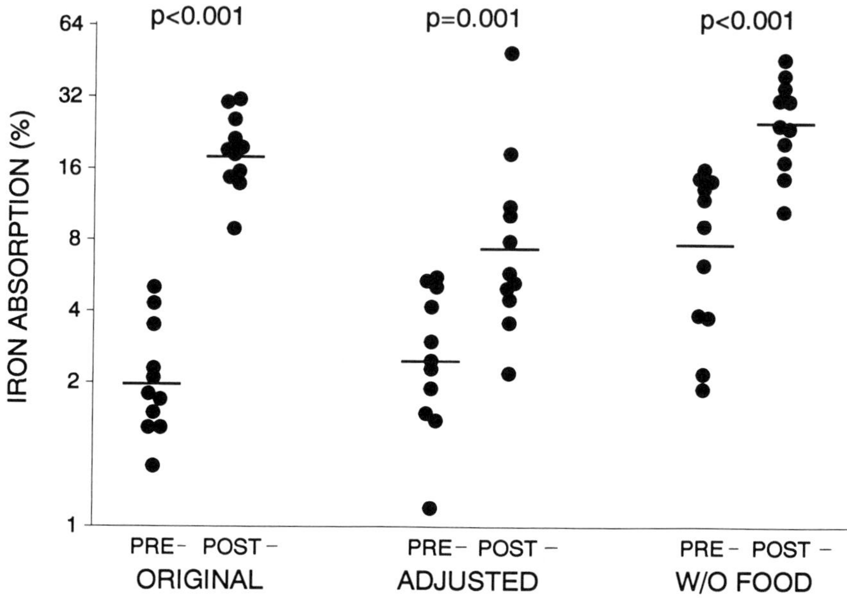

Fig. 3.   Nonheme iron absorption from a 50-mg iron supplement taken both with a meal and by itself pre– and post–erythropoietin administration. The corrected absorption from the iron supplement taken with the meal is also shown.

Effect of EPO Administration on Iron Requirements

As discussed previously, the estimated amount of iron mobilized from stores following EPO administration was 375 mg. This is equivalent to a daily iron requirement of 27 mg over the 14-day period of the study. Extrapolation of the food iron absorption data from the standard meal to an average daily food intake in a Western society indicates that a maximum of only 3 to 4 mg iron per day is likely to be absorbed from the diet while on EPO, far less than the amount required for enhanced erythropoiesis.

Our absorption studies indicate that these enhanced iron requirements can be met by taking oral iron. Since 24.6% of 50 mg iron as ferrous sulfate (12.3 mg iron) was absorbed after EPO, two ferrous sulfate tablets daily (100 mg) taken without food should meet the higher iron requirements on EPO. Because of the inhibiting effect of food on the absorption of ferrous sulfate, higher amounts are needed if the tablets are taken with meals. We found that an average of 9.5 mg of iron was absorbed when taken with the meatless meal. Therefore three tablets, containing 50 mg iron as ferrous sulfate, would be sufficient if all tablets were

Table 2. Time required to absorb sufficient iron to normalize hemoglobin (Hb) concentration in patients receiving EPO[a]

| | | | Time to attain Hb > 13 g/dl (days) | |
| | | | Therapeutic iron | |
Hemoglobin concentration	Hemoglobin iron deficit	Dietary iron	With food	Without food
5	1160	341	40	32
6	1015	298	35	28
7	870	255	30	24
8	725	213	25	20
9	580	170	20	16
10	435	128	15	12
11	290	85	10	8
12	145	42	5	4

[a]For 70-kg male with blood volume 4.3l.

consumed with meals. These amounts of iron are similar to those that have been proposed for maintaining a transferrin saturation >20% in patients on renal dialysis [18].

Our absorption data can also be used to predict the amount of time required to absorb the additional iron required for hemoglobin synthesis from the gastrointestinal tract in anemic patients with depleted iron stores (Table 2). Estimates are given for individuals relying solely on dietary iron and those taking ferrous sulfate tablets with and without food. In a 70-kg individual with a hemoglobin of 10 g%, for example, a hemoglobin iron deficit of 435 mg would require 128 days to replace from the diet alone as compared to only 12–15 days if iron tablets were taken. Any contribution of iron from stores would reduce these iron requirements proportionately.

Conclusions

Significant changes in iron metabolism occur with erythropoietin administration. When iron stores are available, they serve as an important source of iron to meet the increased demands for hemoglobin synthesis. Under the condition of erythropoietin administration in the present study, however, iron stores will be fully depleted over 2 weeks when the baseline serum ferritin is ≤50 μg/l. In this situation, the additional iron requirements must be met by absorption from the gastrointestinal tract. Although there is a striking enhancement in the absorption of nonheme dietary iron following EPO administration, the absolute quantities of iron that can be absorbed from the diet will not meet the increased iron requirements. Our absorption studies indicate, however, that ferrous iron tablets can meet the expanded iron needs during EPO administration in subjects that develop reduced iron stores. It is likely that even with full doses of therapeutic iron, oral iron will not prevent some mobilization from storage iron in those subjects who are initially iron replete.

Acknowledgment

This work was supported by NIH grant DK39246.

References

1 Huebers HA, Finch CA: The physiology of transferrin and transferrin receptors. Physiol Rev 1987;67:520–582.

2 Thorstensen K, Romslo I: The role of transferrin in the mechanism of cellular iron uptake. Biochem J 1990;271:1–10.

3 Huebers H, Csiba E, Huebers E, Finch CA: Molecular advantage of diferric transferrin in delivering iron to reticulocytes: A comparative study. Proc Soc Exp Biol Med 1985;179:222–226.

4 Pootrakul P, Wattanasaree J, Anuwatanakulchai M, Wasi P: Increased red blood cell protoporphyrin in thalassemia: A result of relative iron deficiency. Am J Clin Pathol 1984;82:289–293.

5 Skikne BS, Cook JD: Effect of enhanced erythropoiesis on iron absorption. J Lab Clin Med 1992;120:746–751.

6 McMahon FG, Vargas R, Ryan M, Jain AK, Abels RI, Perry B, Smith IL: Pharmacokinetics and effects of recombinant human erythropoietin after intravenous and subcutaneous injections in healthy volunteers. Blood 1990;76:1718–1722.

7 Huebers HA, Beguin Y, Pootrakul P, Einspahr D, Finch CA: Intact transferrin receptors in human plasma and their relation to erythropoiesis. Blood 1990;75:102–107.

8 Gross G, Ault K, Hitchcock S, Mitchell J, Huebers H, Hillman R: Reticulocyte transferrin receptor expression as a marker of marrow reticulocyte release. Br J Haematol 1992;ISH 24th Congress:76.

9 Skikne BS, Flowers CH, Cook JD: Serum transferrin receptor: A quantitative measure of tissue iron deficiency. Blood 1990;75:1870–1876.

10 Jacob RA, Sandstead HH, Klevay LM, Johnson LK: Utility of serum ferritin as a measure of iron deficiency in normal males undergoing repetitive phlebotomy. Blood 1980;56:786–791.

11 Cook JD, Skikne BS, Lynch SR, Reusser ME: Estimates of iron sufficiency in the US population. Blood 1986;68:726–731.

12 Cook JD, Dassenko S, Skikne BS: Serum transferrin receptor as an index of iron absorption. Br J Haematol 1990; 75:603–609.
13 Cook JD: Adaptation in iron metabolism. Am J Clin Nutr 1990;51:301–308.
14 Bothwell TH, Charlton RW, Cook JD, Finch CA: Iron Metabolism in Man. Oxford, Blackwell Scientific, 1979.
15 Pippard MJ, Callender ST, Warner GT, Weatherall DJ: Iron absorption and loading in beta-thalassaemia intermedia. Lancet 1979;2:819–821.
16 Lynch SR, Skikne BS, Cook JD: Food iron absorption in idiopathic hemochromatosis. Blood 1989;74:2187–2193.
17 Cook JD, Dassenko SA, Lynch SR: Assessment of the role of nonheme-iron availability in iron balance. Am J Clin Nutr 1991;54:717–722.
18 Eschbach JW: Recombinant human erythropoietin (Epoetin Alfa) in patients on hemodialysis: United States; in Erslev AJ, Adamson JW, Eschbach JW, Winearls CG (eds): Erythropoietin: Molecular, Cellular, and Clinical Biology. Baltimore, The Johns Hopkins University Press, 1991, pp 211–226.

Barry S. Skikne, M.D., Division of Hematology, University of Kansas Medical Center, 3901 Rainbow Boulevard, Kansas City, KS 66160-7402 (USA)

Discussion

to the paper by B. S. Skikne and J. D. Cook

Winearls (Oxford): Can you tell me what the signal is to turn on the increased iron absorption? Is it the fall in the serum iron or is it the increase of erythropoiesis?

Skikne: The signal to the bowel mucosal cell that controls iron absorption is one of the major questions that still remain unanswered; what the message is to the bowel mucosal cell at this time is not known.

Kaltwasser (Frankfurt): Addressing your last conclusion, where you mentioned that a certain amount of iron is distributed in the erythropoietic marrow: When your experiment is terminated, do you expect that this iron shifted to the erythropoietic department will be redistributed again to the iron stores?

Skikne: When we measured the ferritin levels 2 weeks following cessation of the erythropoietin administration, the serum ferritin level had risen significantly, so I think when you switch off erythropoiesis suddenly, the iron that has been moved to the erythroid marrow is rediverted back to stores. Also, I suspect that not all the iron that is incorporated into the red cell itself is actually utilized; some of that iron is probably extruded by the cell during erythropoiesis, in the bone marrow, and returns to transferrin for reutilization.

Erslev (Philadelphia): I am very impressed by your data but you have one soft point and that is the calculation of tissue iron from the ferritin. Obviously you must be using some kind of multiplication factor, but I cannot see that you could have all that iron in the erythroid tissue in the bone marrow and then have it released back to the tissue unless there was ineffective red cell production. I think the calculation of total tissue iron just based on ferritin and a multiplication factor is quite erroneous.

Skikne: The calculation is based on a log transformation of serum ferritin level. There may be some error, but I don't think that it is large. We have used this transformation in phlebotomized normal subjects, and the iron stores calculated in this manner from the ferritin levels very closely mimic the amount of iron removed in those subjects.

Birgegard (Uppsala): This was a discussion that we had in the late '70s, and I thought we would not bring it up again. There were studies showing that there was a very close relationship but, among others, we made studies showing that the relationship is not trustworthy. There is a great individual variation, and I think your own data showed there was a tremendous variation between the subjects. So when you calculate a mean for the whole group, that certainly does not go for a lot of subjects that are in the group, and I side with Erslev that it is dangerous to make these calculations from these figures.

Disturbances of Iron Metabolism in the Anemia of Chronic Disorders

Joachim Peter Kaltwasser

Rheumatology Unit, Department of Haematology, Center of Internal Medicine, Johann Wolfgang Goethe-University, Frankfurt a. Main, Germany

Introduction

In a variety of disease processes such as infections, tissue necrosis, surgical procedures, and neoplasias, a very similar type of anemia is observed. The anemia is usually manifested as a normocytic and normochromic or occasionally hypochromic anemia, predominantly in patients with longstanding disease duration. Among hospitalized patients this anemia is probably the most common type of all. The severity of hemoglobin reduction is roughly proportional to the severity of the underlying disease, but usually is "mild in degree and not progressive," as pointed out by Cartwright in his classic 1966 review [15]. The pattern of abnomalities is similar in a variety of diseases, suggesting a common pathogenesis. The anemia is usually called anemia of chronic disorders or diseases (ACD).

Little information is contained in the recent literature about the incidence of ACD in particular disease groups such as connective tissue disease or carcinomas. In patients with rheumatoid arthritis (RA), a moderate anemia is probably the most common extraarticular manifestation of the disease. From epidemiological findings in the late 1960s, a mean hemoglobin concentration of 11 g/dl for women and 12 g/dl for men has indicated an incidence of anemia in RA of as much as about 65% of women and 54% of men (22). A normocytic, mildly hypochromic anemia with a hemoglobin concentration of less than 11 g/dl has also been found at some time in the course of systemic lupus erythematosus (SLE) in 56–98% of cases in several large series of patients [45]. In perhaps 10% of SLE patients, severe anemia with hemoglobin concentration of less than 8.0 g/dl may occur. In contrast, in an analysis of 218 patients from the rheumatology outpatient unit of the University Hospital of Frankfurt, including RA, SLE, and mixed connective tissue disease (MCTD), an incidence of only 7.3% for ACD was calculated [35]. This rather low incidence, which excludes anemias from other causes (e.g., iron deficiency, folate deficiency, or hemolytic anaemias), may be not representative for the whole population of patients with rheumatic diseases because of the restriction of the analysis to the less severe cases of the outpatient unit.

Pathogenesis of ACD

The pathogenesis of ACD is far from being elucidated and has been attributed to multiple pathogenic mechanisms. The roles of the various mechanisms involved is still a matter of controversy. Decreased iron availability for erythropoiesis, decreased red blood cell (RBC) survival, suppressed RBC formation due to decreased erythropoietin levels, and/or a reduced response of the bone marrow to erythropoietin together with the presence of humoral inhibitors of the erythropoiesis are discussed [15, 39, 40, 48].

RBC Lifespan in ACD

A moderately reduced RBC lifespan has been observed in patients with chronic inflammatory diseases and in animals with experimentally induced inflammatory conditions [16, 17, 53]. There is no clear explanation for the reduced RBC survival. Extracorpuscular mechanisms, including increase of osmotic fragility due to slightly elevated temperatures and increased phagocytosis in the reticuloendothelial system, are considered possibly responsible for the shortening of RBC lifespan. ACD is, however, not simply the result of a reduced RBC lifetime but also the result of a negative balance between destruction and adaequate RBC production [39].

Disturbances of Iron Metabolism

Inflammation and neoplasia are characterized by a number of similar effects on iron metabolism, which are summerized in Table 1. The result of profound changes in iron metabolism is a limited availability of iron for erythroid proliferation [20, 39, 40, 48]. There is a decrease in tissue iron release and intestinal iron absorption, leading to hypoferremia and iron-deficient erythropoiesis. These

Table 1. The effect of inflammation on indicators
of iron metabolism

Iron absorption	↓
Serum iron	↓
Total iron-binding capacity	↓
Plasma iron turnover	↓
Hemoglobin	↓
Packed cell volume	↓
Tissue iron release	↓
Tissue storage iron	↑
Serum ferritin	↑
RBC protoporphyrin	↑
Plasma lactoferrin	↑

changes in iron ultimately result in a decreased hemoglobin concentration, a decrease in total iron binding capacity (TIBC) and plasma iron turnover, and an increase in RBC protoporphyrin concentration and serum ferritin and storage iron concentration.

Intestinal Iron Absorption

Studies on iron absorption in subjects or animals with inflammatory or neoplastic diseases are limited in number and conflicting in results. Iron absorption in children with febrile infectious diseases has been found markedly reduced as compared intraindividually to absorption in healthy children [5]. Similar findings have been reported in animals when inflammation was caused experimentally by turpentine or endotoxin injection [18, 31]. In contrast, Heinrich [30] concluded from measurements of an oral ^{59}Fe-test dose, measured by whole body counting, that intestinal iron absorption in patients with infections, lymphogranulomatosis, and cancer follows the same absorption pattern as in normal subjects. Similar results have been published by Boddy and Will [12] in patients with rheumatoid arthritis, although the increase of absorption in anemic patients was considerably less than would be expected from the degree of anemia.

Hypoferremia

Hypoferremia defined as a plasma iron concentration lower than 50 μg/dl is an early and common feature seen not only in infections but also in cancer, rheumatoid arthritis, following trauma and surgery and myocardial infarction [4, 7, 21, 39, 44, 45, 48, 78]. The hypoferremia frequently precedes the onset of fever or other symptoms of infection, and the fall in serum iron concentration correlates well with the severity of the subsequent clinical illness [21, 49]. In contrast to iron deficiency, where hypoferremia signals exhaustion of the mobilizable iron stores, in inflammatory states the amount of tissue storage iron usually is normal or even increased. The mechanism responsible for the fall in serum iron in inflammation and neoplasia is not fully understood. A defective reticuloendothelial release of iron, iron exchange between lactoferrin and transferrin at the site of inflammation, and the interaction with cytokines, especially with the monokine interleukin 1 (Il-1), are regarded as central pathogenetic factors, which will be discussed in detail in the next sections.

Lactoferrin

At the site of an inflammatory reaction the release of chemotactic factors such as complement component C5a attract polymorphonuclear cells (PMNs) and monocytes, which in turn release further chemotactic factors, thus causing an increasing inflammatory response. C5a provokes the discharge of the specific granules of PMNs [39]. Iron-free apolactoferrin, an iron-binding protein similar to but distinct from transferrin, is among the materials released by PMNs at the site of inflammation. Apolactoferrin binds iron avidly at acid pH in contrast to apotransferrin, which releases its iron at low pH. Based on this constellation, Van Snick and coworkers [51] have proposed the hypothesis that apolactoferrin secreted at the site of inflammation could be capable of exchanging iron with transferrin at acid pH and cause the hypoferremia observed in inflammation. The iron-lactoferrin complex is rapidly taken up by the liver and the monocyte-macrophage system. The Van Snick hypothesis has been criticized because minute amounts of endotoxin or Il-1 can also cause a marked fall in serum iron without a corresponding reduction in tissue or plasma pH, where iron remains bound to transferrin in the serum [39]. Baynes et al. (3) have noted that the lactoferrin concentration in plasma mirrors neutrophil counts, and they have claimed that, in patients with neutropenic sepsis, lactoferrin concentration is low in the presence of reduced plasma iron concentration. Similarly, in patients with rheumatoid arthritis, serum ferritin concentrations do not correspond to the variations in plasma lactoferrin. Irrespective of the lack of evidence for the role of lactoferrin in the pathogenesis of hypoferremia, lactoferrin obviously has a role in host defense against bacterial infections, as pointed out by Konijn and Hershko [39] in their excellent 1989 review on ACD.

The mechanism of this protective action is most probably due to a competition of lactoferrin with bacterial siderophores for iron or to a bactericidal effect of lactoferrin. Iron bound to lactoferrin has been shown to augment superoxide anion production by human monocytes [34]. Thus iron-saturated lactoferrin enhances the microbicidal and tumoricidal activity of monocytes.

Tissue Iron Release and Ferritin Synthesis

Iron release from parenchymal cells or cells of the monocyte-macrophage system is characterized by a rapid early phase, followed by a slower late phase of iron release into plasma [27, 31]. The early rapid release accounts for about 60% of iron derived from hemoglobin catabolism and occurs largely during the first 24 h after administration of labeled RBCs. The subsequent release of the remaining label is slower and occurs over 2–3 weeks. The early phase represents release of iron from a labile intracellular pool (Fig. 1), whereas the late release is derived from iron stored in ferritin. In turpentine or endotoxin-induced inflammation in experimental animals a marked reduction occurs in the fraction of iron released in the early phase, probably reflecting a reduction in the "labile iron pool" and an increase in the fraction of iron stored in ferritin as is demonstrated in the hypothetical model (Fig. 1) proposed by H. P. Roeser [48]. The intracellular ferritin is partly denatured to form hemosiderin. Inflammation probably accelerates this process together with an increase in uptake of RBC-iron and lactoferrin-iron complexes. Intracellular mediators of inflammation may be responsible for a discharge of lysosomal enzymes due to destabilization of the lysosomal membranes and may cause enhanced hemosiderin formation from ferritin [39]. The net effect of this process would be a reduction in the proportion of iron available through the labile pool for plasma iron and erythropoiesis.

Administration of heat-damaged ^{59}Fe-labeled RBCs to patients with chronic infections fails to produce the rise in serum iron levels observed in normal or iron-deficient subjects [28, 46]. Using ^{59}Fe-transferrin-antitransferrin immune complexes for labeling of thioglycolate-elicited mouse macrophages, Esparza and Brock [26] and Alvarez-Hernandez et al. [1] have shown that the iron label will be preferentially incorporated in the cells into hemosiderin and soluble compounds other than ferritin. Thioglycolate-elicited macrophages released less iron in vitro than resident macrophages. In thioglycolate-stimulated mouse peritoneal macrophages and in macrophages obtained from turpentin-inflamed mice, transferrin radioiron uptake is four times greater than in macrophages of normal mice [9]. Thus, increased tissue uptake and retention of iron together with reduced intestinal iron absorption may ultimately contribute substantially to hypoferremia and anemia in inflammation and neoplasia. According to Konijn and Hershko [39], the reduction in release of iron from the labile intracellular

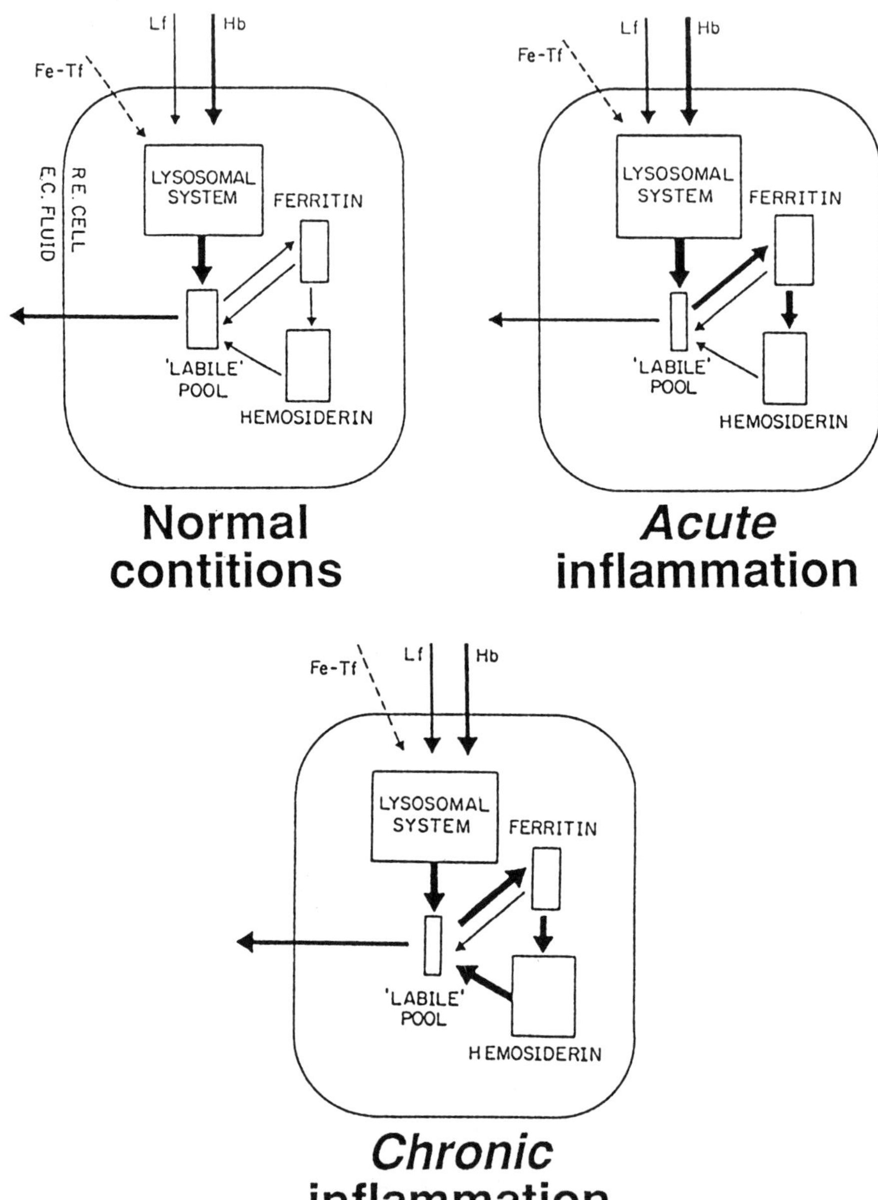

Fig. 1. Suggested scheme for iron turnover in reticuloendothelial cells. Hb, hemo-globin in red blood cells; R.E. cell, reticuloendothelial cell; E.C. fluid, extracellular fluid. [From Ref. 48 with permission.]

iron pool in inflammation and its increased partitioning into ferritin/hemosiderin stores (Fig. 2) can be explained by one or a combination of the following mechanisms:

1. Increased cellular uptake of iron, subsequent expansion of the labile iron pool, stimulating ferritin-synthesis and diversion of the incoming iron to the ferritin stores.
2. A primary membrane effect, blocking the release of cellular iron into the plasma, increasing the labile pool and stimulating ferritin synthesis.

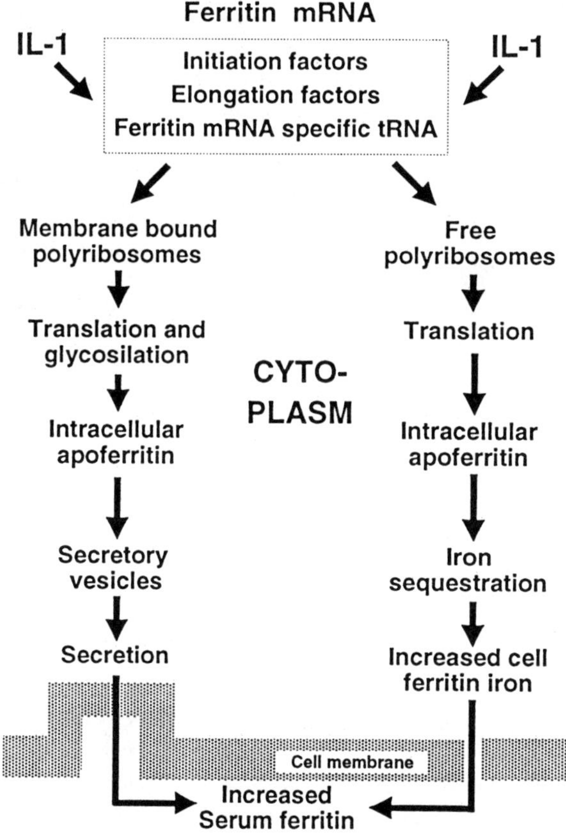

Fig. 2. Proposed scheme for the mechanism of posttranscriptional regulation of apoferritin synthesis in inflammation, the increased intracellular ferritin and serum ferritin, and the role of Il-1. [From Ref. 39 with permission.]

3. A primary enhancement of ferritin synthesis, resulting in the diversion of labile iron into ferritin stores and reducing the pool of iron available for immediate release.

Results of studies of the sequential changes in serum iron and hepatic ferritin synthesis in vivo as well as experiments with cell-free protein-synthesizing systems in vitro are in favor of a primary increased apoferritin synthesis rate, induced in inflammation by a direct stimulation by the inflammatory response, probably through Il-1, by analogy with other acute phase–reacting proteins [39].

Serum Ferritin

Inflammation and neoplasia are also associated with a significant rise in serum ferritin levels [6, 32, 36, 41]. The response of serum ferritin levels to inflammation was found to parallel the acute phase plasma proteins haptoglobin [6] and C-reactive protein [3], suggesting that serum ferritin in inflammation behaves as an acute-phase reactant rather than as an iron storage protein. The degree of rise in serum ferritin concentration is, however, influenced by the iron status of the patient [3].

Serum ferritin is probably a secretory protein since, in contrast to intracellular tissue ferritin, most of the circulating ferritin is glycosylated [19, 55], representing the minor fraction of intracellular ferritin synthesized on membrane-bound polyribosomes [57]. Since the ratio between glycosylated and non-glycosylated forms of ferritin in the serum during inflammation remains constant despite increased ferritin levels [8], it has been concluded that the observed increase in serum ferritin is not the result of a leakage from cells but more likely of increased synthesis and active cellular secretion [39]. The mechanism of induction of ferritin synthesis in inflammation may be different from that of induction by iron in normal unaffected cells, which is mainly on unaffected free polyribosomes [39].

The Role of Interleukin 1 in ACD

The similarity in the pattern of abnormalities in the hematological and acute phase response to inflammation in a variety of disease processes indicates a central role of endogenous mediators in this response. Among the candidates of recently described intracellular mediators, the monokine Il-1 is of particular interest. Il-1 induces fever, leukocytosis, acute phase protein synthesis, and hypoferremia, which together are typical features of acute or chronic infections and inflammatory diseases [29, 42]. Recombinant Il-1β also markedly suppresses colony formation of erythroid progenitor cells [42] and seems to be identical with the leukocyte endogenous mediator (LEM), described by Lee [40] 10 years ago as probably "the final common pathway" that connects the various diseases associated with ACD.

As mentioned earlier, decreased serum iron concentrations during inflammation can be attributed to increased apoferritin synthesis in the macrophage-monocyte system and parenchymal cells [39]. This newly synthesized apoferritin is responsible for the sequestration of iron in tissue [38, 39]. It can be assumed that the changes in iron metabolism mediated by Il-1 action are caused by the induction of apoferritin synthesis simultaneously with other acute phase reactants. The parallel changes in the concentrations of some acute phase reactants and ferritin in the plasma of patients with inflammatory diseases [3, 6] support this assumption. Konijn and Hershko [39] have proposed a scheme of events (Fig. 2) where the increase of apoferritin synthesis in the early phase of inflammation is caused by cell sap factors already present in the cell (elongation factors, ferritin mRNA and tRNA) which are augmenting both free and membrane-bound polyribosomal synthesis of apoferritin in macrophages and liver parenchymal cells. The late wave of increased apoferritin synthesis characterized by increased polysomal as well as cell sap activity may be caused by an Il-1–induced increase in the level of apoferritin mRNA or a derepression of untranslatable "repressed mRNA" according to observations of Zähringer et al. [56]. The increased apoferritin synthesis in addition to increased apolactoferrin secretion due to degranulation of polymorphonuclear leukocytes, caused by Il-1 or complement component C5a, may explain the changes of iron metabolism along the lines proposed by Roeser [48] (Fig. 1).

Preformed apoferritin will "trap" the iron, which enters the cell in the form of RBC-hemoglobin and as lactoferrin-iron, accelerating the diversin of the cellular iron by decreasing by the "labile cellular iron pool." Destabilizing effects of intracellular mediators of inflammation on the lysosomal membranes further cause enhanced formation of hemosiderin, making iron even less available for the labile pool. The overall effect is a reduction in iron availability for release into the plasma iron department and thus a limitation of the iron supply of erythropoiesis. The changes in intracellular iron exchange may also be responsible for the decrease of intestinal iron absorption observed in inflammatory stages. As already mentioned, Il-1 also affects erythropoiesis directly and may be largely responsible for the relative hypoproliferation of the erythropoiesis in ACD, as will be discussed in the last section.

Erythropoietin

Studies on serum erythropoietin (EPO) levels in patients with ACD have yielded conflicting results. Some investigators have shown a blunted EPO response compared to the degree of anemia [2, 33, 50], whereas others have found appropriate serum-EPO concentrations [10, 23]. In a small group of 11 patients with ACD due to inflammatory rheumatic diseases, we also have observed a rather blunted EPO response, relative to the degree of anemia, as compared to serum EPO levels in healthy volunteers undergoing regular phlebotomies [Fig. 3]. Takashina et al. [50] recently showed that serum EPO levels and Hb concentrations in anemic patients with RA and concomitant iron deficiency were significantly negatively correlated, whereas this was not the case in

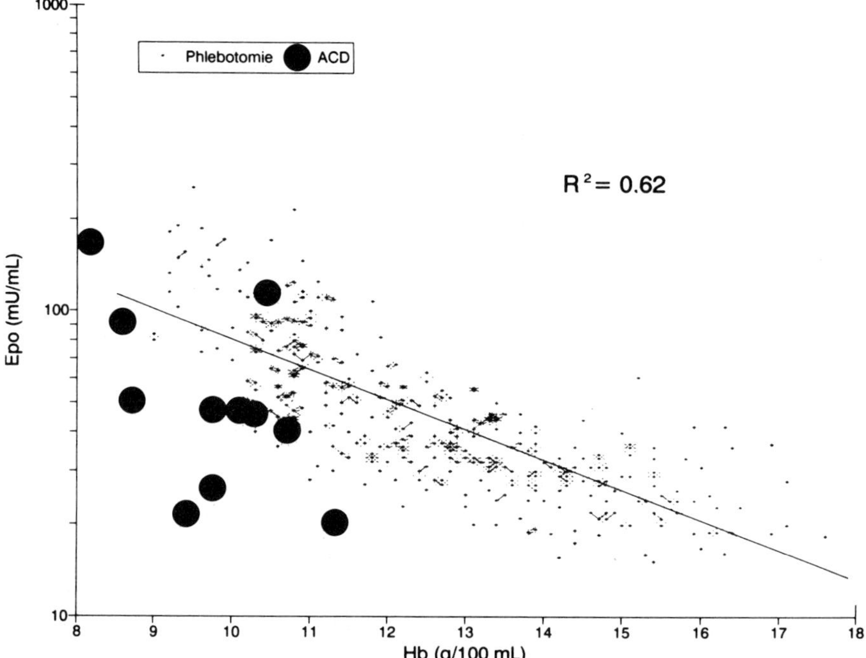

Fig. 3. Hemoglobin-to-serum erythropoietin concentration relationship in 356 erythropoietin determinations of 42 healthy male volunteers during the course of repeated phlebotomies (*), compared to the serum erythropoietin concentration of 11 patients with anemia of chronic disorders (●) due to rheumatoid arthritis (n = 8), systemic lupus erythematosus (n = 2), and mixed connective tissue disease (n = 1).

those with ACD but without iron deficiency (serum ferritin of 20 µg/l or more). The apparent contradiction led to various explanations:

1. EPO secreted in inflammatory diseases may have a normal immunoreactivity but a reduced bioactivity.
2. The marrow response to EPO in chronic disease may be impaired.
3. There may be an inhibitor of erythropoiesis in the serum of patients with chronic inflammatory or malignant diseases.

No data are presently available to confirm or reject the assumption of a reduced bioactivity of EPO in ACD [39]. Most studies addressing the marrow response to EPO in ACD were performed more than 10 years ago and yielded only weak and conflicting evidence for an impaired marrow response [39, 52]. There is, however, certain evidence that an inhibitor of erythropoiesis, derived from constituents of inflammatory tissue response, may be, at least in part, responsible for the inadaequate and hypoplastic marrow response in ACD.

Reid et al. [47] have shown that serum from anemic rheumatoid arthritis patients inhibits BFU-E growth in vitro. Acidic isoferritins secreted from T cells and/or macrophages in leukemia have been shown to inhibit erythropoiesis and colony formation of erythroid (BFU-E) progenitor cells [13, 14].

More recently, Schooley et al. [49] have shown that Il-1 inhibited the action of EPO in EPO-responsive erythroid precursers. Cloned murine as well as human Il-1 inhibited the proliferation response of erythroid precurser cells in culture as much as 17 h after EPO administration, suggesting that Il-1 does not affect binding of EPO to cell surface receptors. The authors have also demonstrated that the inhibitory effect of Il-1 can be overcome with increased concentrations of EPO. Of particular interest in this context is a recent observation by Kimball and Kerman [37] that EPO may also modulate the immune response by decreasing Il-1 production.

Treatment of ACD with Erythropoietin

Since erythropoietin has become available as a recombinant product in 1985, its use as a replacement agent in patients with impaired production due to renal failure has been very successful [24, 25, 54]. Recombinant erythropoietin may, however, also be a useful pharmacological agent in patients with normal but insufficient erythropoietin production, e.g., in patients with ACD. This expectation has proved correct in various preliminary clinical trials (Table 2). EPO doses of 300–600 IU/kg/week, given intravenously or subcutaneously, have been demonstrated to increase hemoglobin concentrations in the majority of

Table 2. Published data on the use of rhEPO in the treatment of ACD

Disease	No. of patients	EPO dose (IU/kgxw)	Route of administration	Duration (weeks)	Hb (g/dl)		Nonresponder	Ref.
					baseline	endpoint		
RA	2	300-450	i.v.	28	32/30%[a]	43/49%[a]	—	43
RA	6	4500-18,000 (total doses)	i.v.	2-11	8.0 ± 0.3[b]	9.2 ± 0.4	2	50
RA	7	250	s.c.	6	9.1 ± 0.95[b]	11.0 ± 0.1	2	11
RA, SLE, MCTD	8	300	s.c.	6	9.7 ± 0.45[b]	11.9 ± 0.7	1	35

[a]Hematocrit.
[b]Mean $\pm$ SEM.
RA, rheumatoid arthritis; SLE, systemic lupus erythematosus; MCTD, mixed connective tissue disease.

patients with ACD and chronic inflammatory diseases such as RA, SLE, or MCTD [11, 35, 43, 50].

In a study with 8 patients with ACD due to various inflammatory rheumatic diseases [35], we administered 150 IU/kg twice a week subcutaneously for 6 weeks. A mean Hb increase of 2.1 g/dl (Fig. 4) was achieved. Seven of 8

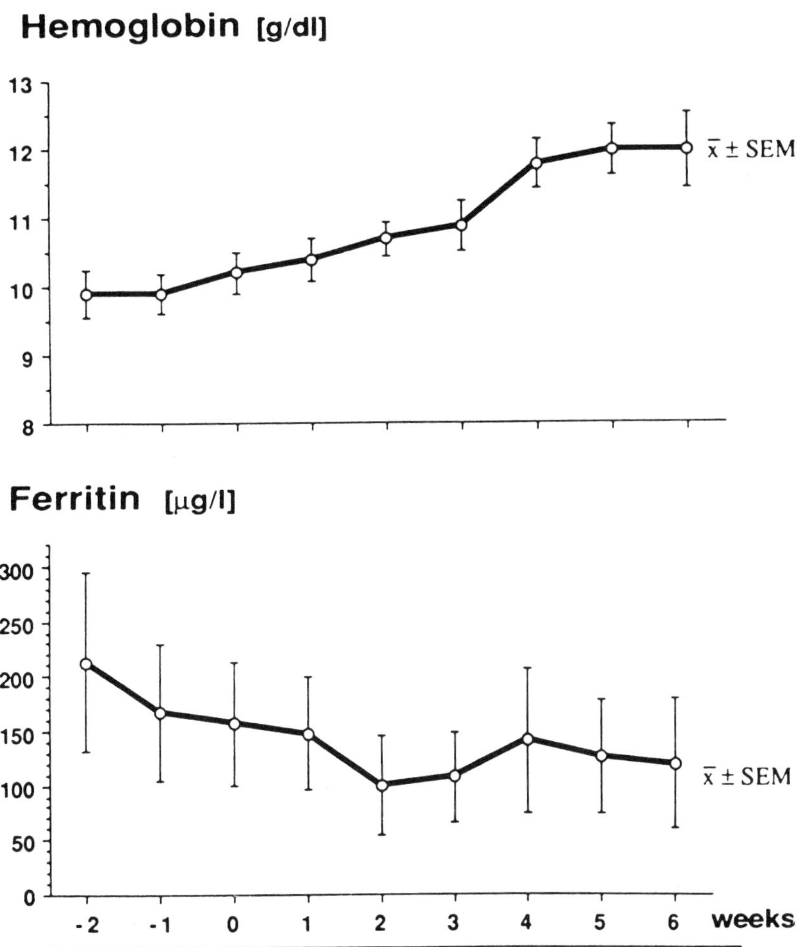

Fig. 4. Course of Hb and serum ferritin concentrations in 8 patients with ACD during subcutaneous application of recombinant erythropoietin in patients with anemia of chronic disorders due to inflammatory rheumatic diseases.

patients clearly responded to the administered EPO dose, whereas 1 patient failed to respond. Serum ferritin decreased during the 6 weeks of EPO treatment from 156 ± 57 µg/l to 120 ± 60 µg/l ($\overline{X}$ ± SEM) (Fig. 4). Reticulocytes also increased slightly from 1.7 ± 0.6% at baseline to 2.3 ± 0.8% after 5 weeks of EPO administration. There were no serious side effects, including increases in blood pressure and frequency of thrombotic events. Our findings are in accordance with those of other investigators, as shown in Table 2. As has been shown by Birgegard et al. [11], the duration of the Hb response to EPO is limited after cessation of treatment and may also be influenced by the course of the inflammatory activity of the underlying disease. The clinical evidence accumulated so far by pilot studies seems, however, to justify the conclusion that ACD responds to rhEPO in a considerable proportion of patients and may therefore be regarded as a new and meaningful therapeutic tool in the treatment of selected cases of ACD. Which patients with ACD require rhEPO and whether restoration of a normal Hb concentration also increases quality of life has, however, yet to be investigated.

Summary

The sequence of changes in iron metabolism occurring in inflammatory and neoplastic diseases is schematically summarized in Figure 5. It is evident that the alterations induced by inflammation in reticuloendothelial cellular metabolism

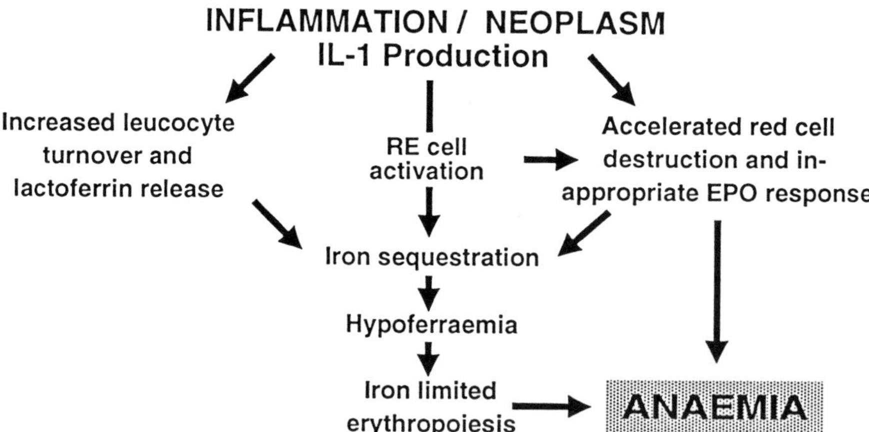

Fig. 5. Suggested sequence of changes affecting iron metabolism following an inflammatory or neoplastic stimulus. R.E. Cell, reticuloendothelial cell; Il-1, interleukin 1; EPO, erythropoietin. [From Ref. 48 with permission.]

and function occupy a central position in the pattern of aberrations of iron metabolism. Cell-derived, locally active mediators such as Il-1 probably play important roles in the induction and maintenance of the alterations of iron metabolism that finally cause a limited iron supply of the erythropoiesis, which together with a reduction in RBC survival and an inappropriate erythropoietin response is responsible for the development of anemia. It may be assumed that these changes are part of an adaptive response designed to enhance the organism's chance of survival during acute and chronic infections [48]. The essential "purpose" of the blockade of iron release and the resultant hypoferremia may be the deprivation of microorganisms in extracellular fluids from ready access to iron, which is an absolute requirement of their viability and proliferation. The viability changes included in the inflammatory response of an organism to infection and tissue injury therefore may be part of an important host defense mechanism where anemia is a minor side effect rather than a central pathological event.

References

1   Alvarez-Hernandez X, Felstein MV, Brock JH: The relation between iron release, ferritin synthesis and intracellular iron distribution in mouse peritoneal macrophages. Evidence for a reduced level of metabolically available iron in elicited macrophages. Biochem Biophys Acta 1986;886:214–222.
2   Baer AN, Dessypris N, Goldwasser E, Krantz SB: Blunted erythropoietin response to anaemia in rheumatoid arthritis. Br J. Haematol 1987;66:559–564.
3   Baynes R, Beswoda W, Bothwell TH, Khan Q, Mansoor N: The non-immune inflammatory response: Serial changes in plasma iron, iron-binding capacity, lactoferrin and C-reactive protein. Scand J Clin Lab Invest 1986;46:695–704.
4   Bennet RM: Haematological changes in rheumatoid arthritis. Clin Rheum Dis 1977;(3):433–465.
5   Beresford CH, Neale RJ, Brooks OG: Iron absorption and pyrexia. Lancet 1971;1:568–575.
6   Birgegard G, Hellgrän R, Killander A, Strömberg A, Venge P, Wide L: Serum ferritin during infection. Scand J Haematol 1978;21:333–340.
7   Birgegard G, Hällgren R, Venge P, Wide L: Serum ferritin during inflammation. A study on myocardial infarction. Acta Med Scand 1979;206:361–366.
8   Birgegard G: The source of serum ferritin during infection. Studies with concanavalin A-sepharose absorption. Clin Sci 1980;59:786–793.
9   Birgegard G, Caro J: Increased ferritin synthesis and iron uptake in inflammatory mouse macrophages. Scand J Haeamtol 1984;33:43–48.
10 Birgegard G, Hällgren R, Caro J: Serum erythropoietin in rheumatoid arthritis and other inflammatory arthritides: Relationship to anaemia and the effect of anti-inflammatory treatment. Br J Haematol 1987;65:479–483.

11 Birgegard G, Gudbjörnsson B, Hällgren R, Wide L: Anemia of chronic inflammatory arthritides: Treatment with recombinant human erythropoietin; in Gurland HJ et al. (eds): Erythropoietin in renal and non-renal anemias. Contribut Nephrol. Basel, Karger, 1991, vol 88, pp 295–303.

12 Boddy K, Will G: Iron absorption in rheumatoid arthritis. Ann Rheum Dis 1969;28:537–540.

13 Broxmeyer HE, Bognacki J, Dörner MH, de Sousa M: The identification of Leukemia-associated inhibitory activity (LIA) as acidic isoferritins in the production of granulocytes and macrophages. J Exp Med 1981;153:1426–1444.

14 Broxmeyer HE, Lu L, Bicknell DC, Williams DE, Cooper S, Levi S, Salfeld J, Arosio P: The influence of purified recombinant human heavy subunit and light subunit ferritins on colony formation in vitro by granulocyte-macrophage and erythroid progenitor cells. Blood 1986;68:1257–1263.

15 Cartwright GR: The anaemia of chronic disorders. Semin Hematol 1966;3:351–375.

16 Cavill J, Ricketts C, Naprer JAF: Erythropoiesis in the anaemia of chronic disease. Scand J Haematol 1977;19:509–512.

17 Cavill J, Bentley DP: Erythropoiesis in the anaemia of rheumatoid arthritis. Br J Haematol 1982;50:583–590.

18 Cortell S, Conrad ME: Effect of endotoxin on iron absorption. Am J Physiol 1978;213:43–47.

19 Cragg SJ, Wagstaff M, Worwood M: Sialic acid and the microheterogeneity of human serum ferritin. Clin Sci 1980;58:259–262.

20 Douglas SW, Adamson JW: The anaemia of chronic disorders. Studies of marrow regulation and iron metabolism.

21 Elin RJ, Wolff SM, Finch CA: Effect of induced fever on serum iron and ferritin concentration in man. Blood 1977;49:147–153.

22 Engstedt L, Strandberg O: Haematological data and clinical activity of rheumatoid disease. Acta Med Scand 1966;180:13–29.

23 Erslev AJ, Caro J, Miller O, Silver R: Plasma erythropoietin in health and disease. Ann Clin Lab Sci 1980;10:250–259.

24 Erslev AJ: Erythropoietin. N Engl J Med 1991;324:1339–1344.

25 Eschbach JW, Egrie JC, Downing MR, Browne JK, Adamson JW: Correction of the anemia of end-stage renal disease with recombinant human erythropietin: Results of a combined phase I and II clinical trial. N Engl J Med 1987;316:73–78.

26 Esparza J, Brock JH: Release of iron by resident and stimulated mouse peritoneal macrophages following ingestion and degradation of transferrin-antitransferrin immune complexes. Br J Haematol 1981;49:603–614.

27 Fillet G, Cook JD, Finch CA: Storage iron kinetics VII. A biological model for reticuloendothelial iron transport. J Clin Invest 1974;53:1527–1533.

28 Freireich EJ, Miller A, Emerson CP, Finch CA: Radioactive iron metabolism and erythrocyte survival. Studies of the mechanism of the anaemia associated with rheumatoid arthritis. J Clin Invest 1957;36:1043–1058.

29 Gordeuk VR, Prithviraj P, Dolinart T, Brittenham GM: Interleukin-1 administration in mice produces hypoferraemia despite neutropenia. J Clin Invest 1988;82:1934–1938.

30 Heinrich HC: Intestinal iron absorption in man; in Hallberg L, Harwerth HG,

Vannotti A (eds): Iron deficiency. Pathogenesis, clinical aspects, therapy. New York, Academic Press, 1970, pp 213–296.

31 Hershko C, Cook JD, Finch CA: Storage iron kinetics. VI. The effect of inflammation on iron exchange in the rat. Br J Haematol 1974;28:67–75.

32 Hershko C, Konijn AM: Serum ferritin in hematological disorders; in Albertini A, Arosio P, Chiancone E, Drysdale JW (eds): Ferritin and Isoferritins as Biological Markers. New York, Elsevier, 1984, pp 143–158.

33 Hochberg MC, Arnold CM, Hogans BB, Spivak JL: Serum immunoreactive erythropoietin in rheumatoid arthritis: Impaired response to anaemia. Arthritis Rheum 1988;31:1318–1321.

34 Ito M, Bognacki J, Broxmeyer H, de Sousa M, Hadden JW: Augmentation of human monocyte chemi-luminescence by iron-saturated lactoferin. Int J Immunpharmacol 1983;5:359–364.

35 Kaltwasser JP, Praeve F, Wigand R, Brune T: The use of recombinant human erythropoietin in the treatment of the anemia of chronic disorders; in Pagel, Weiss, Jelkmann (eds): Pathophysiology and Pharmacology of Erythropoietin. Berlin, Springer Verlag, 1992, p 271.

36 Kim HS, Kaltwasser JP, Roth P: Evaluation of serum ferritin in Leukaemia by two different assays. Tumor Diagn Ther 1984;5:166–170.

37 Kimball PM, Kerman RH: Erythropoietin: A potential immunomodulator? Transplant Proc 1991;23(1):336.

38 Konijn AM, Hershko C: Ferritin synthesis in inflammation I. Pathogenesis of impaired iron release. Br J Haematol 1977;37:7–16.

39 Konijn AM, Hershko C: The anaemia of inflammation and chronic disease; in de Sousa M, Brock JH (eds): Iron in Immunity, Cancer, and Inflammation. Wiley, 1989, pp 111–143.

40 Lee GR: The anaemia of chronic disease. Semin Hematol 1983;20:61–80.

41 Lipschitz DA, Cook JD, Finch CA: A clinical evaluation of serum ferritin. N Engl J Med 1974;290:1213–1216.

42 Maury CPJ: Anaemia in rheumatoid arthritis; role of cytokines. Scand J Rheumatol 1989;18:3–5.

43 Means RT, Olsen NJ, Krantz SB, Dessypris EN, Graber SE, Stone WJ, O'Neil VL, Pincus T: Treatment of the anemia of rheumatoid arthritis with recombinant human erythropoietin: Clinical and in vitro studies. Arthritis Rheum 1989;32:638–642.

44 Miller A, Chodos RB, Emerson CP, Ross JF: Studies of the anaemia and iron metabolism in cancer. J Clin Invest 1956;35:1248–1262.

45 Mowat AG: Connective tissue diseases. Clin Haematol 1972;1(1):573–594.

46 Noyes WD, Bothwell TH, Finch CA: The role of the reticuloendothelial cell in iron metabolism. Br J Haematol 1960;6:43–55.

47 Reid CDL, Prouse PJ, Baptista LC, Gumple JM, Chanarin J: The mechanism of the anaemia in rheumatoid arthritis: effects of bone marrow adherent cells and of serum on in vitro erythropoiesis. Br J Haematol 1984;58:607–615.

48 Roeser HP: Iron metabolism in inflammation and malignant diseases; in Jacobs A, Worwood M (eds): Iron in Biochemistry and Medicine II. New York, Academic Press, 1980, pp 605–640.

49 Schooley, JC, Kullgren B, Allison AC: Inhibition by interleukin-1 of the action of

erythropoietin in erythroid precursors and its possible role in the pathogenesis of hypoplastic anaemias. Br J Haematol 1987;67:11–17.

50 Takashina N, Kondo H, Kashiwazki S: Suppressed serum erythropoietin response to anemia and the efficacy of recombinant erythropoietin in the anemia of rheumatoid arthritis. J Rheumatol 1990;17:885–887.

51 Van Snick JL, Masson PL, Heremans JF: The involvement of lactoferrin in the hypersiderinaemia of acute inflammation. J Exp Med 1974;140:1068–1084.

52 Wallner SF: The anaemia of chronic disorders: Clinical and pathological features; in Dunn CDR (ed): Current Concepts in Erythropoiesis. Chichester, Wiley, 1983, pp 209–231.

53 Weiss DK, Krehbiel JD, Lund JE: Studies on the pathogenesis of anaemia of inflammation: Mechanism of impaired erythropoiesis. Am J Vet Res 1983;44:1832–1835.

54 Winearls CG, Oliver DO, Pippard MJ, Reid C, Downing MR, Cotes PM: Effect of human erythropoietin derived from recombinant DNA on the anaemia of patients maintained by chronic haemodialysis. Lancet 1986;2:1175–1178.

55 Worwood M: Serum ferritin. CRC Crit Rev Clin Lab Sci 1979;10:171–204.

56 Zähringer J, Baliga BS, Munro HN: Novel mechanisms for translational control in regulation of ferritin synthesis by iron. Proc Natl Acad Sci USA 1976;857–861.

57 Zähringer J, Baliga BS, Drake RL, Munro HN: Distribution of ferritin mRNA and albumin between free and membrane bound rat liver polysomes. Biochem Biophys Acta 1977;474:234–244.

Joachim Peter Kaltwasser, Rheumatology Unit, Department of Haematology, Center of Internal Medicine, Johann Wolfgang Goethe-University, 60596 Frankfurt a. Main, Germany

Discussion

to the paper by J. P. Kaltwasser

Krantz (*Nashville*): Commenting on Dr. Kaltwasser's talk I would like to illustrate with three slides. As you have said, interleukin-1 levels are elevated in the anemia of rheumatoid arthritis and elevation is directly proportional to the severity of the anemia. So we added interleukin-1 to normal human marrow cells, which is shown [in Figure 1] by the bottom line, and you see there is an inhibition of human CFU-E development. However, we have learned to purify human CFU-E, and when we add interleukin-1 to the purified CFU-E shown on the top line there is no inhibition. Now, to make a long story short, it appears that there is an accessory cell active here, and we have been able to show that the accessory cell is a T cell and that interleukin-1 acts on the T cells to produce gamma-interferon. It is gamma-interferon that depresses CFU-E development.

[Figure 2] shows you that human gamma-interferon directly depresses purified human CFU-E development in a dose-dependent fashion. Now, Dr. Fuchs in Austria has reported that gamma-interferon levels are elevated in the anemia of AIDS in direct proportion to the severity of the anemia, and just a few weeks ago Dr. Ludwig, doing studies on multiple myeloma, announced at the International Society of Hematology meeting in London that gamma-interferon levels were directly elevated in proportion to the anemia in multiple myeloma. Now [Figure 3]: In the top line you see that if you add erythropoietin to normal human purified CFU-E you can add 1, 2, 4, 8, or 16 units of erythropoietin per milliliter and you never get more response than you get with 1 unit per milliliter. That has been shown for a couple of decades, because you are pretty much saturating all the erythropoietin receptors. However, if you add human gamma-interferon at 100 units per milliliter, shown in the dark line on the bottom, you inhibit CFU-E development down to 60%, and now you can overcome that inhibition with large amounts of erythropoietin up to 16 to 32 units per milliliter to get up to a normal CFU-E level.

Furthermore, if you add more gamma-interferon (1000 units per milliliter) it takes more erythropoietin, so you must add 60 units per milliliter of erythropoietin to overcome the inhibition. So, what I am suggesting is that it is really gamma-interferon that is the direct inhibitor of CFU-E in the anemia of chronic disease, and in vitro we can replicate what we have seen in vivo with human beings.

Kaltwasser: Thank you very much for this comment. I think this is more or less in accordance what I would also like to say. It is difficult now to answer how many of the short-term regulators are involved in this process, and if all the different diseases are following the same pattern or not. But there are also in vitro data—from Schooley and co-

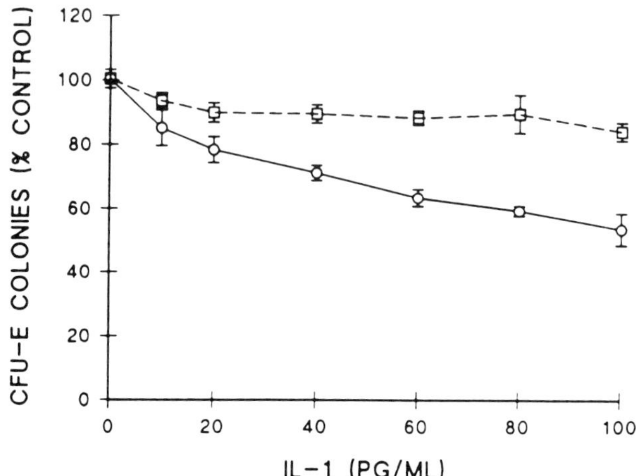

Fig. 1.   Effect of rhIL-1 on CFU-E colony formation by blood BFU-E derived CFU-E and marrow CFU-E. Growth of highly purified CFU-E colonies from three experiments (44.4 ± 32.4% CFU-E) (□) and marrow CFU-E colonies from three experiments (0.36 ± 0.09% CFU-E) (○). Data from each experiment were normalized to CFU-E colony growth without rhIL-1. Results are expressed as mean ± SE.

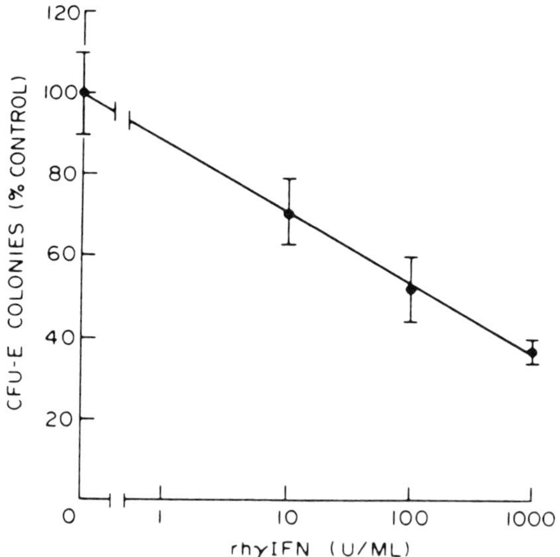

Fig. 2.   Effect of rhγIFN on highly purified CFU-E colony formation. Results of three experiments with CFU-E purity 24.0 ± 3.7% are combined. Data from each experiment were normalized to CFU-E colony growth without rhγIFN. Results are expressed as mean ± SE.

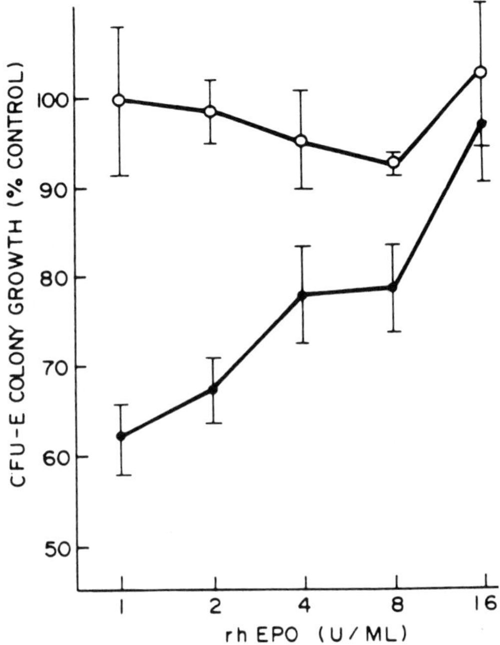

Fig. 3. Effect of varying EPO concentrations on inhibition of highly purified CFU-E colony formation by rhγIFN 100 U/ml. (●) CFU-E colony formation in the presence of γIFN. (○) CFU-E colony formation without γIFN. CFU-E purity in three experiments was 29.2% ± 1.3% (58 ± 3 colonies/clot). Results are expressed as mean ± SE. 100% of control growth is defined as CFU-E colony formation at rhEPO 1 U/ml.

workers, for example, who have shown that recombinant interleukin-1, at least in CFU-E cell cultures, is inhibitory, and they have also shown that this inhibitory effect of IL-1 can be overcome by addition of erythropoietin in the same way you described it here.

Krantz (Nashville): We must understand that interleukin-1 does not act directly on CFU-E.

Kaltwasser: I do not remember Schooley's experimental setting in detail at the moment. Maybe their CFU-E cultures also contained T cells.

Fandrey (Bonn): I would just like to add some in vitro data regarding your observation that you have a blunted erythropoietin response in ACD patients. We performed studies with hepatoma cells that produce erythropoietin and could show that Il-1-alpha and beta and TNF dose dependently inhibit erythropoietin production. In collaboration with Horst Pagel, using the isolated perfused rat kidney, we could confirm these results in the kidney. Direct effects on erythropoiesis have to be considered, but at least these cytokines seem to suppress erythropoietin production in vitro and ex vivo powerfully.

Shaldon (Nimes): I think if one were looking for a logical therapy of chronic diseases associated with anemia, I would look for an antagonist to the cytokine that neutralizes the postulated cause of the anemia rather than just trying to treat the anemia pharmacologically. I think results of phase II studies in the U.S. on interleukin-1 receptor antagonist and soluble TNF receptor in rheumatoid arthritis will answer the question.

Kaltwasser: Thank you for this suggestion. I have another slide prepared which I have not shown, where I have raised this point under the heading of future aspects of the treatment of the anemia of chronic disorders.

Cavill (Cardiff): Could I add that the points made in the last three elegant slides showing the effect of gamma-interferon support the thrust of the kinetic studies which we have carried out. These indicate that the effect of rheumatoid arthritis and other chronic inflammatory diseases is one which is directely effective on the erythroid proliferation and that inhibition or blockage of iron release from the RES cells is a side issue. It is the direct suppressive effect on erythroid proliferation that is the important feature of this disease.

Iron Supplementation of Hemodialysis Patients Receiving Recombinant Human Erythropoietin Therapy

C. Granolleras, R. Oulès, B. Branger, J. Fourcade, S. Shaldon
Department of Nephrology, University Hospital, Nîmes, France

During the first decade of long-term hemodialysis (HD) therapy, it was traditional to transfuse patients to maintain a minimum hematocrit of at least 17 vol%. This resulted in the vast majority of patients receiving regular blood transfusions. During this period, iron deficiency was not a problem. Many patients had transfusional hemosiderosis and associated hepato-splenomegaly.

However, with the demonstration that if blood transfusions were withheld the patient hematocrit fell and then began to rise spontaneously, the problem of the assessment of the iron status of the patient became critical, as functional or total iron deficiency often prevented a successful no-transfusional policy. In 1966 it was demonstrated that the elimination of routine transfusions was possible in 17 patients on long-term hemodialysis who had previously been receiving regular blood transfusions at least monthly for up to 4 years. This cessation of transfusions associated with regular blood loss from the dialysis procedure, laboratory blood examinations, and occult bleeding from the gut due to heparinization during hemodialysis resulted in overt iron deficiency, which was correctable by the administration of i.v. iron. The mean hematocrit fell from 20 to 18 vol% after stopping transfusions and then rose to 26 vol% when i.v. iron was given [1]. The benefit of giving i.v. iron to HD patients on a no-transfusion regime was confirmed at Nîmes. We were able to maintain a mean hematocrit of 24–25% between 1988 and 1992 in a population that did not receive erythropoietin or blood transfusions, but who were treated with 1.5 g of i.v. iron per year (Fig. 1).

A recent literature survey [2] has estimated that blood loss in hemodialysis patients varied between 1 and 7 l of blood per year. Therefore, the need to

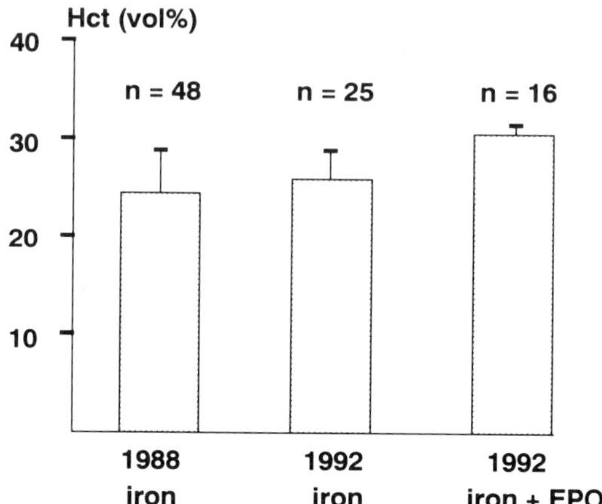

Fig. 1. Data from the study of unselected patients at the Nîmes dialysis center. In 1988, 48 patients received no transfusions or rhEPO but received regular i.v. iron administration of 1–2 g/y as 100 mg per dialysis for up to 10 consecutive dialyses. The mean predialysis Hct was 24 ± 6.5 vol%. In 1992, in 25 patients still on the same regime, Hct was 25.8 ± 4.7 vol%, while a population of rhEPO-treated patients (n = 16) also receiving i.v. iron had a mean Hct of 30.1 ± 2.7 vol%. (Mean ± SD.)

estimate the iron status of hemodialysis patients is crucial if rhEPO therapy is to be effective.

Iron Status in Hemodialysis Patients

Before 1975, iron status was evaluated by measurement of the serum iron concentration and percentage saturation of the plasma iron-binding protein, transferrin. Subsequently, a correlation was established between serum ferritin concentration and so-called indices of iron body stores derived from estimating the iron content of marrow and liver biopsies [3–6]. Other markers for whole body iron status had also been described, such as erythrocyte protoporphyrin and mean red cell corpuscular volume (MCV). However, the specific problem of iron status in the hemodialysis patient was rarely addressed. In 1983, based upon 39 HD patients, including 21 who received regular transfusions, it was concluded from measurement of bone marrow hemosiderin content (as a measure of total iron stores) that serum ferritin was useful in identifying subjects with both increased or reduced iron stores. In contrast, transferrin saturation could only be used for identifying iron overload, MCV for indicating iron deficiency, and erythrocyte protoporphyrin was not useful in either instance [7].

With the initial introduction of rhEPO, a serum ferritin concentration of less than 100 µg/l was suggested as the definitive marker for iron deficiency and hence for iron replacement therapy in HD patients [8]. This was probably an underestimation of effective iron deficiency in HD patients and may have resulted in part in prescription of excessive quantities of rhEPO in order to obtain the target hematocrit.

The reevaluation of iron status in HD patients treated with rhEPO became necessary as the absence of transfusion and the continued variable and largely unestimated loss of several liters of blood per year posed a problem. The problem was how and when to treat patients with iron-replacement therapy.

McDougall et al. in 1989 [9] suggested that erythropoietin could stimulate erythropoiesis to such an extent that the demand for iron could exceed the body's ability to release it from stores. Thus a functional iron deficiency could occur, even when serum ferritin concentrations were normal and iron could be detected in the marrow by staining. He based this observation on 5 patients whose anemia did not respond to oral iron therapy while on i.v. rhEPO. The serum ferritin levels were normal, but the transferrin saturation was less than 20% in all cases. When i.v. iron was given, the anemia improved and the transferrin saturation rose to 24–40%. He concluded that the transferrin saturation of less than 20% was a better indicator of functional iron deficiency than the serum ferritin concentration and implied that the best treatment was i.v. iron rather than oral iron therapy.

With the universal expansion of rhEPO therapy for the rapid correction of anemia in hemodialysis patients, the need to resolve the controversy about the best marker for iron deficiency in the HD patient and the best method for replacing the iron became heightened. Van Wyck et al. [10] proposed a mathematical evaluation of iron stores and needs derived from serum ferritin, serum iron, and transferrin saturation measurements as well as the increment in serum iron following desferoxamine challenge in 27 HD patients prior to receiving rhEPO. They concluded that for replacement of iron by oral therapy: (a) 1 µg/l of serum ferritin corresponds to 10 mg of iron stores (data derived from phlebotomies) and (b) to increase the Hb by 1 g/100 ml one needs 150 mg of iron.

Other methods of evaluating functional iron deficiency have included measurement of circulating transferrin receptors [11]. It has also been suggested that erythrocyte ferritin concentrations were higher in HD patients than in normal subjects with comparable serum ferritin levels, suggesting that erythrocyte ferritin could reflect the reduced utilization of iron by the bone marrow and so the real iron deficiency [12].

Most recently it has been suggested that if more than 2.5% of erythrocytes are judged to be hypochromic by a Technicon H1 automated blood count analyzer in a dialysis patient receiving erythropoietin therapy, a state of functional iron deficiency exists. The latter is correctable with improvement in hematocrit by giving i.v. iron [13].

Thus, it is clear that there is controversy as to the most reliable indicator of the iron status of HD patients receiving rhEPO therapy. In an attempt to arrive at a empirical answer to this problem, we have conducted a multicenter study of 18 HD patients on rhEPO therapy [14].

Material and Methods

Patients:

Eighteen HD patients (dialyzed $3 \times$ week), 8 males, 10 females, mean age 47 years (range 24–67) were studied. They were stable on maintenance subcutaneous rhEPO 3 or 7 times per week with a constant rhEPO dose and a constant Hct of about 30–35 vol% for at least 4 months after attaining their target hematocrit by correction of their anemia with rhEPO.

Study Protocol:

The study compared the hematocrit response and the rhEPO dose in these 18 patients in two phases:

Phase 1: Patients received i.v. iron 1 g (10×100 mg) if the transferrin saturation was under 20% or the serum ferritin concentration was under 100 μg/l.

Phase 2: Patients received 10 mg of i.v. iron per dialysis (1.5 g/y) independently of transferrin saturation or the serum ferritin level unless the transferrin saturation was over 50% or the serum ferritin level exceeded 1000 μg/l.

The study was performed with lyophilized rhEPO (Boehringer Mannheim). 10 mg of iron dextran were given i.v. during the dialysis treatment. The iron was added to 20–40 ml of normal NaCl used to administer heparin continuously by syringe pump. Hematocrit was measured weekly; serum iron, serum ferritin, and tranferrin saturation were measured monthly.

Results

Control values established during phase 1 showed a mean hematocrit of 29 $\pm$ 2.5 vol% and a median rhEPO dose of 66 U/kg/week (Table 1). When the patients received 10 mg of i.v. iron per dialysis, the mean hematocrit rose to 31 $\pm$ 2.1 vol% ($p < 0.05$), and the median rhEPO dose was reduced to 46 U/kg/week ($p < 0.05$). The serum ferritin concentration rose from 321 $\pm$ 246 to 654 $\pm$ 380 ng/ml (NS) and the transferrin saturation from 31 $\pm$ 10.4 to 33 $\pm$ 4.0% (NS).

Table 1. Effect of continuous iron administration on hematocrit, rhEPO dose, serum ferritin, and transferrin saturation

	Transferrin saturation < 20%	4 months after 10 mg iron per dialysis
Mean Hct (vol%)*	29 ± 2.5	31 ± 2.1
Median EPO dose (u/kg/week)*	66	46
Mean ferritin (ng/ml)	321 ± 246	654 ± 380
Mean TS (%)	31 ± 10.4	33 ± 4

*p < 0.05.

Discussion

At least 8 different markers have been proposed for evaluating the iron stores of ESRD patients. No one of these markers is completely satisfying. Our study shows that in spite of normal ferritin and transferrin saturation levels, the administration of continuous iron therapy is able to increase erythropoiesis on rhEPO therapy, allowing a reduction in the rhEPO requirements of about 25%. The estimated iron loss in HD patients is at least 1.5 g/y; the replacement of this loss by 10 mg of iron with each dialysis might eliminate the possibility of iron deficiency.

The adequacy of iron replacement therapy in relationship to a variable and largely unknown or at least unmeasured iron loss in the long-term patient on hemodialysis poses a problem. How does one avoid iron overload, which is an ever-present risk? However, the improvement in quality of life with correction of anemia and the economic benefits from reducing the rhEPO dose must also be considered. In our population, the serum ferritin level increased moderately during one year of continuous iron treatment.

The oral administration of iron has also been shown to be efficient, and HD patients behave as normals in not absorbing more than the body needs [15]. This solution would be ideal if the very poor HD patient compliance to the taking of oral iron could be improved.

Conclusion

The absence of a reliable marker of iron deficiency in HD patients and the knowledge that the minimum iron loss is at least 1.5 g/y allows a correction of this iron loss by empirical administration of i.v. iron in the amount of 10 mg per dialysis. However, the oral route of administration is probably preferable if the patient is compliant.

References

1 Shaldon S: Chronic dialysis without transfusion. Lancet 1967;1:783–784.
2 Muller-Wiefel DE, Scigalla P: Specific problems of renal anemia in childhood. Contrib Nephrol 1988;66:71–84.
3 Jacobs A, Path FRC, Worwood M: Ferritin in serum: Clinical and biological implications. Med Prog 1975;292:951–956.
4 Mirhamadi KS, Wellington MP, Winer RL, Dabir-Vaziri N, Byer B, Gorman JT, Rosen SM: Serum ferritin level. Determinant of iron requirement in hemodialysis patients. JAMA 1977;238:601–608.
5 Esbach JW, Cook JD, Scribner BH, Finch CA: Iron balance in hemodialysis patients. Ann Intern Med 1977;87:710–719.
6 Aljama P, Ward MK, Pierides M, Eastham EJ, Ellis HA, Feest TG, Conceiado S, Kerr DNS: Serum ferritin concentration: A reliable guide to iron overload in uremic and hemodialyzed patients. Clin Nephrol 1978;10:101–104.
7 Moreb J, Popovtzer MM, Friedlander MM, Konijn AM, Hershko C: Evaluation of iron status in patients on chronic hemodialysis: Relative usefulness of bone marrow hemosiderin, serum ferritin, transferrin saturation, mean corpuscular volume and red cell protoporphyrin. Nephron 1983;35:196–200.
8 Eschbach JW, Egrie JC, Downing MR, Browne JK, Adamson JW: The safety of epoitin-alpha: Results of clinical trials in the United States. Contrib Nephrol 1991;88:72–80.
9 McDougall IC, Hutton RD, Cavill I, Coles GA, Williams JD: Poor response to treatment of renal anaemia with erythropoietin corrected by iron given intravenously. Br Med J 1989;299:157–158.
10 Van Wyck DB, Stivelman JC, Ruiz J, Kirlin LF, Katz MA, Ogden DA: Iron status in patients receiving erythropoietin for dialysis associated anemia. Kidney Int 1989;35:712–716.
11 Skikne B, Flowers CH, Cook JD: Derum transferrin receptor: A quantitative measure of tissue iron deficiency. Blood 1990;75:1870–1876.
12 Brunati C, Poperno A, Guastoni C, Perrino ML, Civati G, Teatini U, Perego A, Fiorelli G, Minetti L: Erythrocyte ferritin in patients on chronic hemodialysis treatment. Nephron 1990;54:219–223.
13 McDougall IC, Cavill I, Hulme B, Bain B, McGregor E, McKay P, Sanders E, Coles GA, Williams JD: Detection of functional iron deficiency during erythropoietin treatment: A new approach. Br Med J 1992;304:225–226.
14 Granolleras C, Oulès R, Shaldon S, Pollock M, Baldamus CA, Nonnast-Daniel B, Koch KM: (abstract) Nephrol Dial Transplant 1991;6:824.
15 Gokal R, Millard PR, Weatherall DJ, Callender STE, Ledingham JGG, Oliver DO: Iron metabolism in haemodialysis patients. Quart J Med 1979;191:369–391.

S. Shaldon, 86 Rue de Grezac, Montpellier 34080, France

Discussion

to the paper by C. Granolleras et al.

Winearls (Oxford): Was this a crossover study?

Granolleras: This was a crossover study. They started three times a week, then seven times a week and three times a week again, or seven times, three times, seven times. It was a crossover study in the different phases. But I just showed the pooled data on the patients when they were on three times a week and then on seven times a week.

Winearls: What was the period of time they were on each phase?

Granolleras: At least 12 weeks.

Joven (Reus): Can you comment on the side effects of the iron replacement, if any, and why this route of administration?

Granolleras: The iron was administered with continuous heparin. That is the way we [have been] administering iron for 15 years, and we have never had any adverse reaction with this way of administration.

Breymann (Zurich): Instead of giving iron continuously, why don't you normalize transferrin saturation and ferritin values and then start treatment? And then you check the values and then start again to give high amounts of parenteral iron. Do you think that is a good approach?

Granolleras: I don't think so, because if you have looked at the table and the results, when we started intravenous iron continuously, our ferritin levels were normal, about 300 micrograms per liter, and our transferrin saturation was normal—and in spite of this normal transferrin saturation and ferritin levels we increased the hematocrit and we reduced the erythropoietin dose. That means that the transferrin saturation is not a good indicator; that means that the ferritin is not a good indicator.

Winearls: What formulation of iron are you using? In the U.K. and in the U.S. one formulation of iron dextran has been withdrawn by the manufacturer.

Granolleras: Iron dextran.

Breymann: I think the solution is to take iron saccharate. We treat women with postpartum anemia with saccharated iron, not dextran iron. And we did not see any side effects or anaphylactic reactions and we treated about 200 patients and we only used saccharated iron; you can use it even in higher concentrations without any problems. So not iron dextran: saccharate.

Wardrop (Cardiff): Surely, in long-term management with EPO, when the patient is stabilized, there should be no need for repeated injections of iron because the patient perhaps will be in neither negative nor positive iron balance; or do they have major chronic losses of iron in long-term management?

Granolleras: In a recent survey of the literature published in *Contributions to Nephrology* 2 years ago, some authors estimated the blood loss to more than 1.5 liters and [up to] 6 liters per year, so you have to correct the 6 liters per year.

Kokot (*Katowice*): You mentioned that there is no reliable marker of functional iron deficiency. What is your recommendation for the practitioner in patients who are treated with erythropoietin? Should we supplement every patient on EPO therapy or should we not?

Granolleras: I think that we have to supplement everybody, but what I did not tell is that of course we stop the intravenous iron if the ferritin was over 1000 nanograms per milliliter and if the transferrin saturation was over 50%.

Adamson (*New York*): I think we may be confusing two issues here: there is the use of ferritin values and the serum iron and total iron binding capacity to indicate true iron deficiency and the status of total body iron stores. What has been revealed through a variety of studies is that with the advent of recombinant human erythropoietin therapy and the concern that we have enough iron to sustain hemoglobin synthesis, we are finding some effects that frankly were not anticipated. That is, in a variety of studies, aggressive iron supplementation appears to provide a more effective response to the exogenous erythropoietin. And so I think that the parameters that were worked out in the past for diagnosing iron deficiency anemia are not the parameters to be applied to the clinical observation that iron supplementation appears to enhance the response to a given dose of erythropoietin.

Granolleras: I agree completely.

Shaldon (*Nîmes*): I would like to make one comment to Dr. Adamson. In his study with Dr. Eschbach of a dialysis patient who required Imferon, if I recollect correctly your data, you suggested that although this patient had total body scores in excess, the availability of that iron was in some way inadequate to respond rapidly enough to the erythropoiesis created with the erythropoietin, and therefore you gave the iron parenterally. Now my question is: is that implying that there is some form of block between—in certain uremic patients—in mobilizing their iron stores as rapidly as in normals?

Adamson: No, I don't wish to imply that the renal failure patient mobilizes iron less well than a normal individual, but I think you can create a state of relative iron deficiency depending upon the responsiveness of the marrow to a given dose of erythropoietin. I think it is more common with higher doses. You know in our early studies we went up as high as 1500 International Units per kilogram three times a week in looking at response parameters, and relative iron deficiency was the rule. The individual that you referred to had a transferrin saturation of 13%, which I think all of us would agree is probably an inadequate amount of readily available iron. But the phenomenon is not confined to renal failure patients. Mercuriali, in studies of autologous blood donors at his orthopedic hospital in Milan, has demonstrated clearly that aggressive parenteral iron supplementation along with phlebotomies resulted in an increase in the number of units of red cells that could be predeposited by his control patients. I think what we are seeing is a rather unexpected but very real phenomenon in several clinical conditions.

Nephrology

At which PCV, hemoglobin, or hematocrit should rhEPO therapy be started in patients with the anemia of chronic renal failure?

Eschbach (Seattle): In my opinion, it should be when the patient is symptomatic of anemia, which usually is when the hematocrit decreases to below 30, or a patient has angina, or is requiring red cell transfusions.

Shaldon (Nîmes): I think that is a very desirable statement. I fully endorse it. However, in certain European countries the recommendations are different. Patients start EPO therapy when their hemoglobin is 8 grams per 100 milliliter. The target hemoglobin is usually 10–12 grams per 100 milliliter. Patients who fall between the start value and the target do not receive EPO.

Eschbach (Seattle): Who made that decision?

Shaldon (Nîmes): The government, with the advice of the medical profession.

Winearls (Oxford): What is the rationale to chose a target hematocrit of 30 instead of 28 or 32?

Eschbach (Seattle): In my experience of taking care of patients with the anemia in progressive renal failure, most patients adapt to their anemia fairly well until the hematocrit gets to 30 or below. Some patients cannot tell any difference when the hematocrit gets down below 30, but then when their hematocrit increases from EPO up to 35 and 38 they are aware of how much better they feel. I think that it is reasonable to choose a hematocrit of 30, or perhaps even higher, as the point of beginning EPO therapy.

Winearls (Oxford): There is a firm belief among some nephrologists in the U.K. that patients cannot tell the difference between a hematocrit of 30 and 35 so there is no purpose in starting treatment if the hematocrit is greater than 30.

Second, there is the view that unacceptable side effects of EPO are common when the hematocrit is greater than 35. Until these prejudices can be countered by data contradicting them, many patients will be treated to a hematocrit which still leaves them with the effects of anemia. Finally, there is also the subtle pressure to avoid using EPO for financial reasons.

Shaldon (Nîmes): Yes, I totally agree with you; I think it is a cost-effective deal between the medical profession and the governments. When you set up a medial paradigm it takes at least 5 years to establish it. How long do you think it will be before you can educate your colleagues to change their minds?

Winearls (Oxford): My colleagues will change their minds when they see convincing data demonstrating the safety and benefit of a target hematocrit of greater than 35.

Eschbach (Seattle): We will try to address part of your question at the end of our session when we talk about the target hematocrit.

Joven (Reus): I do not agree that we need any number to begin treatment with EPO, or indicate transfusions; as it happens among people engaged in transfusion medicine, what we need is a thorough assessment of the clinical background. Therefore, this question is probably not well stated and what we need is a clear indication for the use of EPO. For instance, in Spain there are at least half of the patients on EPO while there are regional variations (in Cataluña, less than 30%) with similar patients. How about your countries?

Shaldon (Nîmes): Very briefly, I would like to say that there is clearly no association with mortality that has yet been proven in this issue, but I think in terms of quality of life based by standard questionnaires or objectively with oxygen consumption, there is no question that you are correcting a pathological state, and the better your correct it—if you have no adverse tradeoff—the fitter the patient. The concept of ''positive health'' is only recognized after you have corrected the anemia. The adaptation to sickness by a defense mechanism employed by the patient with chronic disease is well known. I do not think you are right at all in your attitude towards the use of EPO; you have an anemia and the question is how well you should correct the anemia without harming the patient by side effects.

Erslev (Philadelphia): For years I tried unsuccessfully to talk my fellows into undergoing some phlebotomies so we could find out how normal people would respond. However, Frank Bunn has been more successful in Boston. He reports that when healthy young men are chronically bled down to a level of about 32 to 34 they became very symptomatic. They had no idea that life would be gray and depressing at a hematocrit which they had thought was pretty adequate in patients.

What is the indication for treatment of patients with preterminal renal insufficiency—benefits and risks?

Eschbach (Seattle): We have conducted clinical trials in the U.S. with the anemia of progressive chronic renal failure, and a number of you have been involved in these trials as well. Therapy was initiated when the hematocrit decreases to 30. Clearly there is a better quality of life for the patients and they can continue to work. Interestingly, some of the symptoms that we used to consider as uremia disappear when the hematocrit is increased to 35 to 40, and these patients are able to continue working until they require dialysis therapy. In fact, some patients are not symptomatic from uremia and it may be difficult to convince them to start dialysis. I think the risk of EPO is very minimal. There is no increased rate of deterioration in renal function, as was suspected from animal experiments, which has now been observed in many studies. The goal should be to prevent the complications of this anemia. We should treat these patients with EPO so their red cell mass is optimal so that we can keep them rehabilitated once dialysis begins.

Shaldon (Nîmes): Joe, I think you are covering up a major problem here—it is going to recur later on as well—tell me, in these patients do you have to use more antihypertensive drugs or ever initiate antihypertensive therapy?

Eschbach (Seattle): The incidence of increasing blood pressure following EPO therapy is similar to that observed in the hemodialysis population. Usually it is not difficult to control the blood pressure, if it increases, with medication.

Shaldon (Nîmes): That was not my question. I asked you: do you have to use more antihypertensive medication or initiate drug therapy in this population when you are treating their anemia before they enter dialysis therapy?

Eschbach (Seattle): The problem is that there were not enough controls to answer that question. As renal failure progresses, the need for more antihypertensive medication increases regardless of whether the patients are anemic or not.

Wideroe (Trondheim): Before you are starting, I think you have to take proper care of the metabolic disorders related to advanced renal failure as phosphate accumulation and acidosis by adequate dialysis dose and controlled nutrition.

Eschbach (Seattle): I agree entirely. Prior to beginning EPO therapy, iron deficiency should be excluded as well as other factors that are contributing to the anemia; the blood pressure should be controlled; and the patient metabolically stabilized. Sorry, I did not make that clear. Your point is quite correct.

Shaldon (Nîmes): I would like to come back, though, if there are no other emerging questions on the problem of blood pressure control and a study where a patient is getting particularly careful attention for another parameter such as correction of renal anemia. You stated that the renal function didn't progress more rapidly than normal. What were your controls for that statement?

Eschbach (Seattle): The patients were their own controls. The rate of decline in renal function did not change, using either serum creatinine or creatinine clearance data, between the year before the onset of EPO therapy and over 1 year of therapy.

Krantz (Nashville): In that study sponsored by Ortho Biotech in the USA, there were 117 predialysis patients. They were randomized between placebo, 50 IU/kg intravenously three times a week, 100 IU/kg, and 150 IU/kg. Altogether, 26 patients had an increase in blood pressure. In the three groups between placebo and 100 IU/kg, the number of patients with an increase in blood pressure was spread out evenly between the placebo group, the 50 IU/kg group, and the 100 IU/kg group, with no increase due to EPO. Only at 150 IU/kg was there an increase in the number of patients with enhanced blood pressure, and that increase was not statistically significant. So, in the predialysis group of patients, if you keep the EPO at 100 IU/kg i.v. three times a week or less there should be no increase in the incidence of enhanced blood pressure.

What are the main advantages/disadvantages of s.c. versus i.v. administration of rhEPO?

Shaldon (Nîmes): I think the answer to this is very simple. Had the demonstration of efficacy and safety not been in hemodialysis patients, there would not be any i.v. EPO; this was opportunism on Joe Eschbach's part. He would agree with me that there is clearly an economic benefit based on the superior bioavailability analysis of the area under the curve of plasma EPO concentrations following subcutaneous EPO compared to i.v. EPO. The disadvantage is simply the inconvenience of a subcutaneous injection, which may or may not have some pain associated with it depending on the product you use. But apart from that I don't think it is a question of much debate.

Eschbach (Seattle): When the first clinical trial was initiated, it was decided to treat hemodialysis patients because giving EPO intravenously assures that the patient gets 100% of the dose. At that time we had no idea whether EPO was going to work, nor what dose was necessary to get a response, and so we needed to make sure that there was optimal delivery of the drug. I would like to ask Dr. Shaldon a question: If subcutaneous therapy is clearly more effective, why don't we make an effort to get all the dialysis patients on subcutaneous injections?

Shaldon (Nîmes): I have a feeling that there is a registration problem in some countries, but protocol violators are notorious in the population of dialysis doctors. I suspect that the subcutaneous EPO is being used in a larger percentage throughout Europe, I am not familiar with the practice in the U.S. and the legal associations. I believe there is some reimbursement problem in the U.S.

Eschbach (Seattle): In the U.S., Medicare will not reimburse a kidney center if EPO is given subcutaneously to a patient dialysed in a center. The only way EPO can be given subcutaneously and still be reimbursed is if the patient dialyses at home either by hemodialysis or with CAPD.

Breymann (Zurich): Maybe it is also important to point out that it is not only a question of which product we use but also at which temperature we use it. I don't know whether everybody is aware that if you use EPO at room temperature there is a big difference compared to using it after you take it out of the fridge. If you use it at room temperature, the pain is much less in subcutaneous application.

Shaldon (Nîmes): Well, I don't want to get into this argument too deeply, but there are several well-documented scientific studies with placebo control included showing a clear difference between Epoetin alpha and Epoetin beta. It has nothing to do with EPO; it is probably the formulation difference that is responsible. The temperature was controlled in these studies and I think there is a difference.

What is the optimal dose frequency of rhEPO—one, three, or seven times a week—in view of its clinical efficacy?

Shaldon (Nîmes): I think, on the basis of the last discussion, we will not enter into the intravenous field in discussing frequency, and simply I would like to show you one slide [Figure 1], where, in a recent study which Dr. Granolleras reported in part yesterday, you will see there is no difference in the EPO dose or hematocrit achieved in a steady-state population switched between three times and seven times weekly s.c. dose in a randomized fashion so far in an ABA multicenter study with regular maintenance i.v. iron therapy 10 milligrams per hemodialysis. I think you are allowed to conclude from this that the bio-availability of three-times-a-week s.c. EPO would suggest optimal utilization and lowest amounts of EPO given, and that seven times a week probably has no applicable future. We have no data as yet analyzed on once-a-week in this study and I don't think there is any good data where adequate iron replacement has been allowed for.

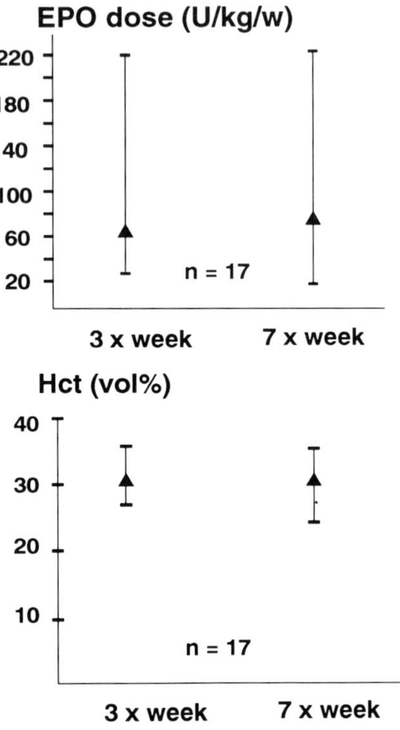

Fig. 1.   The mean hematocrit and weekly rhEPO dose of 17 patients switched from 3 or 7 × week SCEPO to either 7 or 3 × week, while receiving 10 mg i.v. iron therapy per dialysis. To be included, patients had to have been stable on SCEPO 3 or 7 × week for at least 12 weeks prior to inclusion in the study.

Eschbach (Seattle): I would like to confirm Dr. Shaldon's data. We also did a crossover study between three-times-a-week subcutaneous versus daily subcutaneous injections in 12 patients. After 6 months of therapy for each frequency, we could not show any difference in total weekly EPO dose. We concur that there is no benefit in going to daily subcutaneous therapy. Although most of you here are not from the U.S., I do want to make a comment about i.v. therapy. In the U.S.—as I mentioned—i.v. therapy is the predominant route, and unfortunately some of our colleagues are using it weekly, intravenously, and the stated reason is that it is less work for the nurses. However, it is probably 25% less effective that way, as shown by a Canadian study. Therefore, the best way to use it intravenously is two to three times a week. If given subcutaneously, the frequency could be thrice weekly, twice weekly, or even weekly. An occasional patient can benefit from every-other-week subcutaneous therapy.

When is iron supplementation necessary, and which parameters are most suitable to monitor adequate iron supplementation?

Shaldon (Nîmes): I think Dr. Eschbach in one of these meetings said that iron would be the Achilles heel of EPO therapy and, as so often, he was right. But it is also the Achilles heel of hemodialysis therapy because this is a blood-loss disease. We have known that for 25 years, and somewhere along the line the message got lost. People who are regularly losing blood need iron supplementation; I think that is normal clinical medicine. So the answer is iron supplementation is routinely necessary in the non-polytransfused hemodialysis patient. How you judge whether you are giving the iron adequately is clearly controversial in terms of the period of correction of the anemia. One must bow to the knowledge that the low iron binding saturation and the serum iron clearly show the need when the ferritin levels are still found to be high. We had some data presented yesterday suggesting that even the transferrin saturation and the serum iron levels may not indicate the optimized iron needs. We have seen increases in hematocrit following i.v. iron where iron saturation was indicated by transferrin saturation of more than 30 to 40% and serum ferritin levels were greater than 500 nanograms per milliliter. This response is not fully understandable at this moment. So I think routinely one needs to monitor transferrin saturation, and if that gets below 20%, one needs to look at the patients who are presumably on regular oral iron therapy and perhaps consider giving parenteral iron, as these are obviously noncompliant patients.

Eschbach (Seattle): Dr. Shaldon, do you have any recommendations on the frequency of measuring the iron parameters?

Shaldon (Nîmes): Measuring proteins in a routine laboratory, you need to measure them rather more frequently than less frequently to get outside of the coefficient of variation of the measure, and, in my experience, there is certainly an enormous variability in what comes back from the laboratory in transferrin saturation. So I think if you get a low one, you should repeat it before you start running in with extra iron, but I would have thought once a month.

What are the benefits of long-term rhEPO treatment, especially with respect to the progression of cardiovascular disorders?

Eschbach (Seattle): I would like to couple this with one or two other questions. To which value should the PCV or hematocrit be increased under EPO therapy; in other words, what should the target hematocrit be? I would like then to try to address this question, which I think is one of the issues for the future, with some slides and some data. In terms of cardiovascular improvement—to answer that particular question—there are no long-term studies as yet, but to refresh your memory from several other talks we heard yesterday, the cardiovascular improvements that occur, at least with partial correction of the anemia, are:

1. Cardiac enlargement may decrease
2. Angina may decrease
3. Myocardial function may improve
4. Exercise ability increases
5. Blood pressure may increase in hypotensive patients
6. There may be more stable hemodialysis

The issue is: Are these benefits optimal with a hematocrit of 30 to 35 or would they be better at a normal hematocrit? A sub-issue is whether reduction in left-ventricular hypertrophy [LVH] will improve survival in chronic renal failure patients treated with EPO. There is data that suggests that LVH increases the mortality by 3.7 times. LVH consists of two components: One is the dilatation of the heart and the other is the increased wall thickness. Both of these subsets increase mortality. We know that there is a reduction of cardiac output and cardiomegaly, and in some studies a reduction in wall thickness, and so the postulate is: Does a reduction in cardiac size improve survival? If that is the case, what hematocrit would optimize that improvement for our patients? I have arbitrarily defined a target hematocrit as having three components: it is the hematocrit or hemoglobin level that maximizes quality of life, minimizes complications, and is cost-effective. The normal hematocrit is 37 to 50, whereas the clinical trials in the U.S. and in Europe the hematocrit was between 32 and 40; for various reasons that are not totally clear to me, the FDA and the governmental agencies in our country decreed that the hematocrit should only be between 30 and 33 and we are not reimbursed in the U.S. if the hematocrit goes over 36. Despite that, the nephrologists around the world are—in my opinion—undertreating their dialysis patients. The mean hematocrit of patients in the U.S. is 30.7; in Japan it is 28 to 30; in Europe it is 28 to 33—in the majority of patients. We have no objective data as to what should be the hematocrit of dialysis patients. Dr. Erslev just mentioned that when Dr. Bunn phlebotomized some normal individuals, they were symptomatic of anemia at a hematocrit of 32 to 34 and, as Dr. Winearls mentioned, there is concern on the part of nephrologists that complications may occur with higher hematocrits. And yet there is not a lot of data except for the initial trials.

In Seattle, we are involved in a study to address the issue of whether a normal hematocrit provides a better quality of life and whether there are significant adverse effects from a normal hematocrit. Various physiological and subjective measurements are made at a stable hematocrit of 30 to 33 and repeated after at least 4 months at a hematocrit of 40 to 43. These physiological measurements include exercise tolerance, a pulmonary function, leg and hand muscle function, echocardiographic evaluation of cardiac size and wall thickness, red cell survival, choice reaction time (a measurement of speed and accuracy of cognitive response), and subject responses to a standardized quality-of-life questionnaire. Potential complications monitored included blood pressure response, vascular access clotting, iron requirements, and dialysis efficiency. Five of a projected 20 patients have completed the first phase of this study comparing their responses at a normal hematocrit (41 $\pm$ 2) to their baseline (32 $\pm$ 2). The EPO dose increased from 37 $\pm$ 12 to 75 $\pm$ 38 units per kilogram i.v. three times a week. Exercise capacity increased 22%; isometric performance increased 27%; left ventricular end-diastolic diameter decreased slightly in two, and significantly in one, and remained normal in the other two; and red cell survival didn't change. All five patients reported significant subjective improvements. There was not a problem with hypertension or increased vascular access clotting. This is preliminary data on a small number of patients. These patients will be restudied after their hematocrit has returned to their previous baseline.

Shaldon (Nîmes): It is ''brave new world,'' and I have a feeling that you can get away with it in Seattle. I think you could have gotten away with it anywhere in the world 20 years ago. I am really concerned that you would suggest this at a moment in time when patients are receiving shorter and shorter dialysis times and more and more hypotensive drugs. Already, the modern dialysis population is experiencing more and more fluid overload. If you recommend curing their anemia completely under these conditions, I predict that you would be courting disaster in the long run from the progressive effects of viscosity in a patient with fluid overload. In my opinion, if you have a good dialysis center where the patients get well looked after, I think this is feasible, but I think you get very little safety margin from going overboard with the run-of-the-mill patient.

Eschbach (Seattle): I agree with you. Obviously we should be involved in the total care of our patients, and not just concentrate on one aspect of their care, such as the anemia. But their dialysis *and* their anemia therapy should be optimized. In my opinion I do not think that we nephrologists should accept a hematocrit level that hematologists consider anemic. We need to determine how best to use EPO since it is possible that a normal hematocrit will lead to a better quality of life in coping with a chronic disease. In my experience, a hematocrit of 30 to 31 is not optimal unless the patient may be very sedentary (and, unfortunately, this applies to many dialysis patients). Active and/or working patients seem to benefit from a larger hematocrit. Depending on the results of our studies, and hopefully those of other investigators, we may have some objective data to determine how to optimize the hematocrit for individual patients.

Lindsay (Ontario): Can I ask you, Joe, what do you think of the Canadian multicenter study which looked at two different levels of hemoglobin and showed no difference in effect?

Eschbach (Seattle): The Canadian multicenter study studied patients at a hemoglobin of 95 to 110 grams per liter and others at a hemoglobin of 115 to 130 grams per liter. There was no difference between 34 patients with the lower hemoglobin and 33 patients with the higher hemoglobin when they were exercised by an exercise stress test on a treadmill or performed a 6-minute walk. They did these studies at baseline (hemoglobin approximately 70 grams per liter) and 2 and 6 months later. Unfortunately, the baseline values for both of these exercise tests were much higher in the high-hemoglobin group, so I don't know how to interpret the results.

Winearls (Oxford): Although the Canadian placebo-controlled trial was a remarkable study, I do not believe it resolved the issue of the optimal target hemoglobin. There was a considerable overlap in actual hematocrits achieved by patients in the two groups, and the comparison was between change in quality of life. A crossover study comparing higher and lower hematocrits in each patient would have been a better way to distinguish the effect. What did emerge from that study was the higher rate of vascular access failure, specifically Gore-tex grafts, in the EPO-treated patients. If raising the hematocrit to greater than 35 does impose a greater risk to access, nephrologists will be more conservative in their choice of target hematocrit. I know that some patients are routinely given aspirin or persantin. Does Dr. Eschbach agree with this?

Eschbach (Seattle): Clotting of Gore-tex grafts has been a problem even before the advent of EPO therapy. From the data that I have reviewed, there has not been an increase in Gore-tex graft clotting following EPO therapy when large groups of patients are examined. If dialyzer clotting increases, or there is incomplete dialyzer blood return following a rise in the hematocrit, I either increase the heparin requirements or initiate aspirin therapy. I don't think this makes any difference in the incidence of Gore-tex graft thromboses, though.

At what hematocrit or hemoglobin should rhEPO therapy be withheld?

Eschbach (Seattle): I do not think we have sufficient data at this time to answer this question.

Nielsen (*Copenhagen*): When you keep your hematocrit on 42 in your patients: Do they require an increased amount of EPO? Is the maintenance dose increased, or is it just the initial dose that you have to continue?

Eschbach (*Seattle*): The doses I showed on that slide were the maintenance doses, so there is an increase amount as one would expect.

Shaldon (*Nîmes*): Would you put a figure on the percentage increase?

Eschbach (*Seattle*): For the first five patients studied, the dose was approximately doubled.

Intracellular Transduction of Erythropoietin Signal

Isabelle Dusanter, Odile Muller, Michèle Sabbah, Sigmund Fischer,[a] Catherine Lacombe, Patrick Mayeux

ICGM, U 363 and [a]U 332 Hôpital Cochin, Paris, France

Erythropoietin (EPO) stimulates the proliferation and differentiation of erythroid progenitor cells [1]. The specificity of EPO's biological effects is due to the interaction of the hormone with high affinity EPO receptors expressed on the surface of erythroid cells [2].

We studied the structure of the EPO receptor (EPO-R) and were able to show that it was a multimeric complex. Indeed, cross-linking experiments with different cross-linkers showed that three proteins of molecular weight 100, 85, and 66 kd, respectively, were part of the receptor and were not immunologically related [3].

One chain of the EPO-R corresponding to the 66 kd protein has been cloned [4] and is a member of the hematopoietic receptor superfamily, which includes receptors for IL-2 to IL-7, for G- and GM-CSF, for LIF, GH, and prolactin [5].

The exact role of the 100 and 85 kd associated proteins has not yet been determined and the cloned chain of the EPO-R alone, when transfected into various hematopoietic cells, is able to make the cells responsive to the hormone and to trigger their proliferation [6]. The main common feature of all these hematopoietic receptors is that they do not possess in their cytoplasmic domains tyrosine kinase consensus sequences. On the other hand, a large number of growth factor receptors require intrinsic tyrosine kinase activation for cell activation and proliferation; these receptors include the PDGF-R, EGF-R, M-CSF-R, insulin-R, and stem cell factor (SRF).

Until recently, little was known about the biochemical mechanisms responsible for the proliferation upon EPO stimulation. We used a human leukemia cell line, UT7, derived by Komatsu et al. [7] from a megakaryoblastic leukemia, which is induced to proliferate and/or differentiate by GM-CSF, IL-3, EPO, IL-6, and stem cell factor [8].

We have found that EPO specifically induces in this cell line the phosphorylation of several proteins in a rapid and transient manner. The dominant phosphoprotein observed in the EPO-R complex after treatment with EPO was the cloned chain of the EPO-R itself. Another associated phosphotyrosyl protein was phosphatidylinositol 3-kinase (PI 3-kinase), suggesting that tyrosine phosphorylation–dependent activation of PI 3-kinase is a component of the EPO-R signal transduction process.

Materials and Methods

Cell Culture

UT7 cells were grown in alpha medium supplemented with 10% fetal calf serum and 2.5 ng/ml GM-CSF. Before each experiment, the cells were washed and incubated for 18 h in Iscove's modification of minimum essential medium containing 1% bovine serum albumin and 100 μg/ml iron-saturated human transferrin.

For cell stimulation, highly purified recombinant hormones (EPO, GM-CSF, IL-6 IL-3, and SCF) were used.

Antibodies

A monoclonal antiphosphotyrosine antibody and a rabbit polyclonal antiserum raised against a glutathione S transferase–PI 3-kinase (p85) were purchased from Upstate Biotechnology Inc. Anti-EPO antibodies were obtained from rabbits immunized with EPO. Antibodies against the murine EPO-R were obtained by immunizing rabbits against a fusion protein corresponding to the *E. coli* maltose transporter (Mal E) and most of the cytoplasmic part of the murine EPO receptor, as previously reported [3]. Control antibodies included normal rabbit serum and a Mal E rabbit antiserum.

Preparation of Cell Lysate and Immunoprecipitation

Cells were incubated for the indicated times at 37°C with the growth factors. Incubation was stopped by the addition of an excess of ice-cold PBS and immediate pelleting of the cells. Solubilization was then performed by a 15-min incubation in a buffer containing 25 mM Hepes, pH 7.4, 150 mM NaCl, 5 mM EDTA, 10% glycerol, 1% Nonidet P40, 1 mM PMSF, 1 mM *ortho*-phenanthroline 1 mM vanadate, and 10 μg/ml each of aprotinin, leupeptin, and pepstatin. The cell lysates were then centrifuged for 20 min at 25,000 g and the supernatants were mixed with antiphosphotyrosine antibodies. After 1 h on ice, 50 μl of a 1/5 (vol/vol) suspension of protein A Sepharose were added, and the samples were then incubated with agitation for 1 h at 4°.

All the immunoprecipitates were intensively washed before being resuspended in PI 3-kinase buffer (25 mM Hepes pH 7.4, 100 mM NaCl, 5 mM MgCl$_2$, 200 $\mu$$M$ adenosine) or, alternatively, before resuspension in SDS lysis buffer and solubilized by boiling for 10 min. When indicated, the solubilized and denatured immunoprecipitates were further diluted and incubated with a second antibody. Samples were all subjected to SDS-PAGE and electrotransferred onto nitrocellulose filters.

PI 3-Kinase Activity

Immunoprecipitates on protein A Sepharose were resuspended in 50 μl of PI 3-kinase buffer containing 25 μm ATP, 1.5 μCi of (γ^{32}P) ATP, and 0.4 mg/ml of a sonicated mixture of phosphatidylserine and phosphatidylinositol (1/1, W/W). The mixtures were incubated for 15 min at 22°C and the reaction was stopped by addition of 100 μl of 1 N HCl. The lipids were extracted with $CHCL_3/CH_3OH$, and the organic phase was washed twice with $CH_3OH/1$ *M* HCl. The lipids were then separated by thin layer chromatography (TLC) on silica gel plates coated with 1% potassium oxalate using a mobile phase composed of $CHCL_3/CH_3OH/4$ *M* NH_4OH.

Authentic unlabeled phosphatidylinositol 4-phosphate (PI-4-P) was run in an adjacent lane and was revealed using iodine vapors. Phosphate incorporation was determined by autoradiography, and the quantifications were performed by densitometric scanning.

Cross-Linking Experiments

Cross-linking experiments using disuccinimidyl suberate and analysis of ^{125}I-EPO cross-linked complexes were done as previously described [3].

Analysis of Phosphotyrosyl Proteins

Western experiments were performed as previously described [9].

Results

EPO-Induced Phosphorylation of Several Proteins

The activation of members of the hematopoietic receptor superfamily quickly induces an increase in protein tyrosine phosphorylation [10, 11]. We examined signal transduction in UT7 cells after an overnight growth factor deprivation and 10 min of EPO stimulation (1 U/ml). Numerous proteins were tyrosine phosphorylated following incubation with EPO; the principal phosphoproteins revealed by immunoblotting with antiphosphotyrosine antibodies had molecular weights of 140, 120, 95, 75, 60, and 42 kd (Fig. 1). This tyrosine phosphorylation was detected 2 min after EPO stimulation, reached a plateau between 5 and 10 min, and then decreased. This tyrosine phosphorylation was also dependent on EPO concentration and detected using as little as 0.1 U/ml of EPO.

Among Tyrosine-Phosphorylated Proteins Induced by EPO
Is EPO-R Itself

The UT7 cells are responsive to various growth factors such as EPO, GM-CSF, IL-3, IL-6, and stem cell factor. These different growth factors induce different protein tyrosine phosphorylation profiles [9]. It is noteworthy that only EPO specifically induced the phosphorylation of the 75 kd protein.

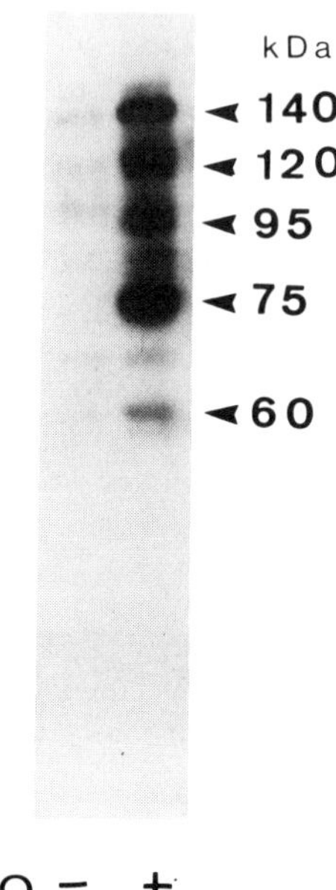

Fig. 1. EPO-induced tyrosine phosphorylation. UT7 cells (10^6/point) were incubated for 10 min at 37°C in the presence of 1 U/ml of EPO, solubilized by boiling in SDS lysis buffer, and subjected to SDS-PAGE under reducing conditions. Proteins were transferred onto nitrocellulose and incubated with antiphosphotyrosine antibodies. Phosphotyrosine proteins were revealed by ^{125}I-labeled antimouse antibody.

In order to test whether this 75 kd protein was the EPO-R itself, UT7 cells were gently solubilized and immunoprecipitated using different antisera. Anti-EPO-R antibodies recognized the 75 kd protein phosphorylated upon stimulation with EPO, even after denaturation of the complex, indicating that this phosphoprotein was the receptor itself (Fig. 2).

To confirm these results, we showed that 30% of the ^{125}I–Epo-R complexes could be immunoprecipitated by the antiphosphotyrosine antibodies. Similar experiments performed on ^{125}I-EPO cross-linked complexes showed that the antiphosphotyrosine antibodies recognized only the 75 kd receptor subunit.

EPO Activates Tyrosine-Phosphorylated PI 3-Kinase

UT7 cells were stimulated for 5 min with EPO (5 U/ml), and the phosphotyrosine-containing proteins were purified by immunoprecipitation with antiphosphotyrosine antibodies. The immunopellets were resuspended in PI 3-kinase reaction buffer containing phosphatidylinositol and (γ^{32}P) ATP. PI 3-kinase

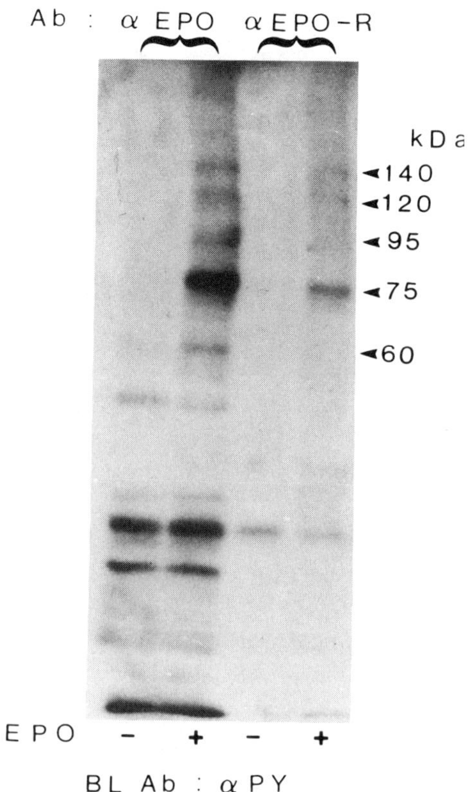

Fig. 2. The major EPO-induced tyrosine-phosphorylated protein. UT7 cells (10^7/point) preincubated with 50 μM *ortho*-vanadate were incubated with or without EPO. Samples were solubilized under mild conditions and immunoprecipitated with anti-EPO antibodies. Alternatively, samples were solubilized by boiling in SDS lysis buffer and immunoprecipitated with anti–EPO-R antibodies. Phosphotyrosine-containing proteins were analyzed by immunoblotting.

activity was determined after a 15-min incubation by detection of (^{32}P) phosphatidylinositol phosphate, which was separated from phosphatidylinositol and (^{32}P) ATP by TLC, autoradiographed, and quantified by densitometric scanning.

As shown in Figure 3, PI 3-kinase activity was detected after only 1 min of EPO stimulation of UT7 cells and reached a maximum level after 5 min of incubation. When UT7 cells were incubated for 5 min with various EPO concentrations, PI 3-kinase activity increased between 1 and 10 U/ml of EPO.

The D 3′ labeling position of phosphate was ascertained by the use of

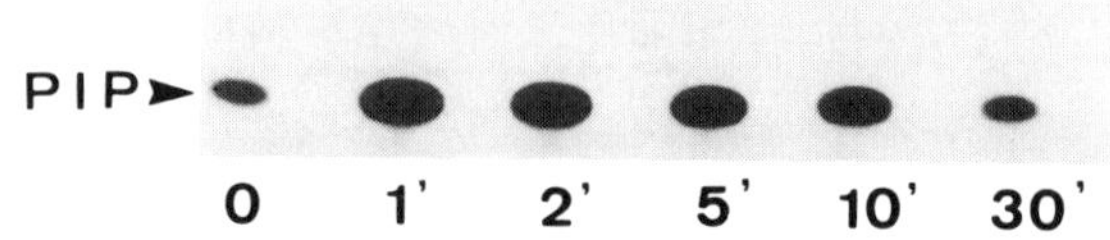

Fig. 3. EPO activates the PI 3-kinase specifically. Cells (10^7/ml) were incubated for the indicated times at 37°C with 5 U/ml of EPO. The cells were then solubilized, cell lysates were centrifuged, and supernatants were mixed with antiphosphotyrosine antibodies. PI 3-kinase activity was determined by detection of (^{32}P) phosphatidylinositol phosphate, isolated by TLC, and autoradiographed.

adenosine to inhibit phosphatidylinositol 4-kinase (PI 4-kinase) and the use of ionic detergents, which inhibited phosphate incorporation into phosphatidylinositol phosphate by inhibition of PI 3-kinase activity as previously described.

Association Between PI 3-Kinase and EPO Receptor

UT7 cells were stimulated with ^{125}I-EPO, lysed, and immunoprecipitated with anti PI 3-kinase antibodies. About 25% of the ^{125}I-EPO-R complexes could be specifically immunoprecipitated by the anti–PI 3-kinase antibodies. Moreover, three ^{125}I-EPO cross-linked proteins were immunoprecipitated by anti–PI 3-kinase antibodies as well as by antiphosphotyrosine antibodies. But these three proteins of 100, 85, and 75 kd were no longer immunoprecipitated by anti–PI 3-kinase antibodies after denaturation of the complexes, indicating that these proteins were associated with but were not part of the PI 3-kinase complex.

Finally, UT7 cells were stimulated with EPO, solubilized, and immunoprecipitated with anti–PI 3-kinase antibodies. After separation on a 10% polyacrylamide gel and detection with antiphosphotyrosine antibodies, various proteins were evidenced. Among them, the 75 kd chain of the EPO-R and a 85 kd protein corresponding to the regulatory subunit of the PI 3-kinase were recognized, whereas three other tyrosine phosphorylated proteins of 110, 97, and 64 kd co-immunoprecipitated by anti–PI 3-kinase antibodies, remained to be identified.

Discussion

In this study, we used the UT7 human cell line, which is growth factor dependent for its proliferation and differentiation. These cells are EPO-responsive and express a large number of endogenous high affinity EPO receptors at their surface (7000 sites/cell), which facilitates the study of the EPO-induced signal transduction.

When cross-linking experiments were performed with disuccinimidyl suberate, three proteins of 100, 85, and 71–75 kd, respectively, were found to be cross-linked to ^{125}I-EPO [9]. One chain of the human EPO receptor has been cloned, contains 508 amino acids, and yields a protein of 66 kd when expressed in COS cells [12]. It seems likely that this chain is further processed in UT7 cells to give a protein of 71–75 kd apparent molecular mass.

We showed that EPO acts on these cells by specifically inducing tyrosine phosphorylation of a set of proteins. Among them, a 75 kd protein corresponds to the cloned chain of the EPO-R, because it is recognized by murine anti–EPO-R antibodies, which are able to cross-react with their human counterpart.

Others reports recently published indicate that EPO induced tyrosine phosphorylation of many proteins [13–16]. However, the molecular weights of the phosphorylated proteins were not identical, and some authors did not report the phosphorylation of the EPO-R itself. These discrepancies can be explained by the different cellular systems utilized: murine or human cells with endogenous or transfected EPO-R.

Because the intracellular portion of the EPO-R does not contain enzymatic activity associated with receptor-mediated signal transduction, this receptor may be associated with one or more protein tyrosine kinase. Linnekin et al. [17] described a 97 kd phosphotyrosylprotein which was also found to bind ATP, a characteristic critical for protein kinases. Moreover, tyrosine kinases of the src family seem to be involved in signal transduction, e.g., the p56 lck and the p59 fyn tyrosine kinases, which form noncovalent complexes with IL-2 receptor and TCR subunits, respectively [18, 19].

Among the tyrosine-phosphorylated proteins that we detected in EPO-incubated UT7 cells, most remain to be identified. They could be proteins belonging to the src family member, or components of the native multimeric EPO receptor complex, or other phosphorylated substrates.

The activation of receptors with tyrosine kinase activity triggers the subsequent phosphorylation of cytoplasmic signaling proteins such as phospholipase C gamma, Ras GTPase-activating protein, and PI 3-kinase. These proteins have a common SH2 (src homology) domain, which allows them to associate with specific tyrosine-phosphorylated sites, and these interactions in turn stimulate intracellular signal transduction pathways.

In contrast, signal transduction events occurring in the hematopoietic receptor superfamily are still poorly understood, but similar intracellular pathways seem to be activated. We showed that in UT7 cells, EPO stimulation induced tyrosine phosphorylation and activation of PI 3-kinase. Indeed, PI 3-kinase was found in antiphosphotyrosine immunoprecipitates and PI 3-kinase associated with the EPO-R after stimulation of responsive cells with EPO; however, the exact location of PI 3-kinase binding on the EPO-R complex is not known.

The activation of PI 3-kinase in IL-2–mediated signal transduction was reported using the IL-2–dependent murine cell line CTLL-2 [21] and human stimulated blood lymphocytes [22]. EPO stimulation of PI 3-kinase activity is at the same level ($4\times$) as that reported for IL-2–stimulated cells. Moreover, GM-CSF also stimulates the production of phosphatidylinositol 3,4,5-triphosphate in GM-CSF–sensitive cells [L. Cantley, personal communication].

Thus, even if the mechanism of action of D 3 phosphoinositides is not understood, the results presented here are consistent with the possibility that EPO-dependent activation of tyrosine kinase and PI 3-kinase activities are important for cellular growth regulation by this cytokine.

Acknowledgments

We acknowledge Dr L.C. Cantley for the communication of results prior to their publication. We are grateful to Jennifer Richardson for critical reading of the manuscript. This work was supported by contract 6327 from the Association pour la Recherche sur le Cancer (ARC).

References

1   Krantz SB: Erythropoietin. Blood 1991;77:419–434.
2   Mayeux P, Billat C, Jacquot R: The erythropoietin receptor of rat erythroid progenitor cells. Characterization and affinity cross-linkage. J Biol Chem 1987;262:13985–13990.
3   Mayeux P, Lacombe C, Casadevall N, Chrétien S, Dusanter I, Gisselbrecht S: Structure of the erythropoietin receptor complex. Characterization of the erythropoietin cross-linked proteins. J Biol Chem 1991;266:23380–23385.
4   D'Andrea AD, Lodish HF, Wong GG: Expression cloning of the murine erythropoietin receptor. Cell 1989;57:277–285.
5   Bazan JF: Structural design and molecular evolution of a cytokine receptor superfamily. Proc Natl Acad Sci USA 1990;87:6934–6938.
6   Li JP, D'Andrea AD, Lodish HF, Baltimore D: Activation of cell growth by binding of Friend spleen focus-forming virus gp55 glycoprotein to the erythropoietin receptor. Nature 1990;343:762–764.
7   Komatsu N, Nakauchi H, Miwa A, Ishihara T, Eguchi M, Moroi M, Okada T, Sato Y, Wada H, Yawata Y, Suda T, Miura Y: Establishment and characterization of a human leukemic cell line with megakaryocytic features: Dependency on

granulocyte-macrophage colony-stimulating factor, interleukin 3, or erythropoietin for growth and survival. Cancer Res 1991;51:341–348.

8 Hermine O, Mayeux P, Titeux M, Mitjavila MT, Casadevall N, Guichard J, Komatsu N, Suda T, Miura Y, Vainchenker W, Breton-Gorius J: Granulocyte-macrophage colony stimulating factor and erythropoietin act competitively to induce two different programs of differentiation in the human pluripotent cell line UT7. Blood 1992; 80:3060–3069.

9 Dusanter-Fourt I, Casadevall N, Lacombe C, Muller O, Billat C, Fisher S, Mayeux P: Erythropoietin induces the tyrosine phosphorylation of its own receptor in human erythropoietin-responsive cells. J Biol Chem 1992;267:10670–10675.

10 Isfort R, Huhn RD, Frackelton AR, Ihle JN: Stimulation of factor-dependent myeloid cell lines with interleukin-3 induces tyrosine phosphorylation of several cellular substrates. J Biol Chem 1988;263:19203–19209.

11 UcKun FM, Dibirdik I, Smith R, Tuel-Ahlgren L, Chandan-Langlie M, Schieven GL, Waddick KG, Hanson M, Ledbetter JA: Interleukin 7 receptor ligation stimulates tyrosine phosphorylation, inositol phospholipid turnover, and clonal proliferation of human B-cell precursors. Proc Natl Acad Sci USA 1991;88:3589–3593.

12 Jones SS, D'Andrea AD, Haines LL, Wong GG: Human erythropoietin receptor: Cloning, expression, and biologic characterisation. Blood 1990;76:31–35.

13 Quelle FW, Wojchowski DM. Proliferative action of erythropoietin is associated with rapid protein tyrosine phosphorylation in responsive B6SUt.EP cells. J Biol Chem 1991;266:609–614.

14 Miura O, D'Andrea A, Kabat D, Ihle JN: Induction of tyrosine phosphorylation by the erythropoietin receptor correlates with mitogenesis. Mol Cell Biol 1991;11:4895–4902.

15 Yoshimura A, Lodish HF: In vitro phosphorylation of the erythropoietin receptor and an associated protein, pp130. Mol Cell Biol 1992;12:706–715.

16 Komatsu N, Adamson JW, Yamamoto K, Altschuler D, Torti M, Marzocchini R, Lapetina EG: Erythropoietin rapidly induces tyrosine phosphorylation in the human erythropoietin-dependent cell line, UT7. Blood 1992;80:53–59.

17 Linnekin D, Evans GA, D'Andrea A, Farrar WL. Association of the erythropoietin receptor with protein tyrosine kinase activity. Proc Natl Acad Sci USA 1992;89:6237–6241.

18 Hatakeyama M, Kono T, Kobayashi N, Kawahara A, Levin SD, Perlmutter RM, Taniguchi T: Interaction of the IL2 receptor with the scr-family kinase p56 lck: Identification of novel intermolecular association. Science 1991;244:551–556.

19 Klausner RD, Samelson LE: T cell antigen receptor activation pathways: The tyrosine kinase connection. Cell 1991;64:875–878.

20 Merida I, Diez E, Gaulton GN: IL-2 binding activates a tyrosine-phosphorylated phosphatidylinositol—3 kinase. J Immunol 1991;147:2202–2207.

21 Remillard B, Petrillo R, Maslinski W, Tsudo M, Strom TB, Cantley L, Varticovski L: Interleukin-2 receptor regulates activation of phosphatidylinositol 3-kinase. J Biol Chem 1991;266:14167–14170.

Catherine Lacombe, ICGM, U 363, Hôpital Cochin, 27 Rue du Fg St Jacques, 75014 Paris, France

Discussion

to the Paper by I. Dusanter et al.

Fandrey (Bonn): Protein kinase C has been implicated to be involved in the signal transduction of EPO. Do you think protein kinase C may play a role in your model?

Lacombe: I cannot exclude that protein kinase C plays a role, but we did not do any experiments for detection of protein kinase C at the moment.

Joven (Reus): Which is the minimum dose in which you find response in your model?

Lacombe: For this kind of experiment?

Joven: Yes.

Lacombe: Usually 0.1 unit per milliliter of erythropoietin added to the culture.

Joven: Have you tried lower concentrations?

Lacombe: Yes, but for this model and this particular cell line the minimum is 0.1 unit per milliliter. But it really depends on the cell line that you use to do this kind of experiment.

Stockenhuber (Vienna): I would like to know whether you also measured an intracellular mediator of EPO, like intracellular calcium?

Lacombe: Not yet; we are on the way to doing it.

Is Erythropoietin a Differentiation Factor, a Mitotic Factor, or a Survival Factor?

Maurice Bondurant, Linda Kelley, Mark J. Koury

Department of Veterans Affairs and Vanderbilt University Medical Centers, Nashville, Tenn., USA

Introduction

Erythropoietin (EPO) regulates the number of erythrocytes produced in animals by the hematopoietic organs. Production of erythropoietin itself is regulated by the oxygen activity (PO_2) around specific cells in the kidney and liver, which is, in normal circumstances, a direct indication of the concentration of erythrocytes in the blood and/or the PO_2 of the air in the lungs. If the specific cells sense a low oxygen activity, they produce erythropoietin, which boosts erythrocyte production and, ultimately, the concentration of erythrocytes in the blood. The resultant increase in oxygen delivered to the environment of the specialized, EPO-producing cells causes them to cease or lower production of EPO, subsequently decreasing the production of erythrocytes. In concise terminology, the production of erythropoietin and the production of erythrocytes are in a feedback loop, which precisely regulates oxygen delivery to the body tissues.

How erythrocytes are formed from specific progenitor cells of the hematopoietic organs has largely been analyzed by in vitro culture of bone marrow or spleen cells in semisolid medium in the presence of EPO [1]. In such cultures, individual ''committed'' progenitor cells undergo multiple rounds of cell division and concomitant differentiation steps over a period of time, finally becoming colonies of erythroblasts and reticulocytes. During culture, colonies of mature erythroblasts and reticulocytes appear at various times over a 2-week period, and, generally, the later the cells in the colonies mature, the more cells the colonies contain. Studies of this phenomenon have led to the concept that the committed erythroid progenitor cells constitute continuous stages of differentiation. Burst-forming units–erythroid (BFU-E) are the most immature of the committed erythroid progenitor cells; they give rise to colonies of thousands of mature erythroblasts in 7 days for murine BFU-E and 14 days for human BFU-E. The BFU-E themselves are generated by restriction or "commitment" to erythroid differentiation of pluripotent hematopoietic cells. Colony-forming units–erythroid (CFU-E) are further along than BFU-E in their degree of differentiation. The CFU-E give rise to colonies of 8–32 erythroblasts after 2 days of culture for murine CFU-E and after 7 days for human CFU-E. The immediate descendants of CFU-E are the proerythroblasts, which are the earliest morphologically recognized erythroid cells and are capable of very limited proliferation.

What role does EPO play in the process of erythroid colony formation in vitro and the formation or erythrocytes in vivo? At some point, probably just before the CFU-E stage, the progenitor cells acquire a dependence upon EPO. If EPO is not added to cultures, no mature erythroid colonies are formed. Thus, operationally, EPO is a colony-stimulating factor (CSF) in the same sense as other hematopoietic CSFs: G-CSF, GM-CSF, CSF-1, and many of the interleukins. Because erythroid colony formation in vitro involves both cell proliferation and maturation, "stimulation" of colony formation has been inferred to be synonymous with initiation of cell cycling and/or induction of a differentiation program in progenitor cells. However, these are not the only possible mechanisms of EPO action.

Three possibly interrelated processes occur simultaneously during colony development: cell growth and replication, extensive differentiation, and maintenance of all functions necessary for cell survival. The last area has only recently been identified as a mechanism of hormonal regulation. EPO might function in a molecular mechanism that is an integral part of one, two, or perhaps all of these processes. It should be emphasized that we do not presently understand to what degree these processes are interconnected and co-regulated in normal hematopoietic progenitor cells. We consider these as separate processes only because of experience with certain continuous cell lines in which cell division, viability, and differentiation can appear to be separated in vitro. Certainly in tissues of animals many differentiated cell types remain alive without dividing. However, it is not clear that separation of cell division, viability, and differentiation applies to hematopoietic progenitors; in fact, there is limited evidence to the contrary.

There is little evidence, or the evidence is mixed, that EPO specifically induces normal erythroid progenitors to enter or progress through the cell cycle. A similar situation exists concerning EPO induction of differentiation. Both concepts imply that significant portions of the committed progenitor cells in an animal exist in a latent state and that EPO triggers cell cycle progression or specific differentiation events. While mitotic or differentiation effects may yet be found to play a role at some stage of EPO-sensitive differentiation, significant evidence indicates that they are not the primary mechanisms by which EPO controls erythrocyte formation. Studies show that EPO is a survival factor for erythroid progenitor cells through its ability to prevent their programmed death (apoptosis) [2–4]. We and others have proposed that erythroid progenitors at relatively late differentiation stages in vivo will undergo apoptosis, which can be prevented only by EPO. We suggest that physiological production of erythrocytes in vivo is controlled by EPO through this mechanism.

To study EPO's function directly, one must have cell systems that respond to EPO. For many types of biochemical experiments, one needs large numbers of EPO-responsive cells that are free of nonerythroid cells and are relatively synchronous in their observed responses. We have developed one such system, the FVA cell system [5], from mice infected with the anemia-inducing strain of the Friend leukemia virus. FVA cells are erythroid progenitor cells explanted from the spleens of mice infected 2 weeks previously with this virus. FVA cells are relatively homogenous in development, approximately at the CFU-E and proerythroblast stages of development, and can be obtained in large numbers ($\approx 5 \times 10^8$ cells). FVA cells proliferate and differentiate into reticulocytes during 48–60 h of in vitro culture—a process that is absolutely EPO-dependent. FVA cells do not constitute a cell line, having no long-term replication potential, and they are not tumorigenic.

Several other erythroid cell systems have been developed which are composed of progenitors derived from explanted hematopoietic tissues. These include mouse cells at about the CFU-E stage derived from animals treated with thiamphenicol to kill all but the earliest hematopoietic progenitors [6]. During hematopoietic recovery, these mice are placed under erythropoietic stress by phlebotomy-induced anemia. The CFU-E derived from this process cannot be obtained in numbers comparable to those from FVA-infected mice—i.e., only about one-tenth as many cells are available. Sawada et al. [7] developed a method of obtaining about 1–2×10^7 human CFU-E by culturing partially purified blood BFU-E for 7–8 days in vitro in the presence of EPO. Explanted cells have been used from mouse fetal livers or from spleens of mice made anemic by treatment with phenylhydrazine. These latter cell populations contain cells at all stages of erythroid differentiation, and they also contain a significant percentage of nonerythroid cells. Thus these last two systems can lead to erroneous conclusions.

Investigators have reported several established cell lines that respond to EPO, although none have been shown to differentiate as completely as do FVA cells [reviewed in Refs. 8, 9]. Some erythroid cell lines naturally express EPO receptors and are EPO dependent for cell survival and growth; others respond to EPO by limited expression of erythroid-specific genes but are not dependent on EPO for survival. Finally, the cloned EPO receptor gene has been transfected into certain nonerythroid cells lines. In this manner, cell lines have been created that express very high numbers of EPO receptors and concomitantly are rendered EPO dependent under appropriate culture conditions. All of these cell systems can potentially reveal part of the picture of EPO's mechanism of action. Each system may have advantages for examining some specific aspect of the process. We will focus the following discussion on the aspects that we have learned about using FVA cells.

Results

Apoptosis in Erythroid Progenitors

Several findings in FVA cells have shaped our view of EPO's role: (a) EPO makes no difference in the rate of DNA synthesis in these cells during the hours of culture when the presence of EPO is critical; (b) most of the DNA synthetic activity in cultures without EPO is fruitless because the DNA is degraded in a constantly increasing proportion of the cells; and (c) a large majority of the cell population dies during 24 h of culture without EPO. These phenomena, which occur upon EPO withdrawal, resemble cell death processes, which are termed apoptosis. Figure 1 illustrates the morphological features that develop in many FVA cells deprived of EPO compared to the morphology of FVA cells that have differentiated into late erythroblasts in the presence of EPO. The apoptotic cells of Figure 1B have undergone a reduction in cell size and a homogeneous "condensation" of chromatin. They do not accumulate appreciable quantities of hemoglobin. The nuclear changes of the EPO-derived cells are distinct in several ways from those observed during normal erythroid differentiation: the nucleus becomes completely homogeneous, lacking any heterochromatin, the nuclear envelope is lost, and the DNA is degraded. None of these changes occurs during EPO-induced differentiation, even in the extruded nuclei derived during reticulocyte formation [L. Kelley et al., unpublished].

Another hallmark of the cell death process in FVA cells cultured without EPO is the degradation of cellular DNA. This degradation is prevented almost completely by EPO. Figure 2 depicts a size analysis by electrophoresis on 1% agarose gels of cellular DNAs from FVA cells cultured for up to 18 h without EPO. In the lanes of DNA from cells without EPO, one sees two DNA size classes: one class is large (>21 kbp) and does not migrate very far, and the

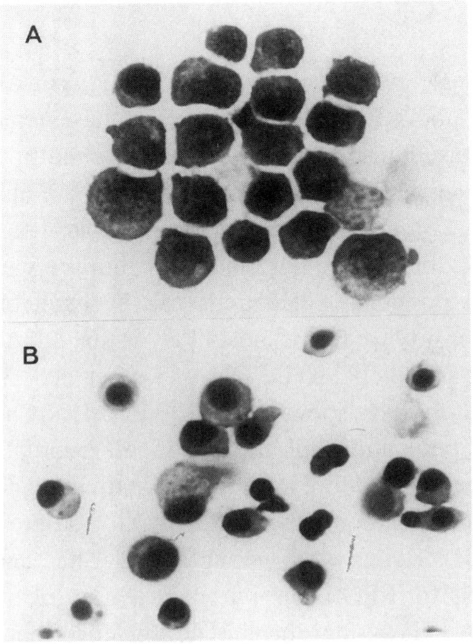

Fig. 1. Morphological changes in FVA cells deprived of erythropoietin. (A) Cells cultured for 20 h in the presence of EPO. (B) Cells cultured for 20 h without EPO.

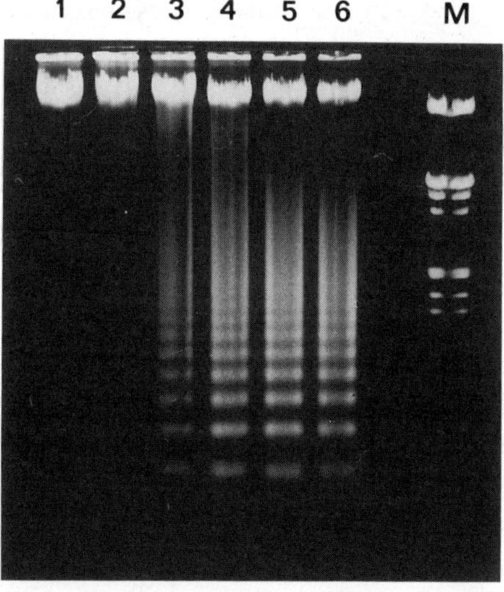

Fig. 2. Progressive degradation of DNA in FVA cells cultured without EPO. Lane 1, freshly isolated FVA cells; lane 2, cells after 2 h of culture; lane 3, cells after 6 h; lane 4, cells after 10 h; lane 5, cells after 14 h; lane 6, cells after 18 h. M marks a lane of DNA marker fragments.

second heterogeneous class, which migrates further, contains a series of bands that are multiples of about 185 nucleotide pairs. A large majority of molecules in the smaller DNA class represent the 185 bp length or multiples of it by a factor of 2 or 3. Various higher multiples of this DNA length are also present. At longer culture times there is a relative paucity of intermediate-length fragments, which reveals that the DNA breaks are not random within the whole DNA of the cell population. Several possible explanations can be envisioned to yield such a pattern, but the possibility we feel is most likely is that DNA of some cells breaks down rapidly and completely, while DNA in other cells is left intact. Recent studies in our laboratory have shown that all FVA cells do not undergo apoptosis synchronously. Subpopulations of the FVA cell population can survive for varying times without EPO. More importantly, individual cells in the population have widely different dose requirements for EPO for progression through growth and differentiation [L. Kelley et al. unpublished]. The concept of varying dose requirements of cells for EPO is an important feature of our model of erythropoiesis. In the FVA cell system there is no evidence that EPO dependence is restricted to a particular phase of the cell cycle. This possibility has not been analyzed thoroughly and is under further investigation in our laboratory. Our preliminary work suggests that cells die during more than one phase of the cycle.

The death of late erythroid progenitors deprived of EPO is not an unusual property of the FVA cell system. A similar process has recently been observed in late human erythroid progenitors [K. Muta and S. B. Krantz, personal communication] and in murine splenic erythroblasts [4] derived without retrovirus infection by the thiamphenicol method described above.

Does EPO Have Mitogenic Activity?

Several reports indicate that EPO may cause certain cell types to initiate DNA synthesis and progress through S phase starting from a latent G_0 or G_1 phase of the cell cycle. Spivak et al. [10] studied an established cell line (HCD-57) that is dependent on EPO for growth in culture. These investigators presented evidence that these cells arrest in the G_0 or G_1 phase of the cell cycle without EPO and that they can be induced to initiate DNA synthesis if EPO is added within 72 h of its initial withdrawal. The cells eventually die without EPO. A study indicates that EPO causes normal BFU-E to enter the cell cycle. Dessypris and Krantz [11] showed that culture of human bone marrow cells with EPO (vs. without EPO) for 24 h caused an increase in BFU-E that were in S phase at the end of the culture period. Interpretation of this latter result is complicated because over half of the BFU-E died during the culture period without EPO. If these cells were dying preferentially in cell cycle phases other than S phase, the apparent stimulation of cells into S phases would be misleading.

Molecular Mechanisms

How does EPO prevent the death of late erythroid progenitors? No detailed mechanism that might be proposed currently has extensive experimental support. There are many molecular effects on erythroid cells induced by EPO, and these are currently being investigated in many laboratories [reviewed in Ref. 9]. Rapid effects of EPO include: (a) induction of tyrosine phosphorylation on several proteins, including the EPO receptor, (b) increased phosphorylation of certain proteins on serine and threonine by an enzyme with properties like protein kinase C, and (c) induction of *c-myc* mRNA accumulation. Slightly later effects include stimulation of total RNA synthesis, maintenance of protein synthesis, and increased glucose transport. Our laboratory is currently analyzing the effects of EPO on expression of a variety of transcription factors for which there is evidence of a role in erythroid development.

The Model of Erythropoiesis

Based on the work of other investigators on the analysis of erythroid progenitors in colony assays and on our observations of the role of EPO as a survival factor in FVA cells, we have proposed a model of erythropoiesis in vivo in which EPO tightly governs red blood cell (RBC) production by preventing apoptosis of EPO-dependent progenitors [3, 12] (Fig. 3). We postulate that there is a period during the differentiation of red cell progenitors during which EPO is required to prevent apoptosis. This period includes the CFU-E and subsequent proerythroblast stages and possibly the predecessors of the CFU-E, the mature BFU-E. We also postulate that individual progenitors within the EPO-dependent population exhibit a range of sensitivities to EPO such that there is an extended dose range of EPO over which individual progenitors may survive and continue proliferation and differentiation. Thus, the level of EPO ultimately controls RBC production by regulating the number of dependent progenitors that survive or die. The postulate of the model that individual progenitors exhibit a range of sensitivities to EPO is drawn partially from the following observation: in in vitro colony assays (e.g., of CFU-E or BFU-E), the number of colonies that develop increases with EPO concentration over a 100- to 1000-fold dose range. The molecular basis for such a variability in EPO sensitivity of progenitors is not known (see further discussion of heterogeneity of responsiveness).

The above model can account for the basic properties of erythropoiesis, including the control of RBC formation at a late stage and the apparent absence

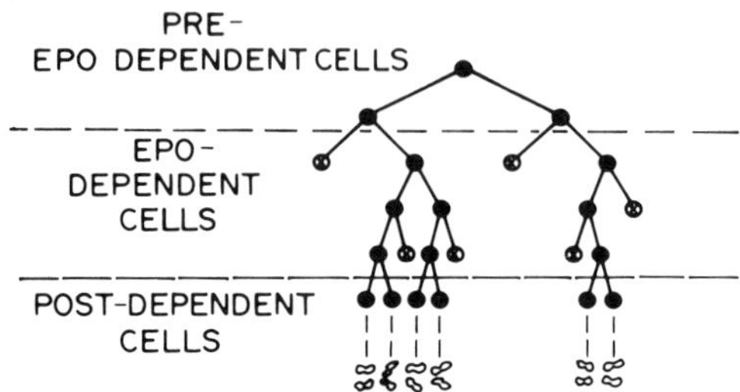

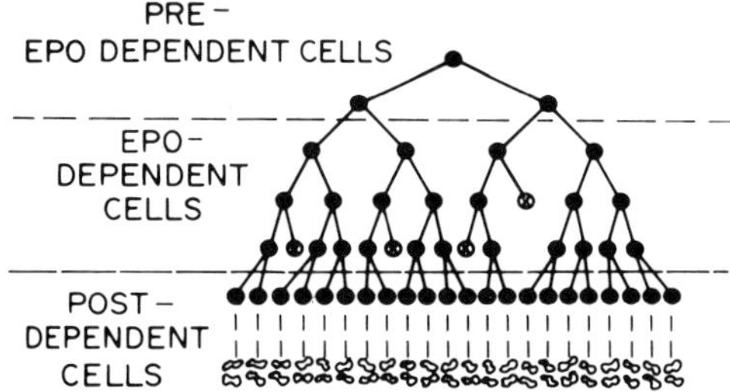

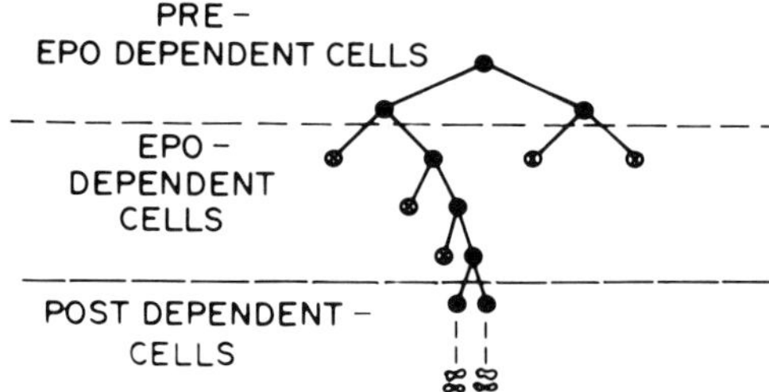

Fig. 3. Model of regulation of erythropoiesis based on EPO prevention of apoptosis. Dark circles represent live erythroid progenitor cells. Circles containing an × represent dead progenitors. The dashed lines bound the stages of erythroid differentiation in which the progenitors are dependent on EPO for survival. Dependence is used to mean that no other factors besides EPO can supply the survival maintenance functions for these stages. [Reprinted with permission from Ref. 12.]

in vivo of a latent state of mature erythroid progenitors. Studies in hematopoiesis have heretofore been very heavily dedicated to analyses of cell division regulation (e.g., regulation of immediate early gene expression, etc.) based on the conceptual frameworks and results from analyses of growth factor requirements and of the phenomenon of contact inhibition in established cell lines. To understand regulation of erythropoiesis and perhaps other systems in which proliferation from a stem cell is accompanied by terminal differentiation, it is necessary to incorporate apoptosis into the conceptual framework. Furthermore, it is worthwhile to recognize that the mechanism of apoptosis may be separate from the mechanisms of cell division or that these processes may be integrated into a linked process in some cells. Our data on FVA cells suggests that these two processes may have control pathways that can operate independently.

The Basis for Cellular Heterogeneity in Responsiveness to EPO

Whether a model of erythropoiesis proposes mitogenesis, cell survival, or differentiation as the basis of action of erythropoietin, one must postulate a heterogeneous response of progenitor cells as a function of EPO dose. The rate of generation of erythrocytes in vivo varies continuously from a normal rate at 10–30 mU of EPO per ml of plasma to a much greater rate at levels of 1–5 U of EPO per ml achieved during severe anemia. Some evidence suggests that the erythrocyte production rate may not be maximum except perhaps at the highest levels of EPO seen in vivo (7–10 U/ml of plasma). In vitro colony assays (CFU-E) at first suggested that, for the mouse, a plateau level of colony number was achieved at about 0.2 U/ml of EPO in the medium [13]. However, assays using recombinant EPO and more purified culture medium ingredients have shown increasing murine CFU-E up to EPO doses greater than 1 U/ml of culture medium [E. Dessypris, unpublished]. Numbers of colonies derived in culture from human CFU-E vary with concentration of EPO at least up to 2–3 U/ml [14]. In mouse FVA cells in culture, we find that EPO provides an increment of additional protection against cellular DNA degradation over a concentration range from 1 to 10 U/ml. We interpret these results to indicate that there is tremendous variation in the dose response of individual cells to EPO—a response range covering 100- to 1000-fold in EPO concentration. In the erythropoiesis model of Figure 3, this variation is illustrated by the concept that at a given level of EPO, some cells die while others survive and progress through differentiation.

What could be the basis for the proposed dose-response variation? One might postulate a time-dependent variation in cellular responsiveness based on cell cycle phase or degree of differentiation of individual cells; for example, a cell cycle dependence of the number of EPO receptors displayed. However, a time-dependent variation of responsiveness for a cell appears unlikely. Since EPO is stable during culture incubation and is ordinarily in excess in unbound form in the medium, one would expect all cells to eventually respond to the continuous presence of a single EPO concentration. We postulate that the different responsiveness of individual cells to EPO is an intrinsic property of the individual cell. Figure 4 shows two general variations of this concept. One possibility is that the degree of responsiveness is a characteristic of a cell that is set and fixed at each cell generation. Thus it would not be inherited, but rather the descendants of a single progenitor would represent the whole range of EPO sensitivity variation. An alternative possibility is a clonal, inherited responsitivity to EPO, which is set at some early progenitor stage and maintained in descendants. In principle it should be possible to distinguish the two possibilities by analyzing the EPO dose responsiveness of populations of CFU-E generated under conditions of high versus low EPO.

The molecular mechanisms for variations of EPO responsiveness are unknown, as are the ways in which the diversity might be generated. Reasonable guesses would be that: (a) there is a wide range of EPO receptor numbers displayed on individual cells, (b) there are variations in receptor subunit structure

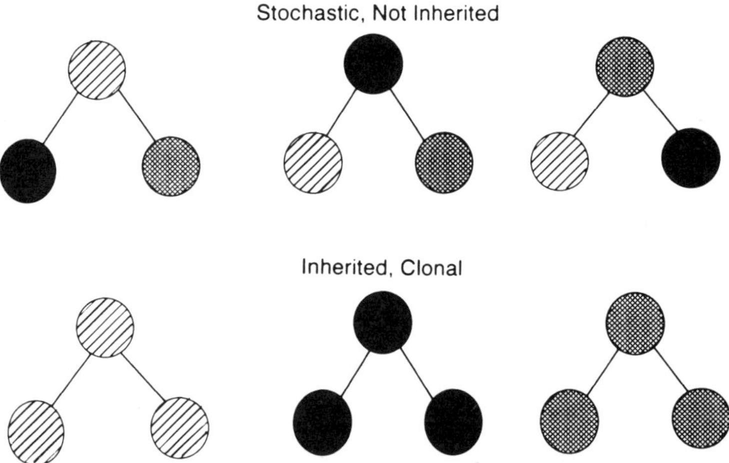

Fig. 4. Alternative models for intrinsic variation of erythroid progenitor responsiveness to EPO. The different patterned circles represent progenitor cells with inherently different dose level requirements for EPO. The top scheme depicts a model in which the variation is reproduced stochastically at each cell generation. The bottom scheme illustrates a model in which the responsiveness variation is generated at some early differentiation stage and afterwards is an inherited property of the descendants of individual progenitors.

in cells or variations in receptor primary structure due to alternative RNA splicing, or (c) there are great variations in internal signal transduction.

References

1 Eaves AC, Eaves CJ: Erythropoiesis in culture. Clin Haematol 1984;13:371–391.
2 Koury MJ, Bondurant MC: Maintenance by erythropoietin of viability and maturation of murine erythroid precursor cells. J Cell Physiol 1988;137:65–74.
3 Koury MJ, Bondurant MC: Erythropoietin retards DNA breakdown and prevents programmed death in erythroid progenitor cells. Science 1990;248:378–381.
4 Boyer SH, Bishop TR, Rogers OC, Noyes AN, Frelin LP, Hobbs S: Roles of erythropoietin, insulin-like growth factor-1, and unidentified serum factors in promoting maturation of purified murine erythroid colony forming units. Blood 1992;80: 2503–2512.
5 Koury MJ, Sawyer ST, Bondurant MC: Splenic erythroblasts in anemia-inducing Friend disease: A source of cells for studies of erythropoietin-mediated differentiation. J Cell Physiol 1984;121:526–534.
6 Nijhof W, Wierenga PK: Isolation and characterization of the erythroid progenitor cell: CFU-E. J Cell Biol 1983;96:386–392.
7 Sawada K, Krantz SB, Kans JS, Dessypris EN, Sawyer S, Glick AD, Civin CI: Purification of human erythroid colony-forming units and demonstration of specific binding of erythropoietin. J Clin Invest 1987;80:357–366.
8 Spivak JL: The mechanism of action of erythropoietin: Erythroid cell response. Hdbk Exp Pharmacol 1992;101:49–114.
9 Koury MJ, Bondurant MC: The molecular mechanism of erythropoietin action. Eur J Biochem 1992; 210:649–663.
10 Spivak JL, Pham T, Isaacs M, Hankins WD: Erythropoietin is both a mitogen and a survival factor. Blood 1991;77:1228–1233.
11 Dessypris EN, Krantz SB: Effect of pure erythropoietin on DNA-synthesis by human marrow day 15 erythroid burst forming units in short-term liquid culture. Br J Haematol 1984;56:295–306.
12 Koury MJ, Bondurant MC: Control of red cell production: The roles of programmed cell death (apoptosis) and erythropoietin. Transfusion 1990;30:673–674.
13 Iscove NN, Sieber F: Erythroid progenitors in mouse bone marrow detected by macroscopic colony formation in culture. Exp Hematol 1975;3:32–43.
14 Iscove NN, Sieber F, Winterhalter KH: Erythroid colony formation in cultures of mouse and human bone marrow: Analysis of the requirement for erythropoietin by gel filtration and affinity chromatography on agarose-concanavalin A. J Cell Physiol 1974;83:309–320.

Maurice Bondurant, Division of Hematology, Vanderbilt University School of Medicine, Medical Center North—Room C3101, Nashville, TN 37232 (USA)

Discussion

to the Paper by M. Bondurant et al.

Goldwasser (*Chicago*): I think it is important to point out what you already know: that these cells as well as the kind of CFU-E that you can purify all come from animals with high EPO titers. So there may be a perturbation in understanding the mechanism of action of EPO because you are already looking at cells hit by EPO.

Bondurant: The animals that FVA cells come from don't have high EPO. But of course these cells are being driven in their development by the virus up to this point. We cannot determine in our system where EPO begins to have an effect because the virus is supplying some activity which mimics EPO, at least up to a certain point. The other CFU-E systems, as Dr. Goldwasser points out, are derived in a very high-EPO environment. This certainly affects attempts to determine the beginning stage of the EPO requirement, and I think that is his point. I believe that, in vivo, control occurs at the period I mentioned based on other earlier studies. Whether or not EPO has effects earlier is still a matter of legitimate investigation.

Caro (*Philadelphia*): As you know, the bcl-2 gene has been proclaimed as being involved in apoptosis. Do you have any evidence that erythropoietin in some way affected the expression of the bcl-2 gene?

Bondurant: At the level of Northern blot analysis, these cells do not express the bcl-2 gene, and we do Northern blots at a sensitive level. Mouse MEL cells, the erythroid cell lines derived from Friend virus infection, do express bcl-2. So I think that this fact is the origin of people saying that bcl-2 is expressed in erythroid cells. Our evidence is that, in later erythroid cells, bcl-2 is not expressed at any level that we can detect. Thus, we do not think that changes in bcl-2 expression mediate the EPO effect.

Bauer (*Zurich*): Dr. Bondurant, you are suggesting somehow that these cells run automatically through the differentiation program provided there is enough erythropoietin? Can you be sure that erythropoietin itself is not helping in differentiation?

Bondurant: I am glad you pointed out something that I did not mention and had intended to. Of course I have not really distinguished between apoptosis, differentiation, and induction of mitosis. It could well be that EPO action is in facilitating or inducing a differentiation event, and that this differentiation event is coupled to the survival of these cells. In other words, erythropoietin could even be functioning, as far as I know, in some aspects of iron metabolism or iron handling inside of the cells which would obviate iron toxicity. So it could be involved in a differentiation step. Likewise one could say that it is inducing mitosis but that one cannot separate mitosis from death, that G_0 is not an option in these cells. No one knows that hematopoietic cells really can go into G_0 normally. So it could be that these processes are inextricably linked, and we will just have to find out how EPO works on a molecular level in the future.

Caro: The heterogeneity in EPO response is a postulate of your model. Do you have any experimental evidence that you do have heterogeneity in the response to EPO?

Bondurant: There is a lot of historical evidence when one looks back. In the colony-forming assay, individual colony numbers increase over a range of 2 to 2.5 logs of EPO dose. So there are individual cells in normal populations which can form colonies at 0.05 units per milliliter of EPO, and it takes well over 1.0 units per milliliter for other colonies to develop. Yes, and we also have evidence from subpopulations of our cells fractionated on Percoll for large differences in dose requirement.

Erythropoietin's Signaling Pathways and Primary Response Genes as Targets for Pharmacological Agents

Arthur J. Sytkowski

Laboratory for Cell and Molecular Biology, Division of Hematology and Oncology, New England Deaconess Hospital, and Department of Medicine, Harvard Medical School, Boston, Mass., USA

The intracellular signal generated by the interaction of erythropoietin (EPO) with its receptor results ultimately in the growth and differentiation of the erythroid progenitor cell. Recent work in our laboratory has been directed towards characterizing the signal transduction elements involved in this process. Additionally, we have sought to identify those genes whose expression is regulated immediately after arrival of the erythropoietin signal in the nucleus.

Our initial work in erythropoietin signal transduction was based upon studies of Friend murine erythroleukemia cells, which showed that the chemical inducer of differentiation—dimethyl sulfoxide (DMSO)—down-regulated the steady-state mRNA levels of the c-*myc* and c-*myb* protooncogenes. Additionally, it had been shown that down-regulation of either of these transcripts was necessary for DMSO-induced differentiation, since interference with this down-regulation precluded hemoglobinization of cells when exposed to the compound [1–6].

Can these findings tell us anything about the mechanism of action of erythropoietin, the natural inducer of erythropoiesis? What is the role of the *myc* and *myb* gene products in the regulation of erythroid growth and differentiation?

While our work was in progress, Todokoro et al. [7] showed that erythropoietin also regulated c-*myc* and c-*myb*, but, in contrast, to DMSO, caused up-regulation of c-*myc*. Both EPO and DMSO caused down-regulation of c-*myb* [7]. Our own results confirmed the findings of Todokoro and demonstrated further that the up-regulation of c-*myc* and the down-regulation of c-*myb* by EPO did not require de novo protein synthesis, thus identifying these two protooncogenes as *primary response genes* or *immediate/early genes* for EPO [8]. This identification of c-*myc* and c-*myb* as EPO primary response genes allowed us to use them as reporter genes for the arrival of the EPO signal at the nucleus. We employed the classical pharmacological tool of molecular blocking agents to identify elements of the signal transduction pathway.

We began with studies of c-*myc* and set out to determine first whether protein kinase C (PKC) was involved in the EPO-gencratcd signal. We selected a group of five inhibitors of PKC. These agents were drawn from among several chemical groups and exhibited different potencies toward PKC in solution. From published studies in a variety of cell types, we assembled a rank order of potency of these molecular blocking agents toward PKC [9–24]. We considered this order—staurosporine > sphingosine ≥ H7 > sangivomycin > H8—to be diagnostic of the PKC-mediated signal. We then tested the ability of each of these molecular blocking agents to block the erythropoietin signal to c-*myc* [25].

Each of the agents exhibited concentration-dependent inhibition of the erythropoietin c-*myc* response. Moreover, the rank order of potencies of these five agents toward the EPO signal was identical to that derived by us from other published studies. Thus, we concluded that PKC activation was involved in the erythropoietin signal to c-*myc*. This conclusion was confirmed by our further observation that both erythropoietin and the PKC agonist 12-O-tetradecanoyl-phorbol-13-acetate (TPA) induced phosphorylation of an 80 kd cytosolic protein substrate, designated pp80 (Fig. 1). The observation that a protein of this molecular size and isoelectric point (pI = 4.8) was phosphorylated when cells were treated with TPA or EPO served to identify it as a member of the p80 or "MARCKS" (myristoylated alanine rich C-kinase substrate) family of PKC

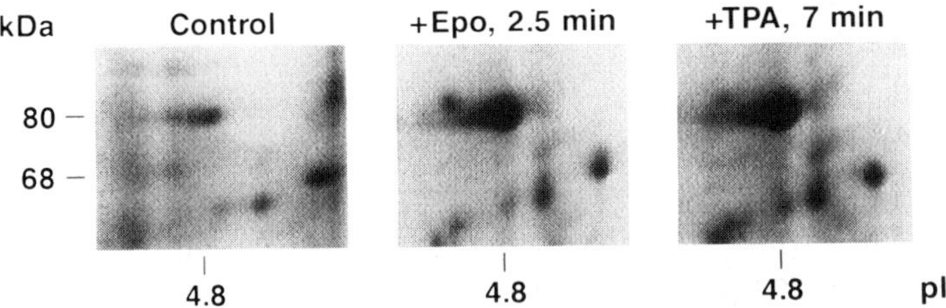

Fig. 1. pp80 phosphorylation is induced by both EPO and TPA in erythroid cells. (Left panel) ^{32}P-labeled phosphoproteins from untreated Rauscher murine erythroleukemia cell cultures analyzed by two dimensional gel electrophoresis. (Center panel) ^{32}P-labeled phosphoproteins from cultures treated for 2.5 min with EPO (10 U/ml). (Right panel) ^{32}P-labeled phosphoproteins from cultures treated with TPA (150 nM) for 7 min. pp80 is clearly induced in both treated cultures. Autoradiograph of two-dimensional electrophoretic separation.

substrates [26, 27]. Interestingly, TPA itself does not up-regulate c-*myc* in erythroid cells, in contrast to its action on c-*myc* in other cell types, such as lymphocytes. There are at least two possible explanations for this difference. First, EPO may activate a TPA-insensitive isoform of PKC. Indeed, recent evidence obtained in studies of thymocytes have demonstrated that PKC epsilon serves just such a role [28]. Second, erythropoietin up-regulation of c-*myc* may require simultaneous activation of a second, independent pathway so that PKC activation is necessary but not sufficient for c-*myc* regulation. At present, we have not yet distinguished between these or among other alternative explanations.

Next, we turned our attention to EPO regulation of c-*myb* [29]. The totally unexpected results of these studies prove that the interaction of EPO with its receptor results in the simultaneous activation of two discrete signaling pathways that regulate c-*myc* and c-*myb* differently. This conclusion was made possible using still another pharmacological agent that specifically blocks the function of a different class of putative signaling elements. This agent, okadaic acid, is a compound that inhibits protein phosphatases of the 1 and 2A classes [30–32]. Importantly, these phosphatase enzymes function in opposition to protein kinase C, namely, by dephosphorylating phosphoserine and phosphothreonine residues in proteins. In comparing erythropoietin's simultaneous up-regulation of c-*myc* and down-regulation of c-*myb*, we found that, whereas PKC inhibitors such as H7 blocked up-regulation of c-*myc*, they had absolutely no effect on down-regulation of c-*myb* (Fig. 2). Rather, okadaic acid blocked down-regulation of c-*myb* while having no effect on up-regulation of c-*myc*. This okadaic acid inhibition of c-*myb* regulation was concentration dependent with an IC_{50} consistent with a specific phosphatase 1,2A inhibition. From these results we concluded provisionally that activation of the erythropoietin receptor generated two simultaneous signaling pathways, a PKC-dependent pathway to c-*myc*, and a phosphatase-dependent pathway to c-*myb*.

In order to explore these mechanisms further, we used the PKC inhibitor H7 and the phosphatase inhibitor okadaic acid to determine whether EPO's regulation of c-*myc* and c-*myb* was at the level of transcription. First, we assessed mRNA stability of c-*myc* and c-*myb* and found that neither EPO treatment alone nor EPO plus inhibitors changed the half-lives of either transcript. Our direct demonstration of transcriptional regulation was based upon similar mechanisms of transcriptional control in both the c-*myc* and c-*myb* genes.

In each gene there is an important transcriptional regulatory site in the first intron [33–36]. This element is responsible for a so-called ''transcriptional arrest'' or ''transcriptional attentuation'' mechanism, presumably due to the

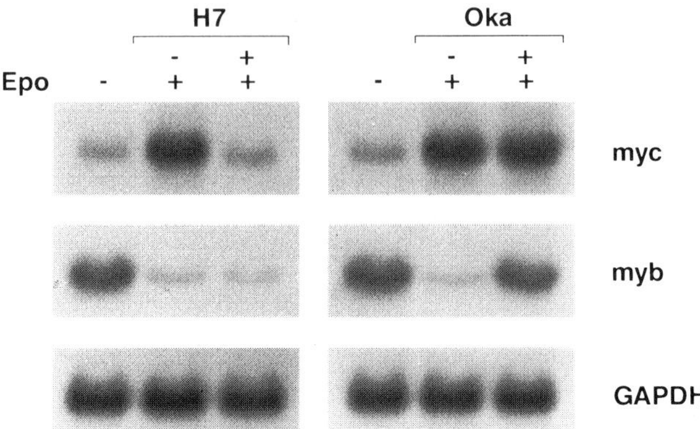

Fig. 2. Effects of H7 or okadaic acid on the c-*myc* and c-*myb* responses to erythropoietin. Northern analysis was performed on RNA isolated from Rauscher cells stimulated with erythropoietin for 2 h in the absence or presence of H7 or okadaic acid (Oka). H7 was used at 50 μ*M*, a concentration that we have shown previously to block the c-*myc* response, and okadaic acid was used at 400 n*M*. Note the inhibition of the c-*myc* and c-*myb* responses by H7 and okadaic acid, respectively.

binding of one or more transcription factors to the element in the respective intron I. Whether these transcription factors are positive or negative regulating is uncertain. After transcription of c-*myc* or c-*myb* is initiated and proceeds through exon I and into intron I, the arrest mechanism must be "released" in order to allow synthesis to continue into exon II, resulting in full-length transcripts such as are detected by conventional Northern analyses. We hypothesized that we could demonstrate this mechanism for EPO by nuclear run-on assays and, additionally, could determine if the EPO signal from PKC to c-*myc* and from phosphatase to c-*myb* operated on these transcriptional regulatory sites.

These experiments demonstrated that erythropoietin regulates transcriptional elongation of c-*myc* and c-*myb* (Fig. 3). In the absence of EPO, transcription of c-*myc* is blocked within intron I, whereas c-*myb* transcription continues into exon II, resulting in full-length transcripts. EPO does not affect the transcription rate of exon I of either protooncogene appreciably. Importantly, EPO induces transcriptional elongation of c-*myc* as evidenced by the increase in exon II. Simultaneously, EPO induces transcriptional arrest of c-*myb*. This is supported by the profound reduction in exon II, which leads to the decrease in steady state c-*myb* mRNA levels. The phosphatase inhibitor okadaic acid reverses the decrease in c-*myb* exon II transcription caused by EPO but does not change c-*myc* exon II transcription. The PKC inhibitor H7 reverses the EPO-induced up-regulation of c-*myc* exon II, while it does not alter c-*myb* transcription. These data confirm

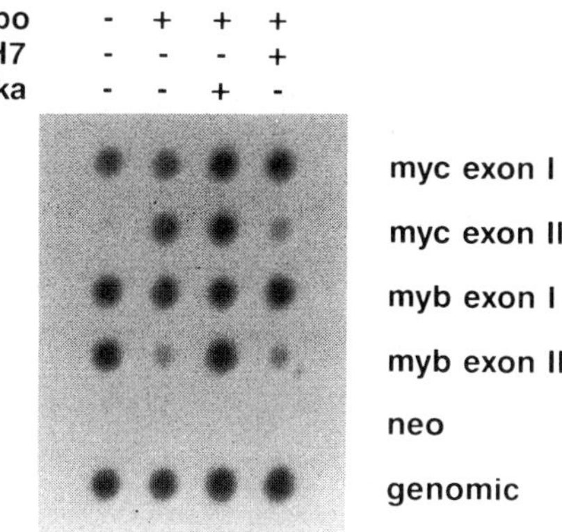

Fig. 3. Effect of erythropoietin on the transcriptional elongation rates and the mRNA stabilities of c-*myc* and c-*myb*. Transcription run-on assays were performed using nuclei isolated from untreated cells or cells treated with erythropoietin for 2 h in the absence or presence of H7 or okadaic acid. ''neo'' indicates neomycin DNA serving as a negative control. Similar results were obtained in two separate experiments.

that okadaic acid and H7 act by inhibiting discrete signaling pathways involved in the transmission of the EPO receptor–generated signals that regulate gene transcription.

The demonstration of a protein phosphatase–dependent signal from the EPO receptor to c-*myb* prompted us to compare Epo's mechanism of action with that of dimethyl sulfoxide. Both the natural inducer and the chemical inducer down-regulate c-*myb* steady-state mRNA levels and lead to terminal differentiation. Earlier studies from our laboratory indicated that these two inducers have different mechanisms of action since EPO-responsive and DMSO-responsive cells could be segregated by cell cloning methodology [37]. As predicted, DMSO down-regulation of c-*myb* was completely resistant to okadaic acid, indicating that DMSO does not regulate c-*myb* through the same phosphatase-dependent pathway as erythropoietin. Also supportive of this conclusion are the results of experiments on the EPO-induced dephosphorylation of pp43, an erythroid membrane–associated phosphoprotein [38, 39]. Whereas, pp43 is rapidly dephosphorylated in the presence of erythropoietin, DMSO is without effect on this protein. Taken together, these results indicate that DMSO regulation of c-*myb* and induction of erythropoiesis occurs independently of EPO receptor activation.

The common effect of both EPO and DMSO on down-regulating c-*myb* expression associated with their action in inducing erythroid differentiation caused us to question whether artificial down-regulation of c-*myb* mRNA levels could mimic some or all of the action of these agents [40]. Indeed, we showed that treatment of Rauscher erythroleukemia cells with an antisense oligodeoxynucleotide to c-*myb* resulted in hemoglobin synthesis to the same degree as that induced by erythropoietin. Interestingly, this induction of hemoglobin occurred without any significant effect on cell proliferation, in contrast to studies of several other hematopoietic cell types in which down-regulation of *myb* is strongly associated with arrest of proliferation [41–43]. However, down-regulation of c-*myb* with antisense oligos did not result in terminal differentiation of the target cell, but rather led to expression of a subset of erythroid specific genes.

It appears that c-*myc* and c-*myb* are but two of a group of primary response genes regulated by EPO which serve as regulators of specific subsets of secondary (erythroid specific) response genes. Recently, we have isolated several up-regulated and down-regulated EPO primary response genes by differential screening of an EPO-induced cDNA library. Preliminary DNA sequencing data of some of these genes has identified one with two zinc finger motifs, suggesting that it may be a new transcription factor, and six other genes that appear to be novel (J. Keutzer and A. J. Sytkowski, unpublished). We propose that the identification of these primary response genes and the characterization of the signal pathways leading to them will provide us with important new targets for pharmaceutical manipulation of hematopoietic cell growth and differentiation.

Acknowledgments

The author acknowledges the collaboration of Drs. Steven Bailey, Yijuang Chern, Hye-Seon Choi, Hiren Patel, and Rudolph Spangler and the excellent editorial work of Rosemary Panza. This work was supported in part by NIH Grant #DK38841 and U.S. Navy Grant #N00014-90-J-1847.

References

1   Lachman H, Skoultchi AI: Expression of c-myc changes during differentiation of mouse erythroleukemia cells. Nature 1984;310:592–594.
2   Coppola JA, Cole MD: Constitutive c-myc oncogene expression blocks mouse erythroleukemia cell differentiation but not commitment. Nature 1986;320:760–763.
3   Dmitrovsky E, Kuehl WM, Hollis GF, Kirsch IR, Bender TP, Segal S: Expression of a transfected human c-myc oncogene inhibits differentiation of a mouse erythroleukemia cell line. Nature 1986;322:748–750.
4   Prochownik EV, Kukowski J: Deregulated expression of c-myc by murine erythroleukemia cells prevents differentiation. Nature 1986;322:848–850.

5   Ramsay RG, Ikeda K, Rifkind RA, Marks PA: Changes in gene expression associated with induced differentiation of erythroleukemia: Protooncogenes, globin genes, and cell division. Proc Natl Acad Sci USA 1986;83:6849–6853.

6   Clarke MF, Kukowska-Latallo JF, Westin E, Smith M, Prochownik EV: Constitutive expression of a c-myb cDNA blocks Friend murine erythroleukemia cell differentiation. Mol Cell Biol 1988;8:884–892.

7   Todokoro K, Watson RJ, Higo H, Amanuma H, Kuramochi S, Yanagisawa H, Ikawa Y: Down-regulation of c-myb gene expression is a prerequisite for erythropoietin-induced erythroid differentiation. Proc Natl Acad Sci USA 1988;85: 8900–8904.

8   Chern Y, Spangler R, Choi H-S, Sytkowski AJ: Erythropoietin activates the receptor in both Rauscher and Friend murine erythroleukemia cells. J Biol Chem 1991;266:2009–2012.

9   Hidaka H, Inagaki M, Kawamoto S, Sasaki Y: Isoquinolinesulfonamides, novel and potent inhibitors of cyclic nucleotide dependent protein kinase and protein kinase C. Biochem 1984;23:5036–5041.

10 Narindrasorasak S, Brickenden A, Ball E, Sanwal BD: Regulation of protein kinase C by cyclic adenosine 3′:5′-monophosphate and a tumor promoter in skeletal myoblasts. J Biol Chem 1987;262:10497–10501.

11 Mary D, Peyron J-F, Auberger P, Aussel C, Fehlmann M: Modulation of T cell activation by differential regulation of the phosphorylation of two cytosolic proetins. Implications of both Ca^{2+} and cyclic AMP-dependent protein kinases. J Biol Chem 1989;264:14498–14502.

12 Sehgal PB, Walther Z, Tamm I: Rapid enhancement of beta 2-expression in human fibroblasts by diacylglycerols and the calcium ionophore A23187. Proc Natl Acad Sci USA 1987;84:3663–3667.

13 Fan X-D, Goldberg M, Bloom BR: Interferon-gamma-induced transcriptional activation is mediated by protein kinase C. Proc Natl Acad Sci USA 1988;85:5122–5125.

14 Doglio A, Dani C, Grimaldi P, Ailhaud G: Growth hormone stimulates c-fos gene expression by means of protein kinase C without increasing inositol lipid turnover. Proc Natl Acad Sci USA 1989;86:1148–1152.

15 Spangler R, Joseph C, Qureshi SA, Berg KL, Foster DA: Evidence that v-src and v-fps gene products use a protein kinase C-mediated pathway to induce expression of a transformation-related gene. Proc Natl Acad Sci USA 1989;86:7017–7021.

16 Zhang H, Buckley NE, Gibson K, Spiegel S: Sphingosine stimulates cellular proliferation via a protein kinase C-independent pathway. J Biol Chem 1990;265:76–81.

17 Tamaoki T, Nomoto H, Takahashi I, Kato Y, Morimoto M, Tomita F: Staurosporine, a potent inhibitor of phospholipid/Ca^{++} dependent protein kinase. Biochem Biophys Res Commun 1986;135:397–402.

18 Vegesna RVK, Wu H-L, Mong S, Crooke ST: Staurosporine inhibits protein kinase C and prevents phorbol ester-mediated leukotriene D4 receptor desensitization in RBL-1 cells. Mol Pharmacol 1988;33:537–542.

19 Winkler JD, Sarau HM, Foley JJ, Crooke ST: Phorbol 12-myristate 13-acetate inhibition of leukotriene D4-induced signal transduction was rapidly reversed by staurosporine. Biochem Biophys Res Commun 1988;157:521–529.

20 Hannun YA, Loomis CR, Merrill AH Jr, Bell RM: Sphingosine inhibition of protein

kinase C activity and of phorbol dibutyrate binding in vitro and in human platelets. J Biol Chem 1986;261:12604–12609.

21 Ghosh TK, Bian J, Gill DL: Intracellular calcium release mediated by sphingosine derivatives generated in cells. Science 1990;248:1653–1656.

22 Faucher M, Girones N, Hannun YA, Bell RM, Davis RJ: Regulation of the epidermal growth factor receptor phosphorylation state by sphingosine in A431 human epidermoid carcinoma cells. J Biol Chem 1988;263:5319–5327.

23 Smal J, DeMeyts P: Sphingosine, an inhibitor of protein kinase C, suppresses the insulin-like effects of growth hormone in rat adipocytes. Proc Natl Acad Sci USA 1989;86:4705–4709.

24 Loomis CR, Bell RM: Sangivamycin, a nucleotide analogue, is a potent inhibitor of protein kinase C. J Biol Chem 1988;263:1682–1692.

25 Spangler R, Bailey SC, Sytkowski AJ: Erythropoietin increases c-myc mRNA by a protein kinase C-dependent pathway. J Biol Chem 1991;266:681–684.

26 Blackshear PJ, Wen L, Glynn BP, Witters LA. Protein kinase C-stimulated phosphorylation in vitro of a Mr 80,000 protein phosphorylated in response to phorbol esters and growth factors in intact fibroblasts. Distinction from protein kinase C and prominence in brain. J Biol Chem 1986;261:1459–1469.

27 Albert KA, Walaas SI, Wang JK-T, Greengard P: Widespread occurrence of "87 kDa," a major specific substrate for protein kinase C. Proc Natl Acad Sci USA 1986;83:2822–2826.

28 Strulovici B, Daniel-Issakani S, Baxter G, Knopf J, Sultzman L, Cherwinski H, Nestor, Jr J, Webb DR, Ransom J Distinct mechanisms of regulation of protein kinase C by hormones and phorbol diesters. J Biol Chem 1991;266:168–173.

29 Patel HR, Choi HS, Sytkowski AJ: Activation of two discrete signaling pathways by erythropoietin. J Biol Chem 1992; 267:21300–21302.

30 Bialojan C, Takai A: Inhibitory effect of a marine-sponge toxin, okadaic acid, on protein phosphatases. Specificity and kinetics. Biochem J 1988;256:283–290.

31 Haystead TAJ, Sim ATR, Carling D, Honnor RC, Tsukitani Y, Cohen P, Hardie DG: Effects of the tumor promoter okadaic acid on intracellular protein phosphorylation and metabolism. Nature 1989;337:78–81.

32 Hartshorne DJ, Ishihara H, Karaki H, Ozaki H, Sato K, Hori M, Watabe S: Adv Protein Phosphastases 1989;5:219–231.

33 Zimmerman K, Alt FW: Expression and function of myc family genes. Oncogenesis 1990;2:75–95.

34 Shen-Ong GLC: The *myb* oncogene. Biochim Biophys Acta 1990;1032:39–52.

35 Watson RJ: A transcriptional arrest mechanism involved in controlling constitutive levels of mouse c-*myb* mRNA. Oncogene 1989;2:267–272.

36 Watson RJ: Expression of the c-myb and c-myc genes is regulated independently in differentiating mouse erythroleukemia cells by common processes of premature transcription arrest and increased mRNA turnover. Mol Cell Biol 1988;8: 3938–3942.

37 Sytkowski AJ, Salvado AJ, Smith GM, McIntyre CJ, DeBoth NJ: Erythroid differentiation of clonal Rauscher erythroleukemia cells in response to erythropoietin or dimethylsulfoxide. Science 1980;210:74–76.

38 Choi H-S, Wojchowski DM, Sytkowski AJ: Erythropoietin rapidly alters phosphorylation of pp43, and erythroid membrane protein. J Biol Chem 1987;262: 2933–2936.

39 Choi H-S, Bailey SC, Donahue KA, Vanasse GJ, Sytkowski AJ: Purification and characterization of the erythropoietin-sensitive membrane phosphoprotein, pp43. J Biol Chem 1990;265:4143–4148.

40 Chern Y, O'Hara C, Sytkowski AJ: Induction of hemoglobin synthesis by down-regulation of MYB protein with an antisense oligodeoxynucleotide. Blood 1991;78:991–996.

41 Gerwitz AM, Calabretta B: A c-myb antisense oligodeoxynucleotide inhibits normal human hematopoiesis in vitro. Science 1988;242:1303–1306.

42 Anfossi G, Gewirtz AM, Calabretta B: An oligomer complementary to c-myb-encoded mRNA inhibits proliferation of human myeloid leukemia cell lines. Proc Natl Acad Sci USA 1989;86:3379–3383.

43 Valtieri M, Venturelli D, Care A, Fossati C, Pelosi E, Labbaye C, Mattia G, Gewirtz AM, Calabretta B, Peschle C: Antisense myb inhibition of purified erythroid progenitors in development and differentiation is linked to cycling activity and expression of DNA polymerase α. Blood 1991;77:1181–1190.

Arthur J. Sytkowski, MD, Laboratory for Cell and Molecular Biology, New England Deaconess Hospital, 21-27 Burl. Building—Room 548, 185 Pilgrim Road, Boston, MA 02215 (USA)

Discussion

to the Paper by A. J. Sytkowski

Bauer (Zurich): It has been reported in the literature that gp55, which is a viral envelope glycoprotein, also can mimic the effect of EPO. Have you had a chance to test this gp55 in your system to see if the intracellular signaling is identical or similar to EPO?

Sytkowski: That's a very important question. We have not studied gp55 per se. However, we have looked at Friend erythroleukemia cells, which are the paradigm for this described interaction. gp55 is a Friend virus–encoded glycoprotein. It appears to bind to the EPO receptor *inside* the cell and it is believed to be the cause of the Friend virus–induced transformation. However, the EPO receptors *on the surface* of the Friend cell act just like Rauscher cell or normal erythroid cell EPO receptors that I have described. You can up-regulate *myc* and down-regulate *myb* with erythropoietin in a Friend cell, although the Friend cell does not hemoglobinize. Whatever signal is being activated by interaction of the EPO receptor with gp55 in the cell is not the same as those generated by erythropoietin at the surface of the cell which regulate *c-myc* or *c-myb*.

Schaffner (Zurich): There is now increasing evidence, for instance from Georg Bornkamm (Munich) with *myc*, that this premature stop of transcription is somehow regulated by the use of either of two promoters in the *myc* gene. So from one promoter there is always read-through; with the other there can be this transcriptional premature termination. Have you checked whether there is a switch in promoter use?

Sytkowski: We have not. That's a very good idea. Thank you.

A Case of Antierythropoietin Antibodies Following Recombinant Human Erythropoietin Treatment

Harald Bergrem,[a] Bo G. Danielson,[b] Kai-Uwe Eckardt,[c] Armin Kurtz,[c] Mats Stridsberg[d]

[a]Department of Medicine, Central Hospital of Rogaland, Stavanger, Norway; [b]Department of Medicine and [d]Department of Clinical Chemistry, University Hospital, Uppsala, Sweden; and [c]Institute of Physiology, University of Regensburg, Germany

Summary

The advent of recombinant human erythropoietin (EPO) for use in clinical medicine has markedly improved the quality of life for patients with renal anemia. Despite a widespread use of EPO, anti-EPO antibody formation seems to be extremely rare. We report a dialysis patient showing strong evidence for the production of anti-EPO antibodies. The patient, a 60-year-old woman with chronic pyelonephritis on chronic hemodialysis since September 1989, had a blood transfusion in December 1989. In May 1990 she was started on EPO treatment (Behringwerke, Marburg, Germany). She responded to EPO, but after 6 months she developed severe anemia. She was investigated for this, and no other cause was found except the presence of anti-EPO antibodies. The presence of anti-EPO antibodies was confirmed by two different radioimmunoassays. Since the patient had also developed HLA antibodies, she was given a series of plasma exchange treatments where both the titer of HLA and anti-EPO antibodies could be reduced. She has been successfully transplanted. One month after transplantation the anti-EPO antibody titer was barely detectable. Even though the formation of EPO antibodies seems to be rare, it has to be considered as a potential risk.

Introduction

The advent of EPO for use in clinical medicine has markedly improved the quality of life for patients with renal anemia, especially patients in hemodialysis [1]. In spite of the fact that recombinant EPO is produced in mammalian cell lines and despite the rapid increase in clinical use, no report has been published on the development of true anti-EPO antibodies [2]. We here report the first patient displaying strong evidence for the production of anti-EPO antibodies.

Case History

The patient is a 60 year-old-woman with chronic pyelonephritis (recurrent upper UTI, IVP showed typical changes) having no history of allergies, joint pains, or rashes suggestive of systemic disease. In January 1989 investigation for a transplant did not show detectable leukocyte antibodies. The patient was put on the transplant waiting list, and hemodialysis was started in September 1989. In December 1989, the patient received 2 units of leukocyte-free blood. Routine screening for leukocyte antibodies in June 1990 showed antibodies against 50–85% of the panel cells. The patient has since remained panel reactive antibody (PRA)–positive. Because of the existing anemia, the patient was included in an EPO study (Behringwerke, Marburg, Germany) in May 1990. Her hemoglobin rose from 61 to 110 g/l during 20 weeks on an average i.v. EPO dose of 75 IU/kg BW, 2 times/week after dialysis (Fig. 1). After 27 weeks, hemoglobin started to fall gradually despite continued EPO treatment and ferritin levels between 200 and 800 μg/l. The patient was admitted and investigated for anemia (no hemolysis, negative gastroscopy, colonoscopy, negative stool tests for blood, normal serum electrophoresis, and no signs of malignant disease or infection). Serum concentrations of EPO measured by radioimmunoassay were in the range of 70–200 U/l. She was put on EPO 175 IU/kg i.v. 2 times/week without response and needed 4 units of blood because of anemia-related angina pectoris during the next 8 weeks. EPO treatment was then discontinued and has not been given since. As no other cause of anemia was found, serum was screened for anti-EPO antibodies in January 1991 (Spectra Lab, Uppsala, Sweden).

Screening for Anti-EPO Antibodies

An assay for detection of antibodies was developed as a modification of the radioimmunoassay for EPO described by Egrie et al. [3]. Serum samples (diluted

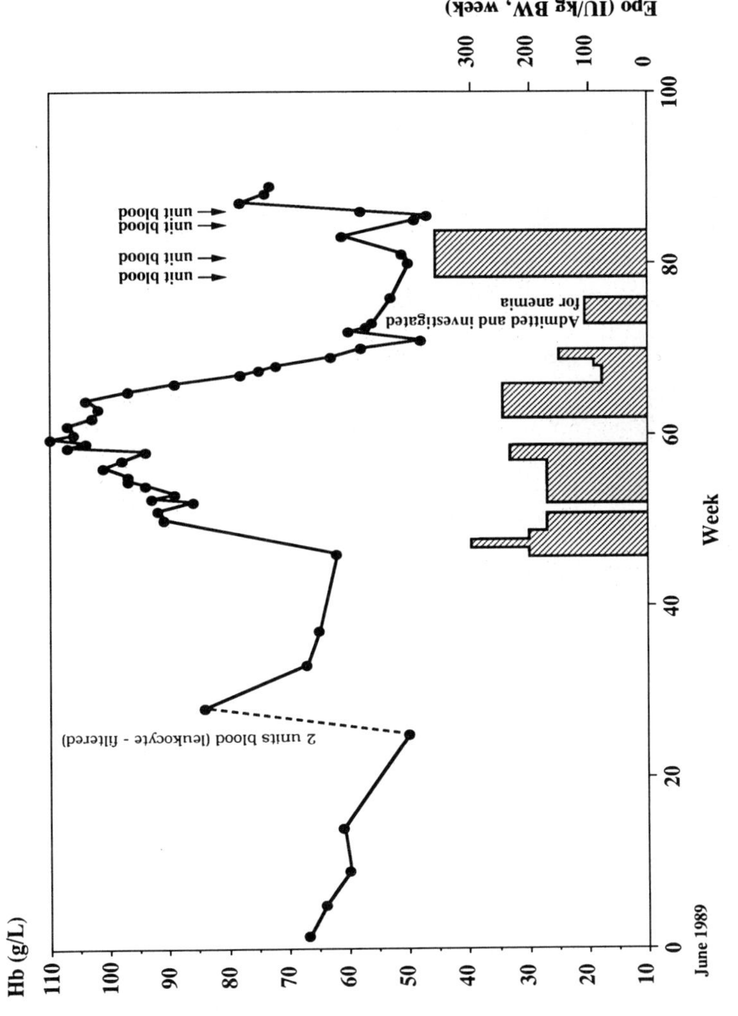

Fig. 1. Hemoglobin levels and the weekly EPO doses given to patient.

1/10) were incubated with ^{125}I recombinant human EPO (Amersham International, UK) for 2 days. IgG fractions were separated from the samples by means of protein A coupled to sepharose beads (Pharmacia, Sweden) and counted in a gamma counter. A sample containing antibodies against EPO bound the labeled Epo and thus was detected as an increased amount of radioactivity. Pooled human sera, free from anti-EPO antibodies, was used as a negative control, and a positive control was prepared by adding a fixed amount of rabbit polyclonal antiserum against EPO (Amgen, California, USA) to the pooled sera. The titer of EPO antibodies was presented in radioimmunoassay units (RU), which is an arbitrary unit specific for this assay [1].

Scatchard Analysis of EPO Binding

100 µl of the patient serum (at a 1:300 dilution) were incubated with graded doses (3–30 fmol) of ^{125}I-recombinant human EPO (spec. activity 600 Ci/mM; Amersham International, UK) in a total volume of 300 µl for 24 h (Fig. 2). Then 100 µl of goat antihuman IgG (Sigma International, Taufkirchen, Germany) were added and 4 h later the samples were centrifuged at 2000 g for 10 min. The

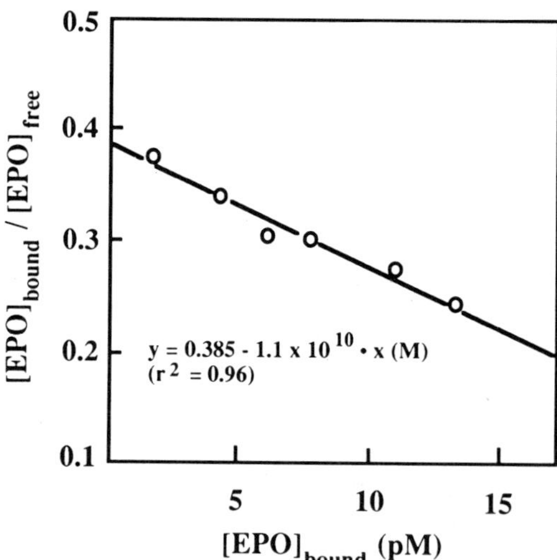

Fig. 2. Scatchard plot of EPO binding by the patient serum. Experiments were done as described in the Methods section.

pellets were counted for radioactivity. Bound EPO concentrations were calculated from the radioactivity after background subtraction. Free EPO concentrations were calculated as the difference of radioactivity precipitable by trichloroacetic acid (i.e., total EPO) and radioactivity of the pellet.

Analysis of Displacement of EPO Binding

To examine whether the binding of EPO (Fig. 3) by the patient serum was competitive, the serum at different dilutions (1:10 to 1:1000) was used as the primary antibody in a radioimmunoassay previously described by us [4]. As the secondary antibody a goat antihuman IgG antiserum (Sigma International) was used. Displacement of radiolabeled EPO was achieved with graded doses of recombinant human EPO (Amersham International, UK) calibrated against the WHO standard (2nd reference preparation B) in our radioimmunoassay [4].

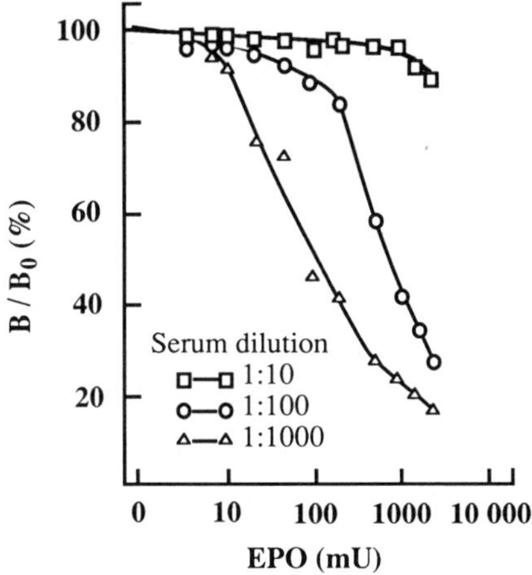

Fig. 3. Displacement of binding of radiolabeled EPO to the patient serum by unlabeled EPO. Patient serum at different dilutions was used as the primary antibody for a radioimmunoassay described in the methods section. B/B_0 gives the ratio of radioactivity bound by the serum in presence of unlabeled EPO over the radioactivity bound in the absence of unlabeled EPO. Total radioactivity of ^{125}I-EPO added per test tube was 10,000 cpm. B_0 was 84, 50, and 12% of total radioactivity at the serum dilutions of 1:10, 1:100, and 1:1000, respectively. EPO in mU gives the amount of unlabeled EPO per ml of solution, 100 μl of which were added to the test tubes.

Results

Approximately 10 weeks after the steep decline of hemoglobin concentrations, the serum of the patient was for the first time screened for EPO antibodies. In fact, a rather high titer of 400 RU IgG antibodies against EPO was found at that time. Scatchard analysis of EPO binding by the serum yielded an affinity constant of 1.1×10^{10} (M^{-1}) and in a binding capacity of 32 nmol EPO per l plasma (Fig. 2). Assuming a specific activity of pure EPO of about 100 000 IU/mg and a molecular mass of around 30 kd, the binding capacity of the serum corresponds to around 100,000 IU/l plasma. The binding of EPO by the antiserum was, moreover, competitive. As shown in Figure 3, bound radiolabeled EPO could be displaced by graded doses of unlabeled EPO.

Since the patient had human leukocyte antibodies, she was given 14 plasma exchange treatments and was started on immunosuppressive treatment with prednisolone and cyclophosphamide from April 1991 (week 88) to reduce these antibodies to increase the chances for a successful kidney transplant. As a result of the plasmapheresis the EPO antibody titer could be reduced (from week 95) (Table 1) and kept low. The patient had no bleeding, infection, inflammation, malignancy, or iron depletion.

Discussion

The initial hemoglobin increase from 62 to 92 g/l in 4 weeks in response to EPO treatment showed that the drug worked as expected and that a dose of 75 IU $\times$ 2/week was suitable for this patient. Because of the good response EPO was

Table 1.   Serum anti-EPO antibody titers

Week	Anti-EPO (RU)
82	400
89	200
94	400
95	70
96	20
97	10
98	10
99	10
100	10

Reference values: <10 RU (no antibodies found).

stopped for 3 weeks but restarted at 125 IU/kg BW. Despite the use of the higher dose, hemoglobin started to fall (Fig. 1). It is unlikely that withdrawing the drug for 3 weeks could cause such a decline in hemoglobin (Fig. 1) [5], and it is clear that the decline had started before the dose was reduced from week 66. Also, the lack of response to 175 IU/kg BW $\times$ 2/week, given for 7 weeks (weeks 78–85) in the absence of any other cause of anemia suggested the possibility of anti-EPO antibodies. The patient had no malignant or infectious disease associated with EPO resistance [2]. Her PTH was slightly elevated, but she had no hypercalcemia. Serum aluminum was also slightly elevated, but it is very unlikely that these factors could cause such a difference in response to EPO within a period of 45 weeks. The patient's serum ferritin was between 200 and 800 μg/l, and she needed several blood transfusions because of angina pectoris. The existence of EPO antibodies as found in this study, on the other hand, would provide a good explanation for the development of anemia and the resistance to recombinant EPO. Since the binding capacity of the serum for EPO is as high as 100,000 IU/l and the affinity of serum for EPO is rather high as typical for antibodies, it can be expected that the concentration of free EPO in the serum is very low. The rather high concentrations of EPO measured in the serum are most likely the result of a technical artefact due to the existence of the antibodies that will compete for tracer binding with the antiserum used for the radioimmunoassay (usually rabbit antihuman EPO).

The serum EPO antibody titer was reduced by the repeated plasmapheresis treatment. The patient was successfully transplanted with excellent renal function, but initially with lack of hemoglobin response. This seems most likely to be due to EPO antibodies, since no other obvious reasons for persistent anemia such as bleeding, infection, malignancy, and iron depletion were present.

Despite a large number of patients having been treated with recombinant EPO in recent years, the recombinant hormone has not yet been reported to be antigenic. Its protein moiety of 165 amino acids is identical to that of human urinary EPO and corresponds to predictions from the human EPO gene [6, 7], except for a terminal arginine residue that is lacking in both recombinant and native EPO isolated from human urine [8]. Extensive glycosylation of the EPO protein, however, results in some heterogeneity of EPO molecules. Differences have been found in the carbohydrate moieties of native urinary EPO among different individuals [9], and some, albeit minor, differences have also been observed between recombinant human EPO produced by CHO cells and human urinary EPO [10]. Notably, the patient studied was treated with recombinant EPO produced by mouse C 127 fibroblasts, and the glycosylation pattern of this preparation has not yet been reported. A recent comparison of specific activities by in vivo bioassays of different preparations of recombinant human EPO, including the one used for treatment of our patient, suggests, however, that glycosylation patterns differ, depending on the cell type used for EPO synthesis [11]. This may have an impact on the antigenicity of different preparations of the recombinant hormone. A contributing factor for the development of EPO antibodies in this patient could have been that she may be immunologically very active, as she formed antibodies towards panel cells after two transfusions of filtered blood.

Even though the formation of EPO antibodies seems to be rare, it must be considered as a potential risk, which may result in severe complications to be taken into account when several new hemopoietic growth factors are added to the therapeutic arsenal in the near future.

References

1   Eschbach JW, Egrie JC, Downing MR, Browne JK, Adamson JW: Correction of the anemia of end-stage renal disease with recombinant human erythropoietin. Results of a combined phase I and phase II clinical trial. N Engl J Med 1987;316:73–78.

2   Spivak JL: Introduction and overview, in Overview of the Literature Related to Erythropoietin 1990. Excerpta Medica 1991, vol 2, pp 1–6.

3   Egrie JC, Lane J, Gaines Das RE, Tam RC: Development of radioimmunoassays for human erythropoietin using recombinant erythropoietin as tracer and imunogen. J Immunol Methods 1987;99:235–241.

4   Eckardt KU, Kurtz A, Hirth P, Scigalla P, Wieczorek L, Bauer C: Evaluation of the stability of human erythropoietin in samples for radioimmunoassay. Klin Wochenschr 1988;66:241–245.

5   Taylor JE, Henderson IS, Mactier RA, Stewart WK: Effects of withdrawing erythropoietin. Br Med J 1991;302:272–273.

6   Jacobs K, Shoemaker C, Rudersdorf R, Neill SD, Kaufman RJ, Mufson A, Seehra J, Jones SS, Hewick R, Fritsch EF, Kawakita M, Shimizu T, Miyake T: Isolation and characterization of genomic and cDNA clones of human erythropoietin. Nature 1985;313:806–810.

7   Lin F-K, Suggs S, Lin C-H, Browne JK, Smalling R, Egrie JC, Chen KK, Fox GM, Martin F, Stabinsky Z, Badrawi SM, Lai P-H, Goldwasser E: Cloning and expression of the human erythropoietin gene. PNAS 1985;82:7580–7584.

8   Recny M, Scoble HA, Kim Y: Structural characterization of natural human urinary and recombinant DNA-derived erythropoietin. J Biol Chem 1987;262:17156–17163.

9   Tsuda E, Goto M, Murakami A, Akai K, Ueda M, Kawanishi G, Takahashi N, Sasaki R, Chiba H, Ishihara H, Mori M, Tejima S, Endo S, Arata Y: Comparative study of N-linked oligosaccharides of urinary and recombinant erythropoietins. Biochemistry 1988;27:5646–5654.

10 Takeuchi M, Takasaki S, Miyazaki H Kato T, Hoshi S, Kochibe N, Kobata A: Comparative study of the asparagine-linked sugar chains of human erythropoietins purified from urine and the cell culture medium of recombinant chinese hamster ovary cells. J Biol Chem 1988;263:3657–3663.
11 International collaborative assay of candidate international standards for a recombinant DNA analogue of human erythropoietin. WHO.

Bo G. Danielson, MD, Department of Medicine, University Hospital, S-751 85 Uppsala, Sweden

Discussion

to the Paper by H. Bergrem et al.

Krantz (Nashville): Just one comment: There have been a couple of patients who have developed a spontaneous red cell aplasia due to autoimmune antibodies to erythropoietin, so just for the sake of completeness I guess we need to consider that this could be an autoimmune disease that just happened to occur this time. Did the patient have any other autoimmune manifestations?

Danielson: No, not other than the formation of HLA antibodies. When we were preparing this paper there was a short note in the French Presse Medicale that there was a French patient who seemed to have developed EPO antibodies as well. But we have no further details on that patient.

Adamson (New York): To follow up on Dr. Krantz's point, that some patients develop autoimmune disorders with red cell aplasia: In fact, did your patient have red cell aplasia? One would predict that there should be zero reticulocytes in your patient at the time that the antibody appeared.

Danielson: I do not have the reticulocytes available here, but I think she had at least a very low level. But I do not have the data here myself.

Winearls (Oxford): Can you tell us anything about the glycosylation of the Behringwerke EPO?

Danielson: I would like to refer that question to the people of Behringwerke in the audience.

Heinrichs (Behringwerke): We preincubated the patient serum with the CHO-derived recombinant EPOs and with our erythropoietin, and we found that all three EPOs blocked the reaction the same way. This result does not point to a specific glycosylation difference.

Samtleben (Munich): Was this patient on dialyzer reuse program?—because this is known to induce antibodies.

Danielson: She was not.

Cavill (Cardiff): Perhaps I could add a second case to this series, where Macdougall et al. have a report in press of a lady who had the anemia of chronic renal failure associated with sickle cell disease. She failed to respond to fairly active erythropoietin therapy (epoietin beta, not alpha), but a subsequent transplantation resulted in her regaining a normalized hemoglobin concentration and, unfortunately, her original sickle cell disease.

Goldwasser (Chicago): Was this patient's serum tested in an in vitro assay to see if it in fact does inhibit EPO activity?

Danielson: It was.

Sytkowski (Boston): I wonder if I can ask whether deglycosylated EPO also bound these antibodies.

Danielson: I cannot answer this question.

Heinrichs: Due to a very restricted supply of available patient serum, it was not possible to perform these experiments.

Bauer (Zurich): After the patient was successfully transplanted, the kidney must have produced erythropoietin. Later on there was no sign of antibody formation?

Danielson: No.

Bauer: Are you sure?

Danielson: I mean, with the assays available, we could not find any formation of new antibodies.

The Effects of Red Blood Cell Transfusion on Host Immune Function

T. Hirose,[1] S. Pepkowitz, A. Jacobs, S. Nichols, S. Lee, T. Hodgson, C. Inducil, R. Gray, S. Kelly, C. Etzler, S. Epling, K. Miller, D. Goldfinger

Division of Transfusion Medicine, Department of Pathology and Laboratory Medicine, and the Division of Cardiology, Cedars-Sinai Medical Center, Los Angeles, Calif., USA

Summary

Clinical immunosuppression following blood transfusion (Tx) has been associated with improved allograft survival, increased postoperative tumor recurrence, and wound infection. To begin understanding the physiological alterations responsible for these phenomena, we utilized a cohort of cardiac surgery patients who received either autologous or no Txs or allogeneic Txs. We compared baseline immunological status to that one week after surgery through 3 in vitro assays, which included: (a) flow cytometric analysis of absolute numbers of lymphocytes (CD2, 3, and 20) and subsets (CD4 and 8), activation markers (CD25, transferrin, HLA-DR), natural killer cells (CD56 and 16), and monocytes (CD14); (b) mitogenic response to interleukin 2 (IL-2) and concanavalin A (ConA); and (c) a functional assay of tumoricidal activity using ^{51}Cr release from Daudi (T-cytotoxic–sensitive) and K562 (NK-sensitive) tumor cell lines.

	Allogeneic Tx, % Lysis (N = 8)		Autologous or No Tx, % Lysis (N = 4)	
	PreOp	PostOp	PreOp	PostOp
Daudi	4.3 ± 2.7	1.4 ± 1.3	2.6 ± 3.8	4.5 ± 6.4
K562	13.2 ± 6.5	5.9 ± 6.3	3.6 ± 3.8	5.4 ± 8.3

[1]*Current affiliation*: Department of Pathology, New England Deaconess Hospital, Boston, Mass., USA

Allogeneic Txs produced a marked, statistically significant decrease in tumoricidal capacity (p = 0.009) and a decrease in absolute numbers of lymphocytes (CD2 and 3; p = 0.04), T helper (CD4; p = 0.007), and activation markers (CD 25 and HLA DR; p = 0.02), as compared to the autologous/no Tx group. Mitogenic response to IL-2 and ConA did not demonstrate a difference between the two groups. Results of the tumoricidal capacity assay and flow cytometric analysis support the theory that functional immunomodulation follows allogeneic Txs and that these alterations may be a factor in the immunosuppression observed clinically.

Introduction

Clinical immunosuppression following blood transfusion has been associated with improved allograft survival as a positive effect but an increase in both postoperative tumor recurrence and wound infection as negative sequellae [1–4]. Currently, few clinical studies document the immune-modulating effects, if any, of autologous transfusions. To initiate an understanding of any differences in the physiological alterations secondary to either autologous or allogeneic transfusion, we studied a cohort of cardiac surgery patients utilizing 3 in vitro assays, which included:

1. Flow cytometric analysis of absolute numbers and activation markers of leukocytes
2. Mitogenic response to interleukin 2 and concanavalin A
3. A functional assay of tumoricidal activity using ^{51}Cr release from Daudi (T-cytotoxic–sensitive) and K562 (NK-sensitive) tumor cell lines

Baseline immunological status before surgery was compared to that 1 week after transfusion. These methodologies allowed us to quantify several aspects of immune function, thereby exploring possible in vitro assays, which may be used in the future to monitor immune modulation and to contribute to the expanding medical database concerning the safety and efficacy of autologous transfusion.

Methods

Patient Population

Eighteen cardiac patients (8 of which were able to predonate autologous blood) undergoing coronary artery bypass graft or valve replacement were followed through surgery and stratified into 2 groups depending on their perioperative transfusion needs:

1. A group (N = 8) that required only autologous transfusions (N = 5) or no transfusion (N = 3)

2. A group (N = 10) that required allogeneic blood transfusions (N = 8), allogeneic platelets only (N = 1), and allogeneic fresh frozen plasma (N = 1)

The median age of the 2 groups (66 years) was not statistically different. Entry exclusion criteria included previous transfusion, a history of malignancy, autoimmune disease, current use of immunosuppressive medications, active systemic infection, and a history of pregnancy (Table 1).

Sample Collection

Venous blood was drawn into 2 10-ml sodium heparin tubes and another aliquot into a 7-ml EDTA tube or a 10-ml ACD tube. The sodium heparin samples were utilized for the chromium release and mitogen assays. The EDTA/ACD samples were collected for flow cytometric analysis.

Chromium Release Assay

Mononuclear cell separation from the peripheral blood collected in sodium heparin was performed manually by a standard Ficoll-Hypaque method. The extracted product, including both the lymphocytes and natural killer cells (NK cells), were washed and centrifuged 4 times (400 g × 10 min) with complete media (RPMI 1640 with L-glu-

Table 1. Patient population statistics

Patient	Age	M/F	Transfusion requirement
Autologous/No transfusion:			
1	63	M	No transfusion
2	66	M	No transfusion
3	34	F	3 units whole blood
4	66	M	2 units whole blood
5	51	M	No transfusion
6	49	M	3 units whole blood 1 platelet pheresis
7	66	M	1 unit whole blood
8	72	M	2 units whole blood
Allogeneic transfusion:			
1	73	F	1 unit packed RBC 2 units FFP
2	59	M	2 units FFP 2 units auto whole blood
3	67	M	2 units packed RBC 1 platelet pheresis
4	64	M	1 unit packed RBC
5	65	M	1 unit packed RBC
6	79	M	3 units platelets
7	66	M	3 units packed RBC
8	62	M	2 units packed RBC
9	74	M	1 unit packed RBC
10	66	M	1 unit packed RBC

tamine, 10,000 units penicillin/streptomycin; 10% fetal bovine serum and phenol pH indicator), resuspended to 4×10^6 cells/ml in complete media, and then incubated for 24 h at 37°C with 5% CO_2. The cytotoxic assays were run in triplicate on a sterile, round-bottom, 96-well microtiter plate. The target cells were chromium-labeled Daudi or K562 tumor cells. The numbers of lymphocytes and NK cells were serially diluted to achieve the following 4 different responder (lymphocyte, NK cell)-to-target ratios: 40:1, 20:1, 10:1, 5:1. The target cell number per well was kept constant at 1×10^5 tumor cells/ml. The assay was incubated for 6 h (37°C with 5% CO_2). The plates were centrifuged (100 g $\times$ 5 min), and 100 lambda of the supernatant was removed for gamma count (using the ^{131}I gamma window).

^{51}Cr Labeling of Target Cells

The target monoclonal tumor cell lines consisted of Daudi (ATCC CCL 213) and K562 (ATCC CC L243). They were chosen for their well-characterized limited responder cell sensitivity: Daudi cells are lysed by T-cytotoxic cells and K562 by NK cells. Labeling was effected by incubation of 6×10^5 tumor cells with 100 lambda of ^{51}Cr (DuPont NEZ-030 chromium-51), with subsequent washing 4x and centrifugation in an Eppendorf centrifuge (5000 rpm for 5 sec). The wells were then incubated a second hour, washed, and resuspended to 1×10^5 cells/ml with complete media. Three 100-lambda aliquots each of Daudi and K562 were gamma counted to determine the total possible release of chromium and to screen out cell suspensions that may have aggregated to form cellular clumps. Tumor viability before each assay was kept above 90% and was monitored by Trypan blue dye exclusion as counted on a hemocytometer.

Thymidine Uptake Assay

The mitogenic response assay was performed in triplicate using peripheral blood mononuclear cells, 4×10^6 cells/ml for each assay. The lymphocytes and NK cells were placed in a round-bottom, sterile 96-well microtiter plate and run concurrently with a triplicate control, without mitogenic stimulation. Five U/ml of interleukin 2 (Sigma human recombinant IL-2) was added to the first triplicate assay, 25 U/ml of interleukin-2 to the second, and 12.5 μg/ml of concanavalin A to the third assay. One lambda of tritiated thymidine (Sigma ^{3}H thymidine) was then added and allowed to incubate with the cells for 4 h. The cells were then harvested on standard glass filters utilizing a skatron microharvesting collector and counted with a beta scintillation counter. Beta emission from the unstimulated control cells were subtracted as background. One lambda of tritiated thymidine was measured for the total possible beta count. The percent uptake was expressed as assay count over total beta count.

Flow Cytometry

Samples for flow cytometry were first analyzed by a Technicon H1 to obtain the absolute white blood count, lymphocyte percentage, and the absolute lymphocyte number. The rest of the sample was then analyzed on a Coulter Epics Profile II flow cytometer following standard whole blood sample lysis preparation. Fluorescent monoclonal antibodies for lymphocytes, monocytes, NK cells, and for the isotypic controls from Coulter Cytometry, Hialeah, FL included: CD45 (HLE-FITC), CD14 (M3-Rd), CD25 (IL2R1-

Rd), CD16 (Leu 11a-FITC), HLA-Dr-FITC and transferrin receptor-FITC. Those from Becton Dickinson, Mountain View, CA included: MsIgG2a-FITC, MsIgG1-Rd, CD20 (B1-FITC), CD2 (T11-Rd), MsIgG1-FITC, MsIgG1-Rd, CD8 (T8-FITC), CD4 (T4-Rd), MsIgG-FITC, MsIgG2a-Rd, CD3 (T3-FITC), MsIgG2a-FITC, MsIgG1-Rd, CD56 (NKH1-Rd).

Instrument alignment and calibration was accomplished at standard intervals (every day) using Coulter DNA check beads; HPCV: less than 4.00 for all parameters analyzed; peak channel: within ± 10% of the previous days value for all parameters analyzed; profile II amps: ± 0.5% A from the previous day's value; adjusted flow rate of DNA check beads: 70–100 events per second. After 10,000 beads have been counted, the HPCV and peak channel green fluorescence (LF1) and orange-red fluorescence (FL2), red fluorescence (FL3), and forward light scatter (FS) parameters were calibrated.

Statistical Analysis

Within each group, autologous/no transfusion versus allogeneic transfusion, postoperative values for each variable were compared to the corresponding preoperative values using paired *t*-tests. Comparisons between the groups were made on average postoperative minus preoperative difference for each variable, using 2-sample *t*-test. Tests for which the p-value was less than 0.05 were reported as statistically significant.

Results

Flow Cytometric Analysis

Allogeneic transfusion produced a marked statistically significant decrease in the absolute numbers of lymphocytes (Fig. 1) with a mean decrease in total T

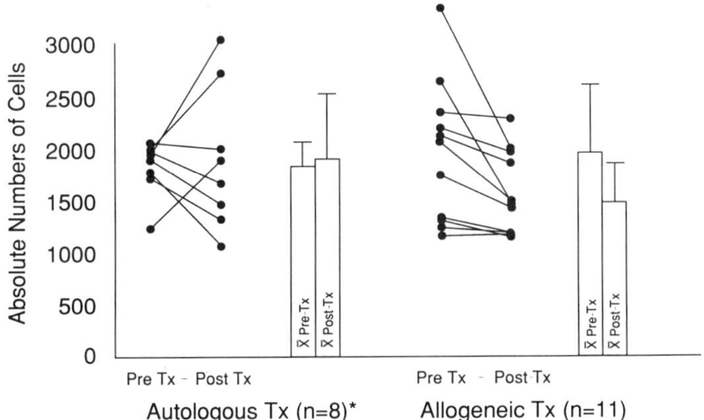

Fig. 1. Alteration in lymphocyte absolute number. Tx = transfusion; * autologous or no Tx.

cells, CD2- and CD3-positive cells 1659 to 1192 and 1492 to 1030, respectively (Table 2, Figs. 2,3) (p = 0.005, p = 0.01). Within this group, the mean T-helper population, CD4 (Fig. 4), also had a statistically significant decline from 1029 to 726 (Table 2, Figs. 2,3) (p = .007). In contrast, the autologous/no transfusion group did not have a decline or statistically significant change in pretransfusion vs. posttransfusion absolute value of lymphocytes or their subsets (Table 3). Activation markers CD25, the interleukin 2 receptor (Fig. 5), and

Table 2.   Flow cytometric data: allogeneic transfusion (n = 10)

| | Absolute cell count | | | | *t*-Test |
	pre-TX mean	SD	post-TX mean	SD	(pre-TX vs. post-TX)
WBC	7949	1295	8955	1503	p = 0.01
ALC	2039	659	1503	414	p = 0.04
CD2	1659	521	1192	328	p = 0.005
CD3	1494	556	1030	202	p = 0.01
CD4	1029	465	726	248	p = 0.007
CD8	545	251	368	168	p = 0.008
CD20	286	144	226	112	p = 0.14
CD16	140	105	124	77	p = 0.60
CD56	333	170	252	175	p = 0.01
HLA-DR	498	265	401	162	p = 0.16
CD25	1660	733	981	260	p = 0.01
Transferrin	26	25	71	114	p = 0.27

WBC, white blood cell; ALC, absolute lymphocyte count; TX, transfusion; SD, standard deviation.

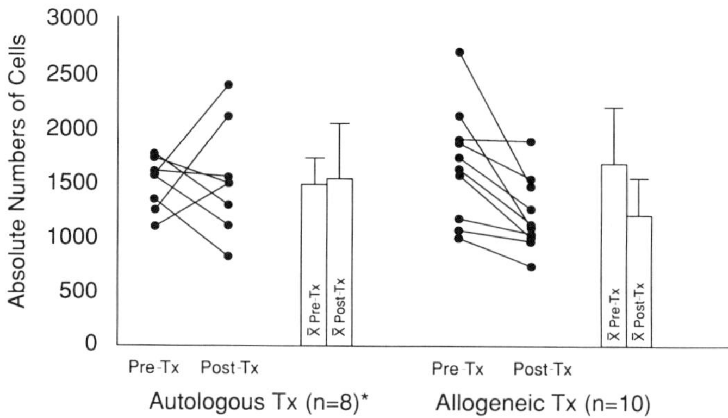

Fig. 2.   Flow cytometric evaluation: T-cell absolute number CD2.

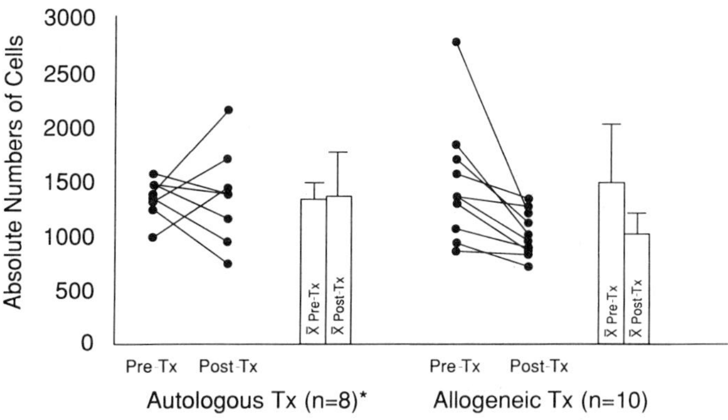

Fig. 3. Flow cytometric evaluation: T-cell absolute number CD3.

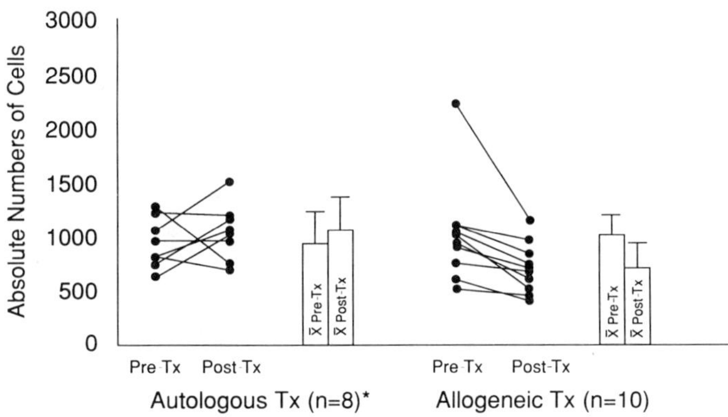

Fig. 4. Flow cytometric evaluation: T-helper/inducer absolute number CD4.

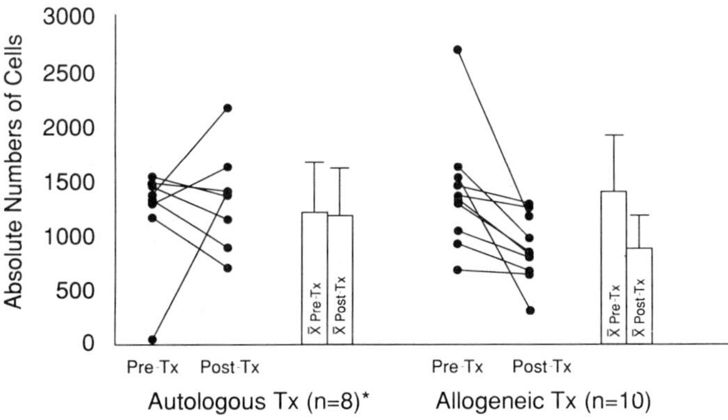

Fig. 5. Flow cytometric evaluation of T-lymphocyte activation interleukin 2 receptor (CD25).

HLA-Dr (Fig. 6) fell in the allogeneic group from 1660 to 981 (p = 0.01) and from 498 to 401, respectively (Table 2) (p = 0.01). Activation value changes were not statistically significant in the autologous groups and had a positive trend in the HLA-Dr expression (Table 3). The monocyte population (CD14) and total B-cell population (CD20) did not vary significantly in either patient group (Tables 2, 3).

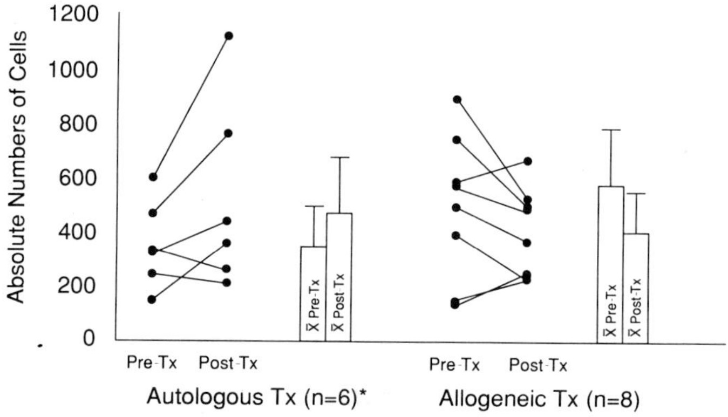

Fig. 6. Flow cytometric evaluation: T-lymphocyte activation HLA-Dr.

Table 3. Flow cytometric data: autologous/no transfusion (n = 8)

| | Absolute cell count | | | | t-Test |
	pre-TX mean	SD	post-TX mean	SD	(pre-TX vs. post-TX)
WBC	7600	1256	8538	2480	p = 0.14
ALC	1830	259	1901	676	p = 0.77
CD2	1470	231	1513	509	p = 0.84
CD3	1355	176	1377	433	p = 0.09
CD4	954	232	1077	244	p = 0.30
CD8	472	202	470	230	p = 0.98
CD20	273	175	310	201	p = 0.27
CD16	151	101	107	52	p = 0.18
CD56	219	131	167	64	p = 0.19
HLA-DR	351	160	525	347	p = 0.11
CD25	1269	518	1459	506	p = 0.49
Transferrin	61	31	57	45	p = 0.87

WBC, white blood cell; ALC, absolute lymphocyte count; TX, transfusion; SD, standard deviation.

Tumor Cytotoxic Assay

Allogeneic transfusions produced a marked statistically significant decrease in T-cytotoxic tumoricidal capacity from a mean value of 4.3% tumor cell lysis to 1.4% (Table 4, Figs. 7, 8) (p = 0.01). NK-cell function was also diminished following allogeneic transfusion with a cytotoxic capacity falling from 29 to 25% (p = 0.02). These changes were not seen in the autologous transfusion group (Table 5).

Mitogen Response Assay

Mononuclear response to the two different concentrations of interleukin 2 and concanavalin A did not reveal a statistically significant activation or suppression of mitogenic response in either the autologous or the allogeneically transfused patients (Tables 6, 7 and Figs. 9–11).

Discussion

This prospective study of a similar population of cardiac patients demonstrates a quantitative alteration in host immune function. Allogeneic transfusion

Table 4. Tumor cytotoxic assay data: allogeneic transfusion (n = 7)

	Percent tumor cell lysis				*t*-Test
	pre-TX mean	SD	post-TX mean	SD	(pre-TX vs. post-TX)
Daudi	4.3	2.7	1.4	1.3	p = 0.01
K562	29	25	25	6.3	p = 0.02

TX, transfusion; SD, standard deviation.

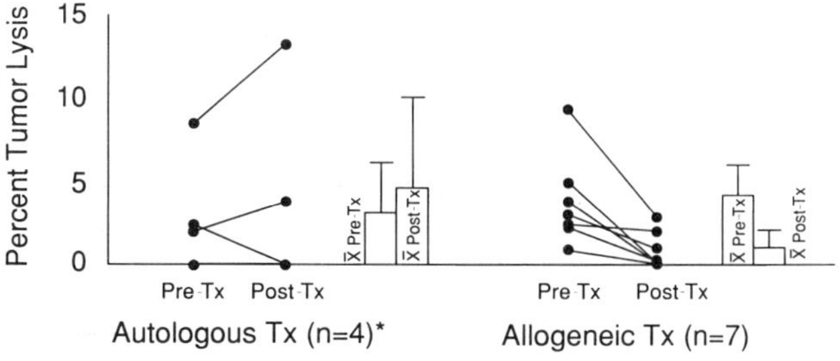

Fig. 7. Tumor cytotoxic assay Daudi.

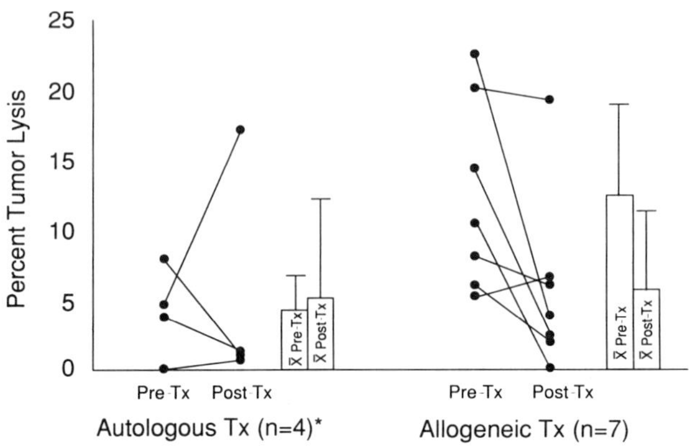

Fig. 8. Tumor cytotoxic assay K562.

Table 5. Tumor cytotoxic assay data: autologous/no transfusion (n = 4)

	Percent tumor cell lysis				*t*-Test (pre-TX vs. post-TX)
	pre-TX mean	SD	post-TX mean	SD	
Daudi	2.6	3.8	4.5	6.4	p = 0.25
K562	3.6	3.8	5.4	8.3	p = 0.69

TX, transfusion; SD, standard deviation.

Table 6. Mitogenic response data: allogeneic transfusion (n = 7)

	Beta counts per minute				*t*-Test (pre-TX vs. post-TX)
	pre-TX mean	SD	post-TX mean	SD	
5 U/ml IL-2	32	26	24	23	p = 0.10
25 U/ml IL-2	29	25	25	75	p = 0.11
12.5 μg/ml ConA	220	227	152	139	p = 0.52

TX, transfusion; IL-2, interleukin 2; ConA, concanavalin A; SD, standard deviation.

Table 7. Mitogenic response data: autologous/no transfusion (n = 4)

	Beta counts per minute				*t*-Test (pre-TX vs. post-TX)
	pre-TX mean	SD	post-TX mean	SD	
5 U/ml IL-2	20	23	21	32	p = 0.88
25 U/ml IL-2	36	58	63	58	p = 0.22
12.5 μg/ml ConA	232	238	15	20	p = 0.27

TX, transfusion; IL-2, interleukin 2; ConA, concanavalin A; SD, standard deviation.

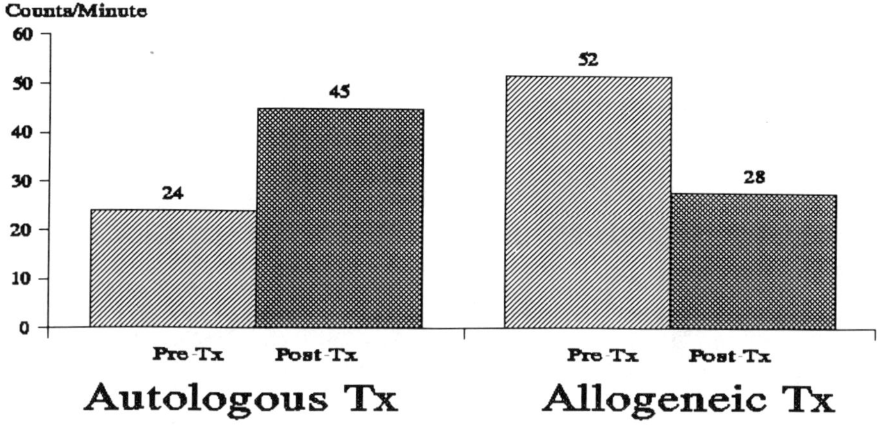

Fig. 9. Mitogenic assay: ^{3}H uptake 25 U/ml interleukin 2 (sample/control).

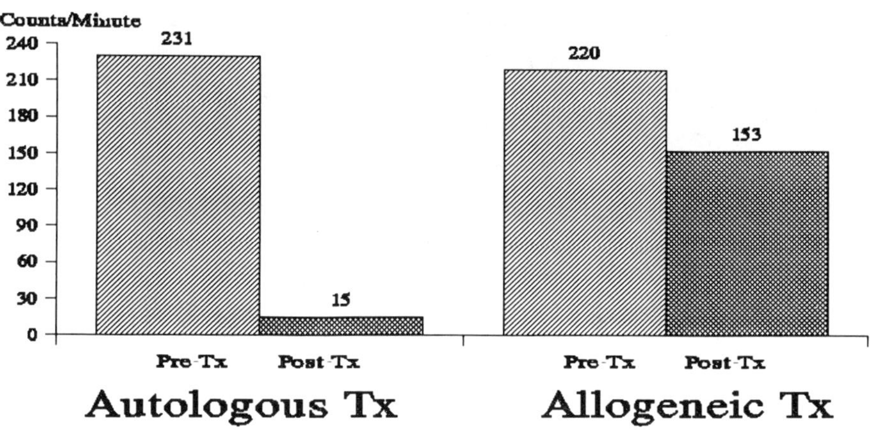

Fig. 10. Mitogenic assay: ^{3}H uptake 12.5 μg/ml concanavalin A.

produced a marked decreased in tumoricidal capacity for both the T-cytotoxic and NK-cell populations in our patients. Comparison of pretransfusion cytotoxic values to that of posttransfusion values was statistically significant in the allogeneically transfused patient, while an immune alteration due to autologous transfusion was not demonstrated by our assays. Further statistical analysis utilizing group comparison *t*-test revealed that allogeneic transfusion produced a marked and highly statistically significant decrease in T-lymphocyte cytotoxic capacity and a trend towards suppression of natural killer cytotoxic capacity when compared against the autologously transfused patients (T-cytotoxic alteration [p = 0.009] and NK cell alteration [p = 0.067]).

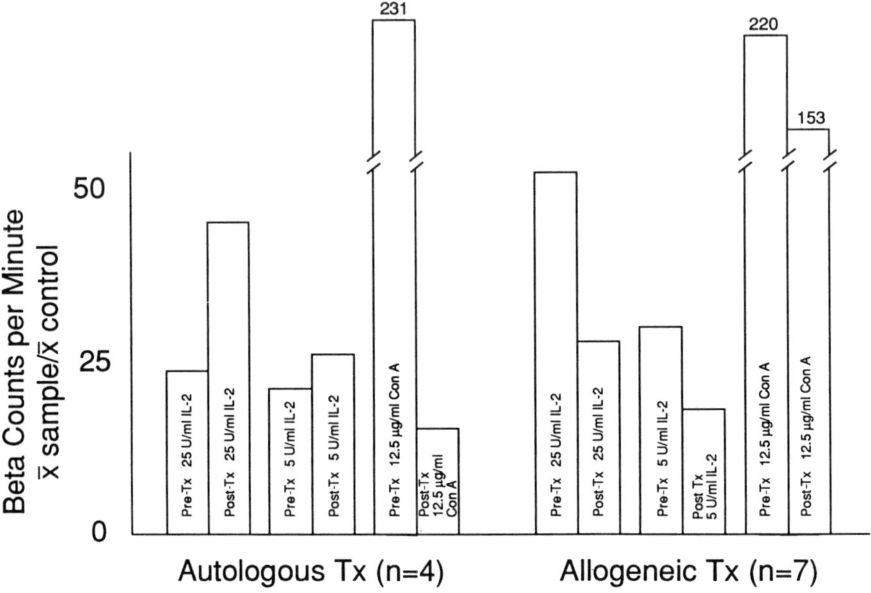

Fig. 11. Mitogenic assay: ^{3}H uptake interleukin 2.

Flow cytometric evaluation provided a further method for determining and quantifying immune modulation. Allogeneic transfusion induced a immune-modulating effect on the baseline circulating immune cell population with a statistically significant decline in the absolute numbers of lymphocytes. Although the total WBC count was higher in this group, the percentage of lymphocytes dramatically fell as did the absolute number of mononuclear subpopulations including the T-helper, T-suppressor (Fig. 12, p = 0.008), and NK-cell populations (Fig. 13, p = 0.01). Despite this fall in lymphocyte count, alteration in the absolute number of B cells was not statistically significant. These changes may indicate an as yet uncharacterized, selective immunological alteration directed towards certain mononuclear cell populations and subpopulations.

Activation of T lymphocytes was depressed following allogeneic transfusion as measured by flow cytometric evaluation of CD25 and HLA-Dr. Group comparison *t*-test of the HLA-Dr receptor change revealed significant decline in expression found with allogeneic transfusion (p = 0.02). In contrast, autologous transfusion or no transfusion did not induce any statistically significant changes in postsurgical immune function or in the absolute numbers of the WBC subpopulations. Our study did not demonstrate any immune modulation due to the cardiac bypass procedure per se. Cardiac bypass without allogeneic blood expo-

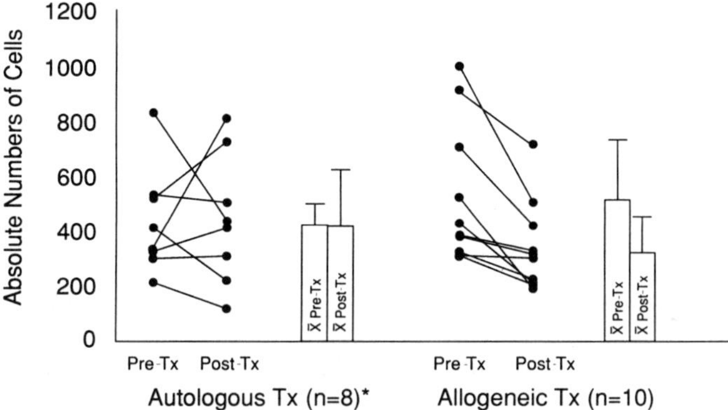

Fig. 12.   Flow cytometric evaluation: T-suppressor/cytotoxic absolute numbers CD8.

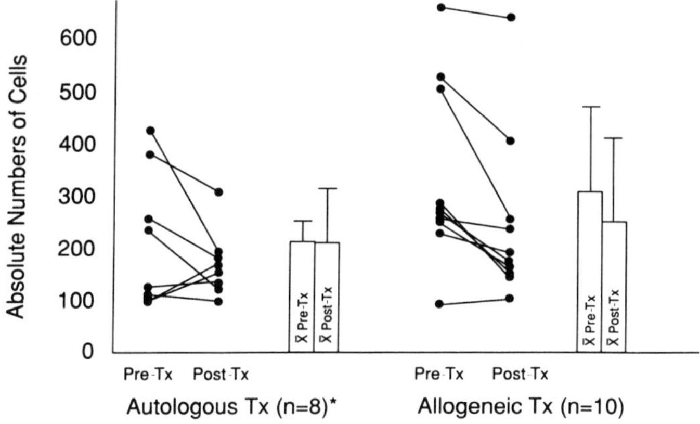

Fig. 13.   Flow cytometric evaluation: natural killer cell absolute numbers NKH-1 CD56.

sure did not demonstate the marked immunosuppression seen with allogeneic transfusion.

Our study was unable to demonstrate a difference in response to mitogenic stimulation between the two groups. Perhaps this was in part due to the marked individual variability in tritiated thymadine response, which contributed to a wide coefficient of variability and standard deviation in both groups. In addition, the quantity of concanavalin A used to induce the mitogenic response was large and any immune suppression/alteration by either allogeneic or autologous transfusion may have been masked.

This study suggests that the immune modulatory effects of blood transfusions are not due to cellular changes during storage or to products leached into the transfusion product from the container or delivery system, but rather are due to host response immunological alterations induced by allogeneic blood components. If future studies reveal this to be the case, it would provide further support for use of autologous transfusion.

Acknowledgment

This work was supported in part by a grant from the Rita and Taft Schreiber Foundation.

References

1 Lagaaij EL, Henneman PH, Van Rood JJ, et al.: Effect of one HLA-Dr-antigen-matched and completely HLA-Dr-mismatched blood transfusion on survival of heart and kidney allografts. N Engl J Med 1989;321:701–705.
2 Van Twuyver E, Mooijaart RJ, De Waal LP, et al.: Pretransplantation blood transfusion revisited. N Engl J Med 1991;325:1210–1242.
3 Murphy P, Heal JM, Blumberg N. Infection or suspected infection after hip replacement surgery with autologous or homologous blood transfusion. Transfusion 1991;31:212–217.
4 Blumberg N, Heal JM; Transfusion and host defenses against cancer recurrence and infection. Transfusion 1989;29:236–245.

Thomas G. Hirose, M.D., Department of Pathology, New England Deaconess Hospital, 185 Pilgrim Road, Boston, MA 02215 (USA)

Discussion

to the Paper by T. Hirose et al.

Shaldon (*Nimes*): I think that this experimental design needs to look at the point data before you can make a population conclusion. You had patients that went the wrong way in both groups, and your statistics were not impressive to me. Therefore, it is only your bias, in my opinion, that leads to these conclusions. What is the diurnal variation in that population's expression of CD receptors, and what is the coefficient of variation of the measurement by flow cytometry of the CD25 receptor?

Hirose: Many studies have shown that there is diurnal variation, and your point is well taken. We will have to study much larger numbers of patients to make a definitive statement that these immunosuppressions following allogeneic transfusion are the changes that are seen. I think it is remarkable that most of the data, especially as done by flow cytometry, had similar assay, highly statistically significant directional changes in our allogeneic population versus the autologous group, but you are absolutely right. We need to have more patient numbers.

Wardrop: How long do these effects last?

Hirose: That is an interesting question. We drew samples 1 week before, 1 week after, and 6 weeks after transfusion and we see that the baseline, flow cytometric, and tumor cytoxic capacity returned to normal in 50% of our patients. The other 50% remained suppressed or had a decreased level, and the question is whether they just did not have enough time to normalize or whether there is some kind of immunological memory involved, but this is just speculation.

Wardrop (*Cardiff*): I was interested in your data, which accord with other peoples' findings, both in clinical consequences—such as postoperative infections—following allogeneic transfusion and in careful immunological observations like yours. But you have not referred to possible mechanisms, and there are suggestions that material derived from allogeneic white cells might modulate immune function. If you could pin down mechanisms, that might help you to clarify the effects better.

Hirose: Yes, that is a very good point. The mechanisms of immune modulation per se are not known. I would say that there is probably a cellular effect due to the white cells although we did have one patient that received allogeneic fresh-frozen plasma, essentially cellular-free, that had some changes (immunosuppression) following the transfusion, so I think that control studies altering the white-cell populations would be very useful.

Kubanek (*Ulm*): Maybe I missed it, but did you test your heterogeneous blood for CMV, because this may cause the effects you have seen?

Hirose: No, we did not.

Blanchard (*Boston*): Did you compare lucopor blood with either filtered or deglissed frozen blood?

Hirose: That will be the next study, the results of which would be valuable. None of the transfusions (components) in our studies were filtered or otherwise leukodepleted.

Recombinant Human Erythropoietin in the Treatment of the Anemia Associated with Solid Tumors

David H. Henry

Graduate Hospital, Philadelphia, Penn., USA

Introduction

Anemia is common in patients with advanced cancer. The etiology of this anemia is multifactorial, including blood loss, hemolysis, nutritional factors, bone marrow invasion with tumor, and the anemia of chronic disease.

Perhaps the most common of these is the anemia of chronic disease: its diagnosis and clinical characteristics have recently been reviewed [1, 2]. The pathophysiology of the anemia of chronic disease has three features: modest shortening of red cell survival, decreased iron reutilization in bone marrow, and inadequate erythropoietin response to the degree of anemia [3]. In addition, myelosuppressive chemotherapy can either cause or exacerbate the anemia associated with advanced cancer, and cisplatin may further contribute to this anemia by impairing the ability of the kidneys to produce erythropoietin.

Blood Transfusion in Cancer Patients with Anemia

Cancer patients with anemia may require blood transfusions for symptomatic palliation. However, blood transfusion is associated with some risks, including the acute reactions of fever, chills, hives, and the more chronic problems of hepatitis (usually non-A, non-B, non-C), and possibly immunosuppression.

The potential consumption of blood for symptomatic palliation of chemotherapy-related anemia could approach 2 million units per year in the United States [4]. A reduction in transfusion requirement for the anemic cancer patient could significantly decrease the drain on the national blood supply. The availability of recombinant human erythropoietin (rhEPO) has made it possible to test whether this nontransfusional form of therapy can enhance erythropoiesis and

"

thereby decrease the transfusion requirement, increase the hematocrit (Hct), and improve the patient's qualify of life.

Clinical Trials with rhEPO in Anemia Associated with Malignancies

Recently, several phase I/II studies have demonstrated the ability of rhEPO to treat the anemia associated with malignancy, but these studies did not have placebo controls [4–8]. Three large multicenter, double-blind, placebo-controlled trials have now been completed in anemic cancer patients: two trials involving patients who received chemotherapy, and a third trial involving patients receiving no chemotherapy [9].

Patients and Methods

In the two chemotherapy studies, patients received either rhEPO 150 U/kg or placebo 3× per week subcutaneously for 12 weeks or until a Hct of 38–40% was obtained, after which point the dose of study medication was titrated to maintain the Hct within the target range. In the first protocol, 132 patients were entered and all were receiving cisplatin-containing, myelosuppressive chemotherapy regimens. In the second protocol, 157 patients were entered and all received myelosuppressive chemotherapy, but without cisplatin.

For the third protocol, 124 patients not receiving concomitant chemotherapy were randomized to rhEPO 100 U/kg or placebo subcutaneously 3× a week for 8 weeks or until a Hct of 38–40% was obtained. Anemia was defined as a hemoglobin $\leq$ 10.5 g/dl or Hct $\leq$ 32%. All patients had biopsy-proven malignancy, but without a primary bone marrow malignancy such as acute leukemia, and all were greater than 30% Karnofsky performance status.

The rhEPO and placebo treatment arms were well balanced at study entry for the parameters of performance status, percent of patients transfused, mean units transfused per month, baseline Hct, and tumor types (Table 1). Also, dose intensity of chemotherapy was equally balanced between the two treatment arms in each protocol.

The Hct change from baseline to final and the blood transfusion requirement were measured during the study. A responder was defined as any patient who increased his or her Hct by 6 or more points, unrelated to transfusion. A complete responder was defined as a patient who normalized his or her Hct to 38% or greater, again unrelated to transfusion. Before and after completion of the double-blind therapy, patients were also asked to rate their energy levels, their ability to perform daily activities, and their overall quality of life.

Results and Discussion

In the cisplatin-containing protocol, the Hct improvement was 4.7 percentage points greater in the rhEPO arm than in the placebo arm. In the noncisplatin chemotherapy protocol, the Hct improvement was 5.8 points greater in the rhEPO arm (Table 2). In the patients not receiving chemotherapy, the Hct improvement was 2.9 percentage points greater for patients receiving rhEPO.

In both chemotherapy protocols, the proportion of patients transfused was less, and the mean units of blood transfused per patient were lower, for those patients receiving rhEPO treatment. These differences, however, were not significant. However, investigators reasoned that at least 1 month might have to elapse for rhEPO-induced erythropoiesis to have a significant impact on the transfusion requirement. When the results from the two 12-week chemotherapy trials were analyzed in this way, the transfusion requirements in the second and third months combined were significantly less for the rhEPO-treated patients than for those on placebo (Table 3).

Table 1. Baseline characteristics

Parameter	rhEPO	Placebo
Percent transfused	44.7	48.4
Mean units transfused/Patient/Month	0.67	0.73
Mean hematocrit (%)	29.1	28.5
Mean neutrophil count (cells/μl)	4163	4017
Endoserum EPO level (mU/ml)		
Mean	146	149
Median	76	85
Mean overall quality of life		
(mm on a 100-mm scale)	50.0	50.4

Table 2. Mean hematocrit (%)

Treatment	N	Baseline	Final	Change
No chemotherapy				
rhEPO	63	29.3	32.1	2.8*
Placebo	55	27.6	27.5	-0.1
Cisplatin				
chemotherapy				
rhEPO	64	29.4	35.4	6.0*
Placebo	61	28.4	29.7	1.3
Noncisplatin				
chemotherapy				
rhEPO	79	28.6	35.5	6.9*
Placebo	74	29.4	30.5	1.1

*p $<$ 0.004.

Table 3.   Transfusion Requirement

Group	N	Month 1 (%) Transfused	Month 1 Units transfused/ patient	N	Months 2 and 3 (%) Transfused	Months 2 and 3 Units transfused/ patient
Cisplatin chemotherapy						
rhEPO	64	43.8	1.71	56	26.8	1.20
Placebo	61	44.3	1.20	55	56.4	2.00
					p < 0.005	p < 0.089
Noncisplatin chemotherapy						
rhEPO	79	25.3	0.69	70	28.6	0.91
Placebo	74	27.0	0.71	68	36.8	1.65
						p < 0.056
Both combined						
rhEPO	143	33.6	1.09	126	27.8	1.04
Placebo	135	34.3	0.98	123	45.5	1.81
					p < 0.005	p < 0.009

Finally, responders and complete responders were analyzed (Table 4). In the cisplatin-containing chemotherapy trial, responders (rhEPO 48% vs. placebo 7%) and complete responders (rhEPO 36% vs. placebo 2%) were significantly more common in the rhEPO treatment arm. Likewise, in the noncisplatin chemotherapy trial, responders (rhEPO 58% vs. placebo 13%) and complete responders (rhEPO 40% vs. placebo 4%) again significantly favored rhEPO therapy. In the group not receiving chemotherapy, responders (rhEPO 32% vs. placebo 11%) and complete responders (rhEPO 21% vs. placebo 4%) were significantly greater in the rhEPO-treated arm.

These responses continued in the open-label phases of all three trials. After a total of at least 6 months on study, the percentage of patients still requiring transfusions decreased to 10% (no chemotherapy trial), 13% (noncisplatin chemotherapy trial), and 11.5% (cisplatin-containing chemotherapy trial).

Pretreatment serum erythropoietin levels in the chemotherapy trials did not predict which patients would be responders, but less than 5% of patients had erythropoietin levels greater than 500 mU/ml. There was a correlation in the no-chemotherapy trial between lower pretreatment EPO levels and tendency to respond.

Table 4. Responders

Group	N	Responders (Hct increase $\geq$ 6%)	Complete responders (Hct $\geq$ 38%)
No chemotherapy			
rhEPO	63	31.7*	20.6*
Placebo	55	10.9	3.6
Cisplatin chemotherapy			
rhEPO	64	48.4*	35.9*
Placebo	61	6.6	1.6
Noncisplatin chemotherapy			
rhEPO	79	58.2*	40.5*
Placebo	74	13.5	4.1

*$p < 0.008$.

Recombinant human erythropoietin therapy was remarkably well tolerated without any significant adverse effects. Quality-of-life scores from baseline to final evaluation improved more for the rhEPO-treated patients than for the placebo-treated patients. When only the rhEPO responders were compared with the placebo groups, improvements were significantly greater in all three areas of quality of life measured. (See also Chapter 22.)

Summary

In summary, rhEPO can be safely and effectively administered to anemic cancer patients. A dose of 100 U/kg three times per week subcutaneously can increase the Hct in anemic cancer patients not receiving chemotherapy. A dose of 150 U/kg three times per week subcutaneously can significantly increase Hct and, after a 1-month lag phase, can decrease the transfusion requirement in anemic cancer patients receiving chemotherapy. Continuation on rhEPO for 6 months or more can cause further responses in all three patient groups.

References

1   Cash JM, Scars DA: The anemia of chronic disease: spectrum of associated disease in a series of unselected hospitalized patients. Am J Med 1989;87:638–644.

2   Shilling RF: Anemia of chronic disease: A misnomer. 2. Ann Intern Med 1991;
    115:572–573.
3   Miller CB, Joan RJ, Piantadosi S, et al.: Decreased erythropoietin response in patients
    with the anemia of cancer. N Engl J Med 1990;332:1689–1692.
4   Platanias LC, Miller CB, Mick R, et al.: Treatment of chemotherapy-induced anemia
    with recombinant human erythropoietin in cancer patients. J Clin Oncol 1991;9:2021–
    2026.
5   Henry D, Nelson R, Brooks B, et al.: prospective evaluation of transfusion require-
    ment for anemic cancer patient +/− chemotherapy. Proc Am Soc Clin Oncol
    1991;10:340.
6   Ludwig H, Fritz E, Kotzman H, et al.: Erythropoietin treatment of anemia associated
    with multiple myeloma. N Engl J Med 1990;322:1693–1699.
7   Oster W. Hermann F, Gamm H, et al.: Erythropoietin for the treatment of anemia of
    malignancy associated with neoplastic bone marrow infiltration. J Clin Oncol
    1990;8:956–962.
8   Miller CB, Platanias LC, Mills SR, et al.: Phase I-II trial of erythropoietin in the
    treatment of cisplatin-associated anemia. JNCI 1992;84:98–103.
9   Abels RI, Larholt KM, Krantz KD. Bryant EC: Recombinant human erythropoietin (r-
    HuEPO) for the treatment of the anemia of cancer; in Murphy MJ Jr (ed): Blood Cell
    Growth Factors: Their Present and Future Use in Hematology and Oncology. Proceed-
    ings of the Beijing Symposium. Dayton, Ohio, Alpha Med Press, 1991, pp 121–141.

David H. Henry, The Graduate Hospital, Tuttleman Center, 2nd Floor, 1840 South
Street, Philadelphia, PA 19146 (USA)

Anemia Associated with Cisplatin Chemotherapy

Carole B. Miller, Sharon R. Mills

Johns Hopkins Oncology Center, Baltimore, Md., USA

Cisplatin (CDDP [*cis*-dichlorodiammineplatinum (II)]) is a chemotherapeutic agent with significant activity in a wide variety of tumors. Anemia is a common cause of morbidity in patients with cancer receiving cisplatin-containing cytotoxic chemotherapeutic regimens [1–5], with patients frequently requiring red blood cell transfusions. In one series of 31 cisplatin-treated patients with metastatic cancer, 12 developed progressive anemia demonstrated as a decline in hemoglobin concentrations from a mean of 12.9 g/dl to a mean of 9.3 g/dl over an average of 49 days [3]. No hemolysis or gastrointestinal hemorrhage was observed in any of these patients. In a group of 26 cisplatin-treated patients with a variety of malignant neoplasms (11 with malignant melanoma), 30% were observed to have a 1.0–5.0 g/dl drop in hemoglobin levels [4]. Anemia associated with cisplatin therapy has been reported in 60% of 30 patients with advanced non–small-cell lung cancer; 13% required blood transfusions [5].

The anemia associated with cisplatin therapy is a normochromic, normocytic hypoproliferative anemia with an inappropriately low reticulocyte count [2] similar to that seen in patients with chronic renal failure on dialysis and not on dialysis [6]. The etiology of the anemia associated with cisplatin-containing regimens is multifactorial, with direct erythroid suppression and immune mechanisms probably playing roles [2]. However, similar to patients with end-stage renal disease [7] and patients receiving zidovudine for human immunodeficiency virus (HIV) infection [8], inadequate erythropoietin response to anemia also appears to be important in the anemia associated with cisplatin treatment. We previously showed that there is an inadequate erythropoietin response to anemia in patients with cancer and that this response worsens with chemotherapy [9]. In that study, the inadequate erythropoietin response to anemia was seen in patients treated with both cisplatin- and non–cisplatin-containing chemotherapeutic regimens. The erythropoietin response to anemia in cisplatin-treated chemotherapy patients is compared to the erythropoietin response in iron-deficient controls in Figure 1. The inadequate erythropoietin response did not appear in our study to be related to clinical nephrotoxicity as manifested by elevation in serum creatinine. However, chemotherapy (especially cisplatin) may have an effect on erythropoietin-producing cells in the peritubular endothelium without producing clinical nephrotoxicity [2]. Several clinical and animal studies have reported progressive normochromic, normocytic anemia associated with cisplatin therapy in which serum erythropoietin failed to rise as the anemia progressed [10, 11]. In the animal models of cisplatin-associated anemia, treatment with exogenous recombinant erythropoietin (rhEPO) improved the anemia [11].

Therefore, the anemia associated with cisplatin chemotherapy is associated with a relative erythropoietin deficiency. As in other anemias of chronic disease associated with erythropoietin deficiency, such as chronic renal failure [12–15] and HIV infection [16], rhEPO may be effective in improving erythropoiesis in patients receiving cisplatin chemotherapy.

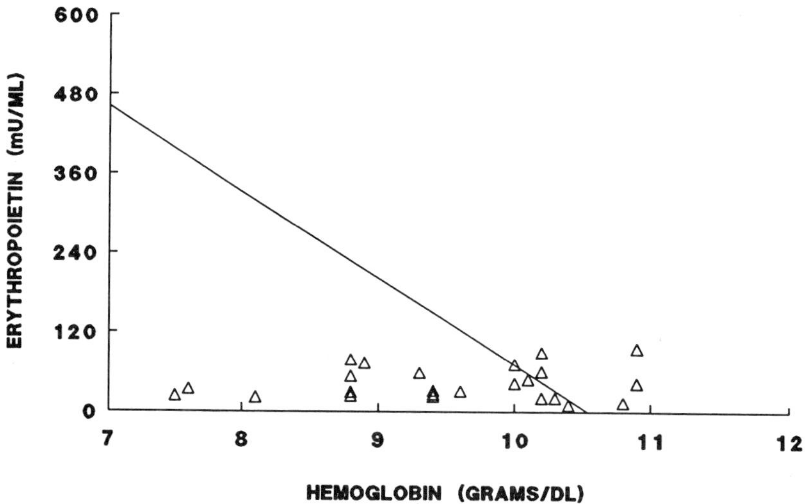

Fig. 1. Erythropoietin response to anemia in patients with cancer receiving cisplatin chemotherapy. Solid line reflects the erythropoietin response to anemia in patients with iron-deficiency anemia. Erythropoietin levels in patients receiving cisplatin-based chemotherapy are designated by (Δ).

Phase I/II Trial of rhEPO in Cisplatin-Associated Anemia

Twenty-one cancer patients (14 men and 7 women; mean age, 51 y; age range, 30–70 y) being treated with cisplatin-containing chemotherapeutic regimens were entered into a multicenter phase I/II study [17]. Five had gastrointestinal tumors; three each had tumors of the lung, brain, or head and neck; one had a breast tumor; and six had other solid tumors.

All 21 patients were receiving cisplatin chemotherapy at entry into the study and all manifested screening hemoglobin levels less than 11 g/dl. None were administered red blood cell transfusions in the 4 weeks prior to their current chemotherapy regimen or had received prior rhEPO therapy. All patients demonstrated adequate bone marrow function. Cisplatin chemotherapy was continued during the study, and oral iron supplementation ($FeSO_4$ 325 mg 3× a day) was administered unless the serum ferritin level was above the upper limit of the normal range.

In this single-arm, dose-escalation study, rhEPO (epoetin beta) was administered intravenously 5 times a week for 4 weeks. Patients were assigned sequentially to 1 of 4 dose groups, receiving rhEPO at 25, 50, 100, or 200 U/kg body weight. Response to rhEPO therapy was defined as an increase in hemoglobin concentration > 1.0 g/dl after 3–4 weeks of therapy without transfusion. Patients requiring transfusions were considered "nonresponders" to rhEPO treatment.

Of the 21 patients entered into the study, 4 required red blood cell transfusions during the study period. Generally, rhEPO treatment was well tolerated in all study subjects. No patient was removed from study because of rhEPO-related toxicity, and no deaths or life-threatening adverse reactions occurred during the trial. Adverse events possibly associated with rhEPO treatment were facial flushing in 2 patients, headache in 4 patients, increased blood pressure in 2 patients, and a deep-vein thrombosis in the right leg of 1 patient. All adverse events were responsive to routine medical management. The frequency of adverse events did not appear to be dose dependent. There was no significant difference in mean systolic blood pressure, but there was a mild increase in diastolic blood pressure (77 ± 15 to 85 ± 15 mm Hg).

Individual patient hemoglobin levels prestudy and after 4 weeks of rhEPO therapy are shown in Table 1. Responses were seen at all dose levels, with hemoglobin levels increasing in a dose-dependent fashion. The ability to respond to rhEPO was independent of pretreatment serum erythropoietin levels, pretreatment hemoglobin levels, pretreatment white blood cell count, pretreatment platelet count, pretreatment ferritin level, or history of transfusion in the 2 months prior to the study.

Table 1. Hemoglobin levels (g/dl) for individual patients prestudy and after 4 weeks of rhEPO therapy

Patient No.	Pre (g/dl)	Post (g/dl)	Change	RBC transfusion
25 U/kg				
1	9.4	12.4	3.0	
2	8.4	TR		NA (2 units day 13)
3	9.9	11.3	1.4	
4	11.1	9.7	−1.4	
5	10.9	10.5	−.4	
6	10.9	10.5	−.4	
50 U/kg				
7	1.2	13.9	1.9	
8	10.9	10.0	−.9	
9	9.5	10.9	1.4	
10	10.6	12.4	1.8	
11	10.1		TR	NA (2 units day 19)
100 U/kg				
12	10.9	12.2	1.3	
13	10.6		TR	NA (2 units day 5; 3 units day 19)
14	9.3	11.2	1.9	
15	9.2	13.1	3.9	
16	10.4	11.8	1.4	
200 U/kg				
17	8.1		TR	NA (2 units day 10; 2 units day 23)
18	10.5	12.6	2.1	
19	8.8	13.2	4.4	
20	7.7	10.7	3.0	
21	10.2	10.5	.3	

TR, red blood cell transfusion; NA, not available.

Mean cumulative changes in hemoglobin levels from baseline are shown in Figure 2. In this analysis, hemoglobin data for transfused patients were included up until the time of transfusion. Hemoglobin levels were significantly increased from baseline in the 200 U/kg group at weeks 2, 3, and 4 and at week 4 in the 100 U/kg group with a trend seen at week 3. The mean hemoglobin was increased by 1.9 ± 1.3 g/dl in the 100 U/kg group and 2.4 ± 1.7 g/dl in the 200 U/kg group after 4 weeks of therapy. Changes were not related to the timing of rhEPO in relation to chemotherapy, as when timepoints in chemotherapy cycles with and without rhEPO were compared, rhEPO had a significant positive effect on hemoglobin levels.

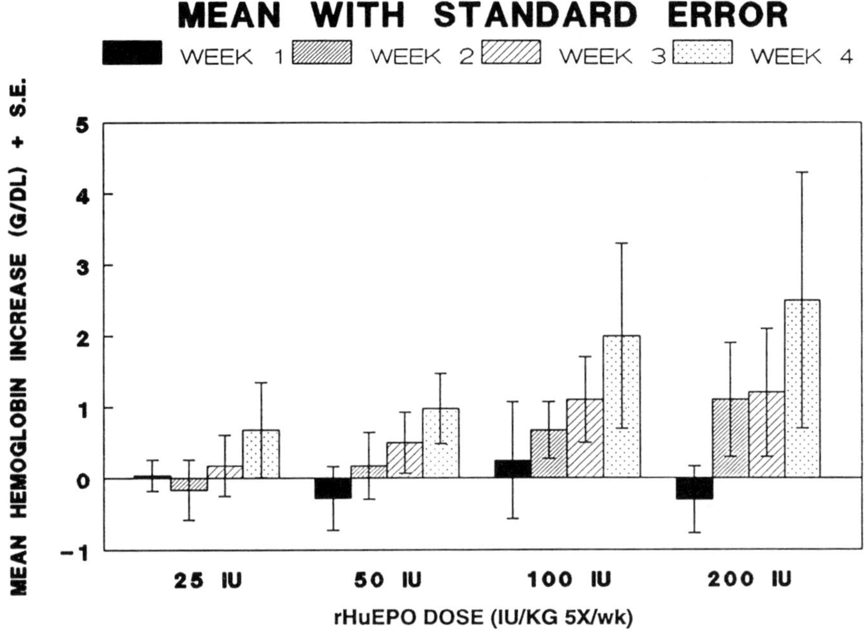

Fig. 2.   Mean hemoglobin change from baseline to end of rhEPO therapy (week 4).

While the transfusion requirement was not statistically evaluable in this phase I/II trial, of the 5 patients who required transfusion during the chemotherapy cycles in the 2 months preceding rhEPO therapy, 3 patients became transfusion independent during the study period despite continuation of chemotherapy.

The results of this preliminary study suggest that rhEPO is well tolerated in anemic patients receiving cisplatin chemotherapy for solid tumors. The dose was not escalated further because of preliminary evidence of efficacy at the 100 and 200 U/kg rhEPO dose levels in patients treated with cisplatin-based chemotherapeutic regimens in this study, as well as in a companion study of rhEPO [18]. In addition, the maximum tolerated dose was not reached during this study. Experience thus far suggests that rhEPO therapy for chemotherapy-associated anemia does not entail the same degree of risk for hypertension as it does for patients with chronic renal failure or end-stage renal disease [17–20].

In the 100 and 200 U/kg dose groups, 70% of all patients treated and 7 of the 8 patients not requiring early transfusion (87.5%) were responders. The mean change in hemoglobin level for all subjects receiving 100 and 200 U/kg was an increase of over 2.2 ± 1.5 g/dl. These data suggest that doses in this range are safe in this patient population and show very preliminary evidence of efficacy, however, a phase III study was needed to confirm efficacy in patients with anemia associated with cisplatin chemotherapy.

Phase III Study of rhEPO in Patients with Cisplatin-Related Anemia

A large multicenter trial of rhEPO in cisplatin-treated patients has been completed [20–22]. One hundred and thirty-two patients with anemia (hemoglobin < 10.5 g/dl) secondary to cisplatin chemotherapy for malignant disease were randomized to receive either rhEPO (epoetin alpha, 150 U/kg) or placebo subcutaneously 3 times a week for 12 weeks. Patients were eligible for the study if they had any malignancy except myeloid leukemia and were receiving cyclic chemotherapy containing cisplatin. Eighteen percent of the patients had hematological malignancies, and 82% had solid tumors. Patients with other causes of anemia (GI bleeding, iron deficiency, folate or B^{12} deficiency) were excluded, as were patients with uncontrolled hypertension, cerebral metastasis, or life expectancy of less than a year. All patients continued on cyclic chemotherapy containing cisplatin.

Primary endpoints for this study were effect of rhEPO on hematocrit, number of red blood cell transfusions required, and quality-of-life measurements. Patients were considered evaluable for toxicity if they received rhEPO and were on study at least 15 days.

One hundred and thirty-two patients were randomized to receive placebo or rhEPO (150 U/kg 3× a week). Baseline hematocrit (29.4 vs. 28.4), percentage of patients requiring transfusion (37.5 vs. 54.1), and baseline erythropoietin level (54 vs. 54) were equal in the 2 groups (rhEPO or placebo, respectively). The intensity of chemotherapy was equivalent in both groups with 83% of the rhEPO-treated patients and 77% of the placebo patients reaching an absolute neutrophil count of fewer than 1000 cells μl and a similar total cisplatin dose (273 vs. 294 mg, rhEPO or placebo, respectively). All patients were evaluable for toxicity; 64 rhEPO-treated patients and 61 placebo patients were eligible for efficacy.

The effect on hematocrit is shown in Figure 3. There was a significant difference in the mean hematocrit at the end of 12 weeks of study (35.4 vs. 29.7). The increase in hematocrit in the rhEPO-treated patients was seen after approximately 2 weeks of therapy, which is approximately the length of time that it takes for erythroid progenitors to mature in vivo from BFU-E to mature

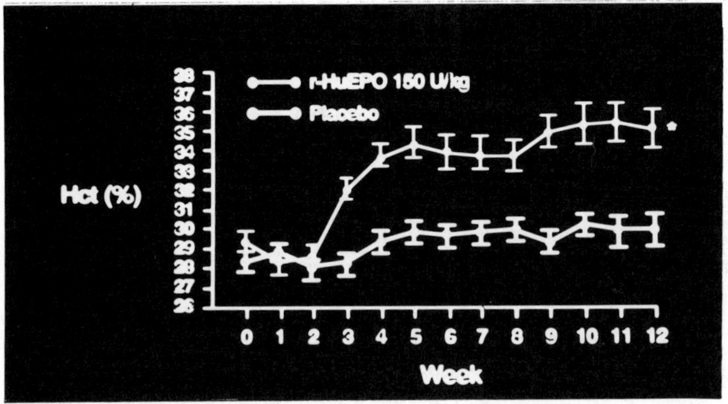

Fig. 3.   Mean weekly hematocrit ± SE in rhEPO- and placebo-treated patients undergoing cisplatin therapy. *p < 0.01.

erythroid cells. Of the rhEPO-treated patients, 48.4% had at least a 6 percentage point increase in hematocrit compared to 6.6% of the placebo-treated patients.

Because of the lag time between the administration of rhEPO and the appearance of mature red blood cells in the periphery, transfusion requirements during month 1 were evaluated separately from transfusion requirements during months 2 and 3. There was no difference in either the percentage of patients requiring transfusion of red blood cells or the number of units required in month 1 (Table 2). However, there was a statistically significant decrease in both the percentage of patients requiring transfusion and the mean number of red blood cell units transfused in the rhEPO-treated patients during months 2 and 3 of the study (Table 2).

Quality of life is an important, though often difficult, parameter to measure in patients with cancer receiving cisplatin chemotherapy. In this study, 3 quality of life parameters—energy level, activity of daily living, and overall quality— were studied using standard scales. Quality-of-life measurements were done pretreatment and at the end of the double-blind period. For analysis, baseline and end-of-treatment measurements were compared within 3 groups: placebo patients, all rhEPO-treated patients, and the subgroup of rhEPO-treated patients who had an increase in hematocrit of at least 6 percentage points during the course of the study (48% of patients). There was a significant increase in energy level in all 3 patient groups, with a significant improvement in activity of daily

Table 2. Transfusion requirements for patients undergoing cisplatin chemotherapy

	Month 1		Months 2 and 3	
	Placebo	rhEPO	Placebo	rhEPO
% transfused	44.3	43.8	56.4	26.8*
Mean units/ patient/month	1.2	1.7	2.0	1.2**

*p < 0.01; **p < 0.09.

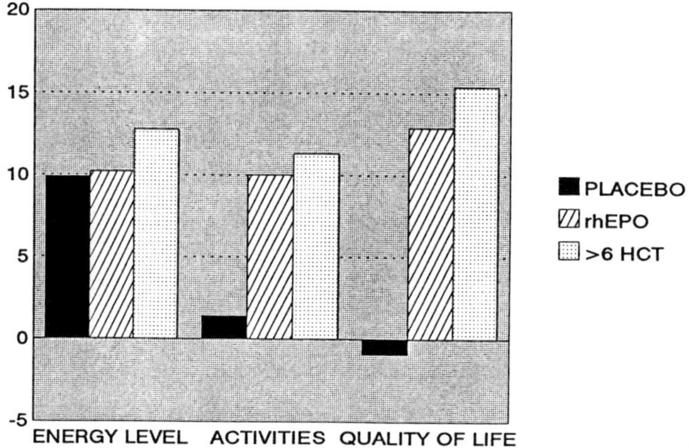

Fig. 4. Changes in quality-of-life measures from baseline to final evaluation in placebo patients, rhEPO-treated patients, and rhEPO-treated patients who had at least a 6 percentage point hematocrit increase during the study unrelated to transfusion. *p < 0.05.

living and overall quality of life seen only in the rhEPO-treated patient groups (Fig. 4).

rhEPO was well tolerated in this study. There was no difference in reported adverse experience between the rhEPO-treated patients and placebo patients with the exception of a decrease in shortness of breath in the rhEPO patients. There was no difference in the incidence of hypertension, seizures, or thrombotic episodes between rhEPO-treated patients and controls.

Effect of Pretransplant Erythropoietin Levels on Response

As the majority of patients with anemia associated with cisplatin therapy had inadequate erythropoietin responses to anemia, we were unable to use pretreatment erythropoietin levels to predict response to rhEPO in the phase I/II trial

[18]. This differs from patients with HIV infection treated with zidovudine, in which pretreatment serum erythropoietin levels can predict response to rhEPO [16]. However, pretreatment serum erythropoietin levels in all the cancer patients treated in the phase I/II trial were lower than the 500 mU/ml level that predicted a poor response to rhEPO treatment in the study of patients with HIV. Therefore, within the range of pretreatment erythropoietin levels seen in that study (<200mU/ml), pretreatment serum erythropoietin levels cannot be used to screen patients for responsiveness to exogenous erythropoietin treatment. The phase III study confirmed that there was no correlation between pretransplant erythropoietin levels and response to rhEPO.

Conclusion

rhEPO (150 U/kg s.c., 3 × a week) appears to improve hematocrit, decrease transfusion requirement, and improve overall quality of life in cancer patients who are anemic secondary to cisplatin chemotherapy. In a phase III trial, almost 50% of patients responded with at least a 6-point increase in hematocrit despite continued chemotherapy. This is especially important as the anemia associated with cisplatin is generally a progressive anemia with successive cycles.

References

1   Cartwright GE: The anemia of chronic disorders. Semin Hematol 1966;3:351–375.
2   Von Hoff DD, Schilsky R, Reichert CM: Toxic effects of cis-dichlorodiammine-platinum (II) in man. Cancer Treat Rep 1979;63:1527–1531.
3   Rossof AH, Slayton RE, Perlia CP: Preliminary clinical experience with cis-diamminedichloroplatinum (II) (NSC 119875, CACP). Cancer 1972;30:1451–1456.
4   Chary KK, Higby DJ, Henderson ES: Phase I study of high-dose cis-dichlorodiammineplatinum (II) with forced diuresis. Cancer Treat Rep 1977;61:367–370.
5   Saito Y, Mori K, Tominaga K: Phase I study of 5-day continuous infusion of cis-diamminedichloroplatinum (II) in the treatment of non-small-cell lung cancer. Cancer Chemother Pharmacol 1990;26:389–392.
6   Eschbach JW, Adamson JW: Anemia of end stage renal disease. Kidney Int 1985;28:1–5.
7   Chandra M, Clemons GK, McVicar MI: Relation of serum erythropoietin levels to renal excretory function: Evidence for lowered set point for erythropoietin production in chronic renal failure. J Pediatr 1988;113:1015–1021.
8   Spivak JL, Barnes DC, Fuchs E, et al.: Serum immunoreactive erythropoietin in HIV-infected patients. JAMA 1989;261:3104–3107.
9   Miller CB, Jones RJ, Piantadosi S, et al.: Decreased erythropoietin response in patients with the anemia of cancer. N Engl J Med 1990;322:1689–1691.

10   Wood P, Nygaard S, Hrushesky WJM: Cisplatin-induced anemia is correctable with erythropoietin. Blood 1988;72(Suppl):A52.
11   Matsumoto T, Endoh K, Kamisango K: Effect of recombinant human erythropoietin on anticancer drug-induced anaemia. Br J Haematol 1990;75:463–468.
12   Eschbach JW, Kelly MR, Haley NR, et al.: Treatment of the anemia of progressive renal failure with recombinant human erythropoietin. N Engl J Med 1989;321: 158–161.
13   Eschbach JW, Egrie JC, Downing MR, et al.: Correction of the anemia of end-stage renal disease with recombinant human erythropoietin. N Engl J Med 1987;316: 73–78.
14   Casati S, Passerini P, Campise MR, et al.: Benefits and risks of protracted treatment with human recombinant erythropoietin in patients having haemodialysis. Br Med J 1987;295:1017–1020.
15   Bennett WM: A multicenter clinical trial of epoetin beta for anemia of end-stage renal disease. J Am Soc Nephrol 1991;1:990–998.
16   Fischl M, Galpin JE, Levine JD, et al.: Recombinant human erythropoietin for patients with AIDS treated with zidovudine. N Engl J Med 1990;322:1488–1493.
17   Miller CB, Plantanias LC, Ratain MJ, et al.: A phase I/II trial of erythropoietin in the treatment of chemotherapy-induced anemia in patients with cancer. J Natl Cancer Inst 1992;84(2):98–103.
18   Plantanias LC, Miller CB, Mick R, et al.: Treatment of chemotherapy-induced anemia in cancer patients with recombinant human erythropoietin. J Clin Oncol 1991;9(11):2021–2026.
19   Miller CB: Erythropoietin in renal and non-renal anemias; in Gurland HJ, Moran J, Samtleben W, et al. (eds): Chemotherapy-Induced Anemia. Contrib Nephrol. Basel, Karger, 1991, pp 248–251.
20   Abels RI, Larholt KM, Krantz KD, et al.: Recombinant human erythropoietin (r-HuEPO) for the treatment of the anemia of cancer; in Martin J Murphy Jr (ed): Blood Cell Growth Factors: Their Present and Future Use in Hematology and Oncology. Alpha Med Press, 1991, pp 121–141.
21   Henry DH, Rudnick SA, Bryant E, et al.: Preliminary report of two double blind, placebo controlled studies using recombinant human erythropoietin in the anemia associated with cancer [Abstract]. Blood 1989;73(Suppl):6.
22   Henry DH, Bennett J, Brooks R, et al.: Recombinant human erythropoietin (rHuEPO) for the treatment of the anemia of cancer, final results of multicenter trials. Blood 1991;78:152a(abstract).

Carole B. Miller, M.D., Oncology Center, Room 167, The Johns Hopkins University, 600 North Wolfe Street, Baltimore, MD 21287-8985 (USA)

Discussion

to the Paper by C.B. Miller and S.R. Mills

Cazzola (*Pavia*): I would like to open the discussion by asking you how big was the problem of functional iron deficiency in your study. We learned from Dr. Skikne's presentation that almost all normal subjects treated with recombinant human EPO will experience functional iron deficiency. Some of your patients have functional iron deficiency before treatment simply because they have systemic symptoms and reticuloendothelial iron block. Did you evaluate this problem? Did you treat patients with iron, and by which route?

Miller: I can only comment on the phase I/II trial. I do not have the iron data for the multicenter trial. In the phase I/II trial we treated patients when their ferritin fell below the lower half of normal. They got treated with oral iron (325 milligrams three times a day). Only less than 10% of the patients in the phase I/II trial required supplementation with iron, as the majority of the patients started off with high ferritin levels. Now, we did not look at the total iron-binding capacity or the serum iron. We relied on ferritin, and I am now learning that we may have to look further at the other iron stores as well. But despite just following ferritins, we were able to see responses in the majority of patients. In both the multicenter trial and the phase I/II trials there was no correlation between the baseline serum erythropoietin level and the response to the human erythropoietin. However, I do have to remind you that the majority of the patients had low endogenous erythropoietin levels.

[*Unidentified*]: Can you tell us a little bit more about the detail of your cohort study, especially at what point of chemotherapy periods were the questions asked? If we really have an increasing quality of life, then it makes sense to increase hemoglobin by rhEPO.

Miller: The quality-of-life questionnaires were done pre-treatment and at the end of the 12 weeks of therapy. Because erythropoietin could be started at any point related to the chemotherapy, there was no standard time related to the chemotherapy that the patient was given the questionnaires. So, the quality-of-life measurements reflect a broad range of times related to chemotherapy and therefore may be difficult to evaluate. The questionnaire was a standard five- to ten-page page questionnaire using analog scales that has been well documented in the cancer literature as being the appropriate scale to look at quality of life in cancer patients. I don't have a lot of details on it, as I didn't participate in that trial.

Breymann (*Zurich*): What happens to patients who developed infections under chemotherapy opportunistic infections and therefore anemia? Do you exclude these from the study, or do you continue with your EPO treatment?

Miller: All the patients who had started on the study and subsequently developed an infection did continue on erythropoietin. They were only excluded if they developed an infection before starting the erythropoietin.

Stockenhuber (Vienna): Did you continue your EPO therapy during the whole study period even if it came to high hematocrit levels of, for instance, more than 40%?

Miller: In a phase I/II trial, as it was a short trial, we did not stop rhEPO early in any patient. However, in the placebo-controlled randomized trial, when the patients reached a target hematocrit of 38, erythropoietin was discontinued. I don't know the percentage of the patients, however, that was able to stop before the 12 weeks were completed.

Recombinant Human Erythropoietin in Hematological Malignancies

Luisa Ponchio, Giovanna Farina, Claudia Pedrotti, Vittorio Rosti, Gaetano Bergamaschi, Mario Cazzola

Department of Internal Medicine and Medical Therapy, University of Pavia and IRCCS Policlinico S. Matteo, Pavia, Italy

Summary

Refractory anemia is frequently observed in hematological malignancies, and rhEPO has been employed for its treatment in some of these disorders. Phase I/II clinical studies indicate that treatment with rhEPO can be effective and safe in ameliorating anemia in patients with monoclonal gammopathies or malignant lymphomas. Treatment is particularly effective in subjects showing blunted endogenous erythropoietin production and may be effective even in those exposed to chemotherapy. Functional iron deficiency may be a cause of nonresponse, and oral or parenteral iron supplementation is required in these cases to obtain response. Patients with hematopoietic stem cell disorders are less likely to respond to rhEPO, but a minority of these subjects may benefit of this treatment. Phase III clinical trials are now required.

Introduction

Recombinant human erythropoietin (rhEPO) has been shown to be effective and well tolerated in correcting the anemia of renal failure [1–3]. In a phase I/II clinical trial, we have recently found that rhEPO can ameliorate the refractory anemia associated with hematological disorders [4]. This article will review the present state of the art on the use of rhEPO in hematological malignancies. These conditions include hematopoietic stem cell disorders (e.g., myelodysplastic syndromes and idiopathic myelofibrosis), monoclonal gammopathies, and malignant lymphomas. Before examining the use of rhEPO in these conditions, we will briefly analyze a rational laboratory approach to be employed in these clinical studies.

Laboratory Investigations Useful for Monitoring the Erythroid Marrow Response to rhEPO

A rational laboratory approach to the patient treated with rhEPO should include the assessment of endogenous erythropoietin production, quantitation of total and effective erythropoietic activity, and evaluation of iron supply to the erythroid marrow.

Endogenous erythropoietin production may be quantitated through serum EPO. Since serum levels increase exponentially as the hematocrit decreases, serum erythropoietin must be evaluated in relation to the degree of anemia. To do this, it is necessary to define a reference range by studying normal subjects and patients with hemolytic or aplastic anemia [5]. The appropriateness of erythropoietin response to anemia can then be evaluated through the observed/predicted log (erythropoietin) ratio (O/P ratio) [4].

Total erythroid marrow activity can be quantitated through the simple measurement of serum transferrin receptor (TfR) [5]. Serum transferrin receptor is a truncated form of surface receptor and is derived from erythroid precursors in the bone marrow. There is a close relationship between serum transferrin receptor and ferrokinetic measurements of erythropoiesis in normal conditions and a variety of disease states [5]. We have found that the serum transferrin receptor assay is a valid method for monitoring the erythropoietic response to rhEPO [4]. Sequential measurements of this parameter proved to be a reliable predictor of response: in fact, responders showed a considerable increase (>40%) in serum transferrin receptor after 2 weeks of treatment, whereas most nonresponders showed no significant change.

The reticulocyte count is required for evaluation of the effective erythropoiesis. By using flow cytometry, different populations of reticulocyte can be recognized [6]. The fraction called high fluorescence ratio (HFR) reticulocytes contains newly released red cells: this represents the most sensitive index of effective erythropoiesis [6]. When the erythroid marrow responds to rhEPO in an effective way, one can observe a combined increase in serum transferrin receptor and reticulocyte count. If serum transferrin receptor increases without any significant variation in reticulocyte count, stimulation of ineffective erythropoiesis is likely.

Adequate iron supply to the erythroid marrow is essential for the erythroid marrow response to rhEPO. Clinical trials on the use of rhEPO have revealed a condition called functional iron deficiency [4], characterized by normal body iron stores but an iron supply to the erythroid marrow that is inadequate for marrow demand. This condition may be recognized by measuring serum iron, transferrin saturation, and serum ferritin: typically, serum iron is lower than 50 μg/dl and transferrin saturation is lower than 16%, whereas serum ferritin is normal to high. A new approach is based on the evaluation of hypochromic red cells (i.e., red cells with Hb concentration < 28 g/dl) [7]. Hypochromic red cells are normally lower than 2.5%: an increase to over 10% during rhEPO indicates functional iron deficiency and the need for iron supplementation [7].

rhEPO in the Treatment of Myelodysplastic Syndromes and Idiopathic Myelofibrosis

Myelodysplastic syndromes are mainly characterized by refractory anemia, which represents one of the most frustrating therapeutic problems for hematologists. There were great expectations for rhEPO, and a great number of phase I/II studies have been carried out in recent years [9–23]. As shown in Table 1, the overall response was 16%. The low efficacy of erythropoietin in myelodysplastic syndromes is likely due both to the low responsiveness of myelodysplastic BFU-E to rhEPO (24) and to stimulation of ineffective erythropoiesis [25]. Although blunted erythropoietin production is not an important mechanism of anemia in myelodysplastic syndromes, patients showing low erythropoietin levels are more likely to respond to rhEPO [25].

Few data are available on the use of rhEPO in the treatment of anemia in idiopathic myelofibrosis [4]. Not only does erythropoietin appear to be ineffective in these patients, but it may also produce symptomatic spleen enlargement, probably due to stimulation of extramedullary erythropoiesis.

rhEPO in the Treatment of Anemia Associated with Multiple Myeloma

Frequency of Anemia in Multiple Myeloma

As stated by Kyle [26], almost every patient with multiple myeloma eventually becomes anemic. Incidence and severity of anemia, however, vary considerably according to the clinical course of the disease. About 62% of a series seen by Kyle at the Mayo Clinic up to 1971 were anemic at clinical onset [27], while half the patients (237 out of 485) entering the third MRC myelomatosis trial had an initial hemoglobin of 10 g/dl or less [28]. In our department about one third of

Table 1. Clinical trials on the use of rhEPO in myelodysplastic syndromes[a]

rhEPO dose (U/kg/week)	Route	Responders	Ref.
130–515[b]	IV	3/8	8
75–1500	IV	0/2	9
700	IV	1/1	10
420–630	SC	2/10	11
240–1920	SC	1/14	12
2400–3200	IV	4/17	13
350	SC	2/16	14
600–3000	IV	3/12	15
150–450	SC	0/12	16
300–1500	SC	1/10	17
250–750	SC	0/4	4
300–1800	SC	1/4	18
1050	SC	3/9	19
300–900	SC	1/17	20
600–900	SC	0/6	21
450–900	SC	5/20[c]	22
3000[b]	IV	0/8	23
		27/170 (16%)	

[a]Response is defined as abolishment of transfusion requirement in transfusion-dependent patients or an increase in Hb $\geq$ 1.5 g/dl in patients without transfusion requirement.
[b]Assuming a mean body weight of 70 kg.
[c]Assuming that half the responders had complete response.

patients showed Hb values lower than 10 g/dl at clinical onset, whereas about 10% had values lower than 8 g/dl and required blood transfusions (Table 2). The Hb concentration on presentation is of strong prognostic value, and is a basic parameter in the Durie and Salmon staging system [29]: stage I patients have by definition values greater than 10 g/dl, whereas all subjects with Hb lower than 8.5 g/dl are classified as stage III.

Pathogenesis of Anemia in Multiple Myeloma

Ting et al. [30] studied 24 untreated patients with myelomatosis in order to characterize their anemia using standard hematological and ferrokinetic techniques, together with measurements of circulating erythropoietin, erythropoietin sensitivity of marrow cultures, and in vitro measurements of heme synthesis. All patients showed an erythroid marrow activity lower than twice normal in the presence of anemia, indicating relative marrow failure as a mechanism of anemia

Table 2.   Frequency of anemia at clinical onset in patients with multiple myeloma followed at the Department of Internal Medicine and Medical Therapy, University of Pavia, Pavia, Italy

Patient presentation	Diagnosis period	
	1972–1986	1987–1989
Multiple myeloma	345	162
Hb < 12 g/dl	210 (61%)	92 (57%)
Hb < 10 g/dl	114 (33%)	49 (30%)
Hb < 8 g/dl	48 (14%)	15 (9%)

[31]. There was a borderline plasma expansion, indicating minor hemodilution, whose physiological relevance was marginal. Erythroid activity was inversely related to renal function, serum erythropoietin, and plasma cell mass: these data would seem to indicate that both impaired endogenous erythropoietin production and tumor cell mass play a role in the pathogenesis of anemia. The relationship between anemia and renal failure had been previously observed by Birgens et al. [32].

Ting et al. [30] also found that a few patients showed a reduced in vitro response of marrow CFU-E to erythropoietin. This has recently been confirmed by Aoki et al. [33], who found a variable response of CFU-E to rhEPO independently of the percentage of plasma cells in the bone marrow. These latter authors have suggested that the number or sensitivity of erythropoietin receptors on the CFU-E may be variably reduced in multiple myeloma and have concluded that treatment with rhEPO may be effective in at least a portion of patients.

The reduced sensitivity of erythropoietin, however, does not necessarily mean that receptors are altered. A number of cytokines seem to play a role in the pathogenesis of multiple myeloma, IL-6 being the most relevant [34]. Interleukin 1 and tumor necrosis factor (TNF), whose release is typically increased in the so-called anemia of chronic disease, both inhibit erythroid marrow proliferation and blunt the normal exponential relationship between hematocrit and serum erythropoietin [35]. In animal models these cytokines have been found to exert suppressive effects on erythropoiesis that can be reversed with exogenous erythropoietin [36, 37]. In some experimental studies, however, erythropoietin failed to reverse anemia in mice bearing tumors that produce high levels of TNF-α [38].

In summary, at least two factors are responsible of anemia in untreated patients with multiple myeloma: blunted endogenous erythropoietin production and reduced sensitivity of erythroid progenitors to erythropoietin. Tumor mass activates both mechanisms by producing the M component responsible of renal damage and a number of cytokines with multiple inhibitory effects.

Clinical Studies on the Use of rhEPO in the Treatment of Anemia in Multiple Myeloma

In 1990, Taylor et al. [39] reported the successful use of erythropoietin in 2 patients with myeloma who were dependent on transfusions and were receiving hemodialysis for renal failure. Ludwig et al. [40] treated 13 patients with myeloma-associated anemia by administering rhEPO. Eleven patients (85%) had steady increases in hemoglobin levels with eventual correction of anemia, whereas no patient had evidence of erythropoietin-related disease progression. It was concluded that rhEPO may be a useful therapeutic tool for treating myeloma-associated anemia.

We employed subcutaneous rhEPO in 4 patients with multiple myeloma and 1 patient with AL amyloidosis, all of them under chemotherapy [4]. All patients showed a blunted erythropoietin production and 4 responded to treatment maintaining Hb above 10 g/dl without transfusion. Finelli et al. [41] performed a pilot study on anemic patients affected by multiple myeloma refractory to first- or second-line chemotherapy. rhEPO was administered subcutaneously at a dose of 150–300 U/kg/day t.i.w. Four of the 10 patients treated did not require blood transfusions: all showed an increase in Hb level after the 8-week treatment, the peak Hb level ranging from 9.3 to 12.9 g/dl. Only 2 of the 6 transfusion-dependent patients in this study showed a response (abolishment of transfusion requirement). The reasons for these less favorable results are not clear, but might be due to selection of patients with more severe disease.

In summary, all the above studies have shown that rhEPO may be effective in ameliorating the anemia associated with multiple myeloma. They also excluded a stimulatory effect on the neoplastic clone by growth factor suspected by Rogers et al. in a particular case [42].

rhEPO in the Treatment of Anemia Associated with Malignant Lymphomas

The mechanisms of anemia associated with malignant lymphomas are largely similar to those of multiple myeloma, except for renal failure, which is quite uncommon in lymphoproliferative disorders and frequent in monoclonal gammopathies. Neoplastic bone marrow infiltration and chemotherapy seem to each play a major role in the pathogenesis of anemia associated with malignant lymphomas. In our study [4], a blunted endogenous erythropoietin production was found in all patients with malignant lymphoma under chemotherapy.

A number of studies [4, 41, 43–45] have shown that pharmacological doses of rhEPO are able to stimulate erythropoiesis and ameliorate anemia in the majority of anemic patients with malignant lymphoma. It should be noted that a management issue in these studies has been the high frequency of functional iron deficiency associated with rhEPO treatment [4]. An impaired iron supply to the erythroid marrow can blunt the erythropoietic response to rhEPO [4] and lead to defining as unresponsive patients who would respond after correction of functional iron deficiency. In our study, two subjects required parenteral iron to correct functional iron deficiency [4].

The above findings suggest that rhEPO could be incorporated in chemotherapy protocols to prevent anemia and, in particular, the need for transfusion.

Conclusions

The available phase I/II clinical studies indicate that treatment with rhEPO can be effective and safe in ameliorating anemia in patients with monoclonal gammopathies or malignant lymphoma. Treatment is particularly effective in subjects showing inappropriate erythropoietin response to anemia and may be effective even in those exposed to chemotherapy. Functional iron deficiency may be a cause of nonresponse: in fact, an impaired iron supply to the erythroid marrow can blunt the erythropoietic response to rhEPO and lead to defining as unresponsive patients who would respond after correction of functional iron deficiency. Patients with hematopoietic stem cell disorders are less likely to respond to rhEPO, although favorable responses may be occasionally observed.

Acknowledgments

This work was supported by grants from Associazione Italiana per la Ricerca sul Cancro, Fondazione Ferrata Storti, and IRCCS Policlinico S. Matteo.

References

1 Winearls CG, Oliver DO, Pippard MJ, Reid C, Downing MR, Cotes PM: Effect of human erythropoietin derived from recombinant DNA on the anaemia of patients maintained by chronic haemodyalysis. Lancet 1986;II:1175–1177.

2   Eschbach JW, Egrie JC, Downing MR, Browne JK, Adamson JW: Correction of the anemia of end-stage renal disease with recombinant human erythropoietin. Results of a combined phase I and II clinical trial. N Engl J Med 1987;316:73–78.

3   Eschbach JW, Kelly MR, Haley NR, Abels RI, Adamson JW: Treatment of the anemia of progressive renal failure with recombinant human erythropoietin. N Engl J Med 1989;321:158–163.

4   Cazzola M, Ponchio L, Beguin Y, Rosti V, Bergamaschi G, Liberato N, Fregoni V, Nalli G, Barosi G, Ascari E: Subcutaneous erythropoietin for treatment of refractory anemia in hematologic disorders. Results of a phase I/II clinical trial. Blood 1992;79:29–37.

5   Cazzola M, Beguin Y: New tools for clinical evaluation of erythron function in man. Br J Haematol 1992;80:278–284.

6   Bowen D, Bentley N, Hoy T, Cavill I: Comparison of a modified thiazole orange technique with a fully aytomated analyser for reticulocyte counting. J Clin Pathol 1991;44:130–133.

7   Macdougall IC, Cavill I, Hulme B, Bain B, McGregory E, McKay P, Sanders E, Coles GA, Williams JD: Detection of functional iron deficiency during erythropoietin treatment: A new approach. Br Med J 1992;304:225–226.

8   Bessho M, Jinnai I, Matsuda A, Saito M, Hirashima K: Improvement of anemia by recombinant erythropoietin in patients with myelodysplastic syndromes and aplastic anemia. Int J Cell Cloning 1990;8:445–458.

9   Stebler C, Tichelli A, Dazzi H, Gratwohl A, Nissen C, Speck: High-dose recombinant human erythropoietin for treatment of anemia in myelodysplastic syndromes and paroxysmal nocturnal hemoglobinuria: A pilot study. Exp Hematol 1990; 18:1204–1208.

10 Hast R, Celsing F, Ekman M, Syenke L: Response to recombinant human erythropoietin treatment in myelodysplastic syndromes (MDS). J Intern Med 1991;229: 381–386.

11 Bowen D, Culligan D, Jacobs A: The treatment of anaemia in the myelodysplastic syndromes with recombinant human erythropoietin. Br J Haematol 1991;77: 419–423.

12 Schouten HC, Vellenga E, van Rhenen DJ, de Wolf JThM, Coppens PJW, Blijham GH: Recombinant human erythropoietin in patients with myelodysplastic syndromes. Leukemia 1991;5:432–436.

13 Stein RS, Abels RI, Krantz SB: Pharmacologic doses of recombinant human erythropoietin in the treatment of myelodysplastic syndromes. Blood 1991;78:1658–1663.

14 Kurzrock R, Talpaz M, Estey E, O'Brien S, Estrov Z, Gutterman JU: Erythropoietin treatment in patients with myelodysplastic syndrome and anemia. Leukemia 1991;5:985–990.

15 Hellström E, Birgegård G, Lockner D, Öst Å, Wide L: Treatment of myelodysplastic syndromes with recombinant human erythropoietin. Eur J Haematol 1991;47: 355–360.

16 van Kamp H, Prinsze-Postema TC, Kluin PM, den Ottolander GJ, Beverstock GG, Willemze R, Fibbe WE: Effect of subcutaneously administered human recombinant erythropoietin on erythropoiesis in patients with myelodysplasia. Br J Haematol 1991;78:488–4931.

17 Verhoef GEG, Zaché P, Ferrant A, Demuynck H, Selleslag D, van Hove L, Deckers F, Boogaerts MA: Recombinant human erythropoietin for the treatment of anemia in the myelodysplastic syndromes: A clinical and erythrokinetic assessment. Ann Hematol 1992;64:16–21.

18 Sherperd JD, Currie CJ, Sparling TG, Krystal G, Eaves AC: Erythropoietin therapy of myelodysplastic syndromes. Blood 1992;79:1891–1893 (letter).

19 Rafanelli D, Grossi A, Longo G, Vannucchi AM, Bacci P, Rossi Ferrini P: Recombinant human erythropoietin for treatment of myelodysplastic syndromes. Leukemia 1992;6:323–327.

20 Razzano M, Caslini C, Cortellazzo S, Battistel V, Rambaldi A, Barbui T: Therapy with human recombinant erythropoietin in patients with myelodysplastic syndromes. Br J Haematol 1992;81:628–630.

21 Mittelman M, Floru S, Djaldetti M: Subcutaneous erythropoietin for treatment of refractory anemia in hematologic disorders. Blood 1992;80:841 (letter).

22 Adamson JW, Schuster M, Allen S, Haley NR. Effectiveness of recombinant human erythropoietin therapy in myelodysplastic syndromes. Acta Haematol 1992;87 (Suppl 1):20–24.

23 Casadevall N, Belanger C, Goy A, Varet B, Lang J, Poisson D. High-dose recombinant human erythropoietin administered intravenously for the treatment of anaemia in myelodysplastic syndromes. Acta Haematol 1992;87(suppl 1):25–27.

24 Merchav S, Nielsen OJ, Rosenbaum H, Sharon R, Brenner B, Tatarsky I, Scigalla P, Wieczorek L. In vitro studies of erythropoietin dependent regulation of erythropoiesis in myelodysplastic syndromes. Leukemia 1990;4:771–774.

25 Cazzola M, Ponchio L. Subcutaneous erythropoietin for treatment of refractory anemia in hematologic disorders. Response. Blood 1992; 80:841–843 (letter).

26 Kyle RA: Diagnosis and management of multiple myeloma and related disorders. Progr Hematol 1986;14:257–282.

27 Kyle RA: Multiple myeloma. Review of 869 cases. Mayo Clin Proc 1975;50:29–40.

28 Medical Research Council: Report on the second myelomatosis trial after 6 completed years of follow-up. Br J Cancer 1980;42:813–822.

29 Durie BGM, Salmon SE: Clinical staging system for multiple myeloma. Cancer 1975; 36:842–854.

30 Ting WC, Cavill I, Jacobs A, Kaaba S, May A, Smith S, Whittaker JA: Anaemia in patients with myelomatosis. Br J Cancer 1982;45:887–894.

31 Cazzola M, Pootrakul P, Huebers HA, Eng M, Eschbach J, Finch CA: Erythroid marrow function in anemic man. Blood 1987;69:296–301.

32 Birgens H, Paaske Hansen O, Henriksen JH, Wantzin P: Quantitation of erythropoiesis in myelomatosis. Scand J Haematol 1979;22:357–363.

33 Aoki I, Nishijima K, Homori M, Nakahara K, Higashi K, Ishikawa K: Responsiveness of bone marrow erythroid progenitors (CFU-E and BFU-E) to recombinant human erythropoietin (rh-Ep) in vitro in multiple myeloma. Br J Haematol 1992; 81:463–469.

34 Klein B, Bataille R: Cytokine network in human multiple myeloma. Hematol/Oncol Clin North Am 1992;6:273–284.

35 Erslev A: Erythropoietin. N Engl J Med 1991; 324:1339–1344.

36 Johnson CS, Keckler DJ, Topper MI, Braunschweiger PG, Furmanski P: In vivo

hematopoietic effects of recombinant interleukin-1α in mice: Stimulation of granulocytic, monocytic, megakaryocytic, and early erythroid progenitors, suppression of late-stage erythropoiesis and reversal of erythroid suppression with erythropoietin. Blood 1989;3:678–683.

37 Johnson CS, Cook CA, Furmanski P: In vivo suppression of erythropoiesis by tumor necrosis factor-α (TNF-α): Reversal with exogenous erythropoietin (EPO). Exp Hematol 1990;18:109–113.

38 Clibon U, Bonewald L, Caro J, Roodman GD: Erythropoietin fails to reverse the anemia in mice continuously exposed to tumor necrosis factor-alpha in vivo. Exp Hematol 1990;18:438–441.

39 Taylor J, Mactier RA, Stewart WK, Henderson IS: Effect of erythropoietin on anaemia in patients with myeloma receiving haemodialysis. Br Med J 1990; 301:476.

40 Ludwig H, Fritz E, Kotzmann H, Höcker P, Gisslinger H, Barnas U: Erythropoietin treatment of anemia associated with multiple myeloma. N Engl J Med 1990;322:1693–1699.

41 Finelli C, Cavo M, Visani G, Bonelli MA, Gamberi B, Fogli M, Cenacchi A, Tosi P, Bertelletti D, Villa R, Tura S: Recombinant human erythropoietin as a treatment for anemia in B cell malignancies; in Cazzola M, Barosi G, Ascari E (eds); Erythropoietin Symposium 1992. Pavia, Ferrata Storti Foundation, 1992, pp 85–93.

42 Rogers S, Russell NH, Morgan AG: Effect of erythropoietin in patients with myeloma. Br Med J 1990; 301:667 (letter).

43 Oster W, Herrmann F, Gamm H, Zeile G, Lindemann A, Müller G, Brune T, Kraemer H-P, Mertelsmann R: Erythropoietin for the treatment of anemia of malignancy associated with neoplastic bone marrow infiltration. J Clin Oncol 1990; 8:956–962.

44 Platanias LC, Miller CB, Mick R, Hart RD, Ozer H, McEvilly J-M, Jones RJ, Ratain MJ: Treatment of chemotherapy-induced anemia with recombinant erythropoietin in cancer patients. J Clin Oncol 1991;9:2021–2026.

45 Longo G, Curci G, Federico M, Bonacorsi G, Donelli A, Fiorani C, Di Prisco AU, Torelli U: Treatment of anemia associated with lymphoproliferative disorders: role of recombinant human erythropoietin; in Cazzola M, Barosi G, Ascari E (eds): Erythropoietin Symposium 1992. Pavia, Ferrata Storti Foundation, 1992, pp 94–101.

Mario Cazzola, Clinica Medica 2, Policlinico S. Matteo, 27100 Pavia, Italy

Discussion

to the Paper by L. Ponchio et al.

Miller (Baltimore): I have a question: In the myelodysplastic patients, was there anything that could predict response in the 20% of patients who responded?

Cazzola: Yes and no. Patients who are heavily transfusion-dependent are unlikely to respond, whereas patients who are at clinical onset are more likely to respond. We have a study going on now in Italy. Using a probe called M27β, it is possible to study a female patient in order to establish whether hematopoiesis is clonal or polyclonal. We are trying to correlate the presence of residual nonclonal stem cells with response, but it is too early to answer your question now.

Horina (Graz): A question that belongs to both of you: You gave evidence that IL-1 overproduction might be a major factor in the pathogenesis of the anemia. Did you have a chance to measure IL-1 in your patients, and did you have a chance to correlate IL-1 and EPO levels?

Miller: No, we did not measure IL-1. That was work from Hep 3B cell lines by Mark Goldberg. We did not correlate IL-1 levels with EPO response.

Cazzola: We did not, but we measured reactive protein C, which may be an indicator of IL-1 production. There is no significant conclusion by now, but patients with higher reactive protein C appear to be unlikely to respond to recombinant human EPO.

Birgegard (Uppsala): You measured transferrin receptor in some of those patients. Maybe I missed it: Was it only in the myelodysplastic syndromes that you saw an increase in transferrin receptor without response in hemoglobin, or did that happen in other patients too?

Cazzola: We measured serum transferrin receptor in all the patients. I showed that patient with primary acquired sideroblastic anemia, a type of myelodysplastic syndrome, to provide you with an example of what stimulation of ineffective erythropoiesis is. If you have an increase in serum transferrin receptor which reflects total marrow erythroid activity and no change in the reticulocyte count, by definition, you have stimulation of ineffective erythropoiesis. In patients with multiple myeloma or malignant lymphoma responding to recombinant human EPO, the increase in the serum transferrin receptor was paralleled by an increase in the reticulocyte count, and we have presented data suggesting that an increase in serum transferrin receptor greater than 40% over baseline associated with an increase in reticulocyte count is a predictor of response to rhEPO.

Birgegard: My question was the opposite. Did you see other patients than MDS patients who increased in transferrin receptor without response in hemoglobin or reticulocytes?

Cazzola: With an increase in serum transferrin receptor and no increase in reticulocyte count? . . . . No, we did not.

Brunner (Berne): At what stage of the disease in myeloma and lymphoma, early or late, did you give EPO and, in addition, did these patients have other treatments or were they without treatment (chemotherapy)?

Cazzola: We treated with rhEPO all patients with hemoglobin levels below 10 grams per deciliter. Your question is important. In fact, we believe that patients at clinical onset are very likely to respond to recombinant human EPO, while patients with advanced disease—and particularly those refractory to second-line treatment—are very unlikely to respond.

Brunner: What about other treatments, because additional chemotherapy also may increase hemoglobin?

Cazzola: Recombinant human EPO was started when the hemoglobin level fell below 10 grams per deciliter irrespective of chemotherapy. Thus, some patients were treated with rhEPO and chemotherapy at the same time; some patients were treated just with rhEPO.

Winearls (Oxford): There was a report of a patient who developed painful splenomegaly after EPO treatment, and this was attributed to extramedullary hemopoiesis. Have you seen this in any of your patients?

Cazzola: Yes, we have. Two of the six patients with idiopathic myelofibrosis had a considerable spleen enlargement during rhEPO, and we have evidence that the stimulation of splenic erythropoiesis is the cause.

Adamson (New York): Could you remind us, was this daily dosing?

Cazzola: It was 5 days per week by s.c.

Adamson: And what was the duration of therapy for the myelodysplastic patients?

Cazzola: We used an escalating dose regimen: 50 units per kilogram, 75, 100, 150. Each dose was given for a 4-week period. Thus, unresponsive patients were treated at least for 4 months.

(Adamson): But 4 months included potentially 3 months of relatively low dosing.

Cazzola: Yes.

Adamson: The point behind the original question is this: Our experience—which was just published in *Acta Hematologica*—with 20 patients with myelodysplasia, suggested that in this group of patients high rhEPO doses are going to be necessary for protracted periods of time, because the marrow is relatively unresponsive. I wonder if we might not rescue more of these patients if we treated at the onset with higher doses of EPO and accepted the fact that we are going to have to treat them for a longer period of time to see a maximum response?

Cazzola: I agree with you. It is possible that higher doses will be effective. But you also have to take into account cost-benefit analysis. We calculated that the annual cost of a transfusion treatment based on 4 units of red cells per month will be approximately $10,000 a year. If you use the rhEPO at a dose of 75 units per kilogram per day 5 days a week you have a cost which is comparable—about $9000 a year—but if you increase your dose to maybe 300 units per kilogram per day, your cost will be about $36,000 a year. That is not cost-effective.

Major (Zurich): How do you count the reticulocytes; is this the flow reticulocytometer?

Cazzola: Until the beginning of this year, it was a conventional technique using a microscope. We are now using a cytofluorometer, and this is a particularly good technique because it is more precise and reliable. It is particularly useful also because we can measure the fraction called high fluorescent rate (HFR) reticulocytes; that probably is the best indicator of effective erythropoiesis.

Major: You said that transferrin receptor is a better parameter for the response to erythropoietin. How is it in comparison with this new method, reticulocyte flowcytometry?

Cazzola: The two parameters reflect two different aspects. The serum transferrin receptor is essentially derived from transferrin receptors on marrow erythroblasts and is a measure of the total erythroid activity, i.e., the number of erythroblasts in the bone marrow. The reticulocyte count or the HFR fraction is a measure of the effective erythropoiesis, and so of the newly released reticulocytes. You have to use the two parameters in order to identify stimulation of effective erythropoiesis or stimulation of ineffective erythropoiesis.

Recombinant Human Erythropoietin Therapy
in Patients with Osteosarcoma and Ewing's Sarcoma

C. Wurnig,[a] M. Keil,[b] R. Windhager,[a] A. Zoubek,[c] J. Krugluger,[a]
E. Schwameis,[a] J. Kirchheimer,[a] F. Stockenhuber[b]

[a]Department of Orthopedics and [b]Department of Nephrology, University
of Vienna, and [c]St. Anna Children's Hospital, Vienna, Austria

Introduction

The well-known myelosuppressive effect of cytostatic drugs is one of the
main side effects of cytostatic therapy [1]. Among these, the appearance of
anemia must also be considered important. Its etiology is multifactorial: it is
mainly a result of the cytotoxic effect of chemotherapeutic substances on the
bone marrow, but it also seems to be caused by low erythropoietin levels and
reduced erythropoietin responsiveness, partly due to elevated levels of tumor
necrosis factor [2–6]. Yet whatever the reasons for this anemia, it becomes a
major problem in the handling of tumor patients, which may result in a delay in
or even the elimination of chemotherapy. Treatment with adriamycin and cisplatin particularly accentuates the anemic effect. Usually the anemia must be
counteracted by substitution of blood, exposing the patients to all the concomitant risks [7–10]. The aim for the future should be a reduction in if not avoidance
entirely of blood transfusions.

To evaluate whether recombinant human erythropoietin (rhEPO) is able to
ameliorate tumor anemia, we investigated the effects of EPO during long-term
chemotherapy. We considered the possibility of decreasing the number of blood
units administered during chemotherapy and increasing the blood levels of Hb
and Hk as well.

Methods

After obtaining informed consent of the patients participating in this randomized
prospective study, these patients received chemotherapy according to the COSS and

CESS protocols, respectively. Two groups of patients undergoing long-term chemotherapy were compared. One group of patients (A) was treated with EPO (Recormon[R], Boehringer Mannheim), whereas the other (B) received a placebo. Erythropoietin substitution was administered i.v. $2\times$ week at a dosage of 600 U/kg body weight [11] in case of Hb levels below 11.5 g/dl until Hb levels had increased to more than 13.5 g/dl.

Chemotherapy Protocols

COSS protocol:

duration: 24 weeks; 3 cycles preoperatively, 4 cycles postoperatively
Substance and dosage per cycle:

high-dose methotrexate	12 g/m^2 (max. 20 g)
adriamycin	2 × 30 mg/m^2
ifosfamide	2 × 3 g/m^2
cisplatin	120 mg/m^2

CESS protocol:

duration: 40 weeks; 4 cycles preoperatively, 10 cycles postoperatively
Substance and dosage per cycle:

etoposide	3 × 150 mg/m^2
vincristine	2 × 1.5 mg/m^2
adriamycin	3 × 20 mg/m^2
actinomycin D	3 × 0.5 mg/m^2

Patients

Seventeen patients were included in this study (13 male and 4 female). The patients' ages ranged between 15 and 52 years (mean 27 years), and their diagnoses were as shown in Table 1. Eight patients were in group A (treatment group) and 9 in group B (placebo group), randomized from the total population. Inclusion criteria were patients receiving long-term chemotherapy according to the COSS or CESS protocols ranging in age between 15 and 60 years. Exclusion criteria were cerebral metastases, liver diseases,

Table 1. Patients undergoing chemotherapy

Histological diagnosis	Number of patients	Protocol
Osteosarcoma	7	COSS
Mesenchymal chondrosarcoma	2	COSS
Giant cell tumor	1	COSS
Fibrosarcoma	1	COSS
Ewing's sarcoma	5	CESS
PNET	1	CESS

essential hypertension, skin exanthema, decreased blood levels of Fe, vitamin B_{12} and folic acid, gastrointestinal bleeding, androgen or steroid therapy, epilepsy, thrombophilia, and cardiovascular diseases.

A routine evaluation was performed before each injection of erythropoietin during the first 2 weeks of treatment and then every week until the end of chemotherapeutic treatment. Each evaluation comprised a physical examination, a complete blood count including leukocyte differential, red cell, reticulocyte and platelet counts, measurement of hemoglobin and hematocrit, determination of serum ferritin and transferrin concentrations, and a blood chemistry profile including serum iron, electrolytes, and indices of renal and liver function. Blood pressure was determined before initiation of chemotherapy and during every chemotherapy cycle. Serum erythropoietin concentration was measured by a specific radioimmunoassay. Substitution therapy was terminated either with the end of the chemotherapy or when the Hb level reached 13.5 g/dl. The mean duration of EPO substitution therapy was 17.5 weeks.

Results

In group A it was possible to keep the Hb value at an average of 11.1 g/dl; in group B this value was 10.6 g/dl (Fig. 1). According to our study protocol, blood

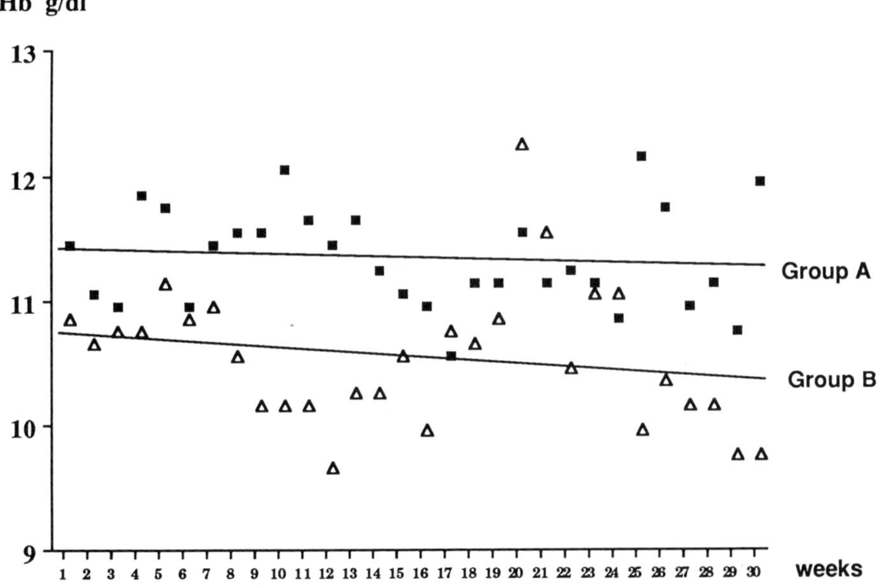

Fig. 1. Course of hemoglobin in group A (n = 8, Epo treatment) and in group B (n = 9, placebo).

units were substituted in case of hemoglobin dropping to less than 9 g/dl. In group A each patient undergoing chemotherapy received an average of 4.25 units of stored blood as compared to 8.7 units in group B (p < 0.01).

Summarizing, we can say that this pilot study shows a difference between the 2 groups of patients. The difference determined for the number of blood units used is statistically significant, whereas it is not significant for hemoglobin, hematocrit, or erythrocyte levels. Pretreatment serum levels of erythropoietin did not exceed 120 U/I in any of the patients. Serum EPO concentrations after intravenous administration increased to 3000 U/I and showed a kinetic profile with a monoexponential decay and a half-life of 6.5 h. As ferrokinetics revealed initially rather low serum iron and ferritin concentrations, patients were treated orally with iron so that no further decrease in serum iron or ferritin could be observed.

No side effects were noticed despite this high dosage of EPO. Symptoms such as hypertension, seizures, or thrombohemorrhagic complications observed in patients suffering from anemia as a result of a chronic renal failure and a consecutive EPO administration [12] did not occur. Patients with chemo-therapeutic-associated anemia showed excellent tolerance of the EPO treatment. They even experienced subjective improvement in their quality of life.

Discussion

This study shows that tumor and chemotherapy-induced anemia can be ameliorated but not avoided in the majority of patients and the demand of blood units can be reduced. We can conclude that under the described regimes of erythropoietin substitution therapy, this kind of anemia does not seem to over-come the myelosuppressive effect completely. We will continue our studies since, on the one hand, these preliminary results cannot be representative of the effectiveness of recombinant human erythropoietin but, on the other hand, these results strongly suggest a positive effect of EPO substitution during long-term chemotherapy in the treatment of tumor-associated anemia in Ewing's sarcoma and osteosarcoma.

References

1   Bray GL, Reaman GH: Erythropoietin deficiency: A compilation of cisplatin therapy and its therapy with recombinant human erythropoietin. Am J Pediat Hematol Oncol 1991; 13:426–430.

2   Miller CB, Jones RJ, Piantadosi S, Abeloff MD, Spivak JL: Decreased erythropoietin (EPO) response associated with the anemia of malignancy. Proc ASCO 1988;8:182.
3   Johnson CS, Cook CA, Furmanski P: Reversal of tumor necrosis factor alpha (TNF-alpha) induced suppression of erythropoiesis in vivo by treatment with erythropoietin (EPO). Proc Am Assoc Cancer Res 1989;30:409.
4   Rothmann SA, Paul P, Weick JK, McIntyre WR, Fantelli F: Effect of cis-diamminedichloroplatinum on erythropoietin production and hematopoietic progenitor cells. Int J Cell Cloning 1985;3:415–432.
5   Cox R, Musial T, Gyde OHB: Reduced erythropoietin levels as a cause of anemia in patients with lung cancer. Eur J Cancer Clin Oncol 1986;22:511–514.
6   Wood P, Hrushesky WJM: Cisplatin-induced anemia: An erythropoietin deficiency syndrome? Proc ASCO 1984;3:22.
7   Kanz L, Lindemann A, Oster W, Herrmann F, Mertelsmann R: Hematopoetin in clinical oncology. Am J Clin Oncol 1991; 14 (Suppl 1) 27–33.
8   Blumberg N, Heal JM: Transfusion and host defence against cancer recurrence and infection. Transfusion 1989;29:236–245.
9   Rosenberg SA, Seipp CA, White DE, Wesley R: Perioperative blood transfusions are associated with increased risks of recurrence and decreased survival in patients with high-grade soft-tissue sarcomas of the extremities. J Clin Oncol 1985;3:698–709.
10 Johnson JT, Taylor FH, Thearle PB: Blood transfusion and outcome in stage III head and neck carcinoma. Arch Otolaryngol Head Neck Surg 1987;113:307–310.
11 Erslev AJ: The therapeutic role of recombinant erythropoietin in anemic patients with intact endogenous production of erythropoietin. Sem Oncol 1992; 19 (Suppl 8): 14–18.
12 Eschbach JW: The anemia of chronic renal failure: pathophysiology and the effects of recombinant erythropoietin. Kidney Int 1989;134–148.

Univ.Doz.Dr. F. Stockenhuber, Department of Nephrology, University Clinic of Internal Medicine III, University of Vienna, Währingergürtel 18-20, 1090 Vienna, Austria

Discussion

to the Paper by C. Wurnig et al.

Adamson (New York): For a non-oncologist, what is the cure rate with these kinds of tumors on these kinds of protocols?

Stockenhuber: The cure rate is very high; it is about 80 to 90%.

Breymann (Zurich): Dr. Miller showed a separation between cisplatin containing chemotherapy and other chemotherapy; you did not. I wonder whether it is very important, whether you should see cisplatin for itself, because it causes proximal tubular damage and proximal tubular, necrosis, and that is also the space where we have EPO production. I would like to know whether you have any indication that you have a damage of peritubular cells too with cisplatin therapy which you don't have in all these other chemotherapeutic agents. I think this is very important.

Stockenhuber: Until now we did not see, but we have a very small number of cases until now and we want to get in each group—Ewing sarcoma and osteosarcoma—at least 30 patients. We just had until now 17 patients, as you have seen.

Cazzola (Pavia): I would comment on the effect of rhEPO on platelet transfusion requirements. There are experimental studies in animals suggesting that short-term treatments with recombinant human EPO can stimulate megacariocytopoiesis and platelet production, whereas the long-term treatments can cause thrombocytopenia. Findings of studies on the use of recombinant human EPO after bone marrow transplantation suggest that recombinant human EPO can reduce platelet transfusion requirements in that particular set. Your experience was the opposite, and this may be due to your long-term use of rhEPO.

Stockenhuber: Yes.

Cazzola: How long did you treat your patients?

Stockenhuber: 26 weeks in the osteosarcoma group.

[Unidentified]: What is the final conclusion of your study? Is it worthwhile to treat with rhEPO or not?

Stockenhuber: I think in this group of patients we have to go on with the study and then I can tell you.

Shaldon (Nimes): I am a little concerned about the randomization of your placebo group. In the slide where you showed the regression lines, there were, it seemed to me, two different populations. You said there was no significant difference, but were these arbitrarily randomized patients?

Stockenhuber: Yes, these patients were really randomized because the study is done by orthopedics and I am the only one who knows who gets EPO and who gets placebo.

Treatment of Myelodysplastic Syndromes with a Combination of Granulocyte Colony-Stimulating Factor and Erythropoietin

Eva Hellström-Lindberg,[a] Gunnar Birgegård,[b] Magnus Carlsson,[c] Jan Carneskog,[d] Inger-Marie Dahl,[e] Ingunn Dybedal,[f] Gunnar Grimfors,[g] Karl Merk,[h] Jon-Magnus Tangen,[i] Ingemar Winqvist,[j] Åke Öst[k]

Department of Medicine at [a]Huddinge University Hospital, Stockholm, [b]University Hospital, Uppsala, [c]Jönköping Hospital, [d]Sahlgrenska Hospital, Göteborg, [g]Karolinska Hospital, Stockholm, [j]Lund Hospital, Lund, Sweden; [h]Radiumhemmet and [k]Department of Pathology, Karolinska Hospital, Stockholm, Sweden; and Department of Medicine at [e]Tromsö Hospital, [f]Trondheim Hospital, and [i]Ullevål Hospital, Oslo, Norway

Summary

In an attempt to obtain a synergistic effect on the hemoglobin levels in anemic patients with myelodysplastic syndromes (MDS), granulocyte colony-stimulating factor (granulocyte-CSF) and erythropoietin were combined in a clinical phase II trial.

Twenty-two patients with MDS (6 with stable anemia and 16 with transfusion-dependent anemia) were included in the study. Granulocyte-CSF (0.3–3.0 μg/kg/day, s.c.) was given alone for 6 weeks and then in combination with erythropoietin (60–120 U/kg/day, s.c.) for the following 12 weeks. The dose of granulocyte-CSF was adjusted to obtain a granulocyte count between 6 and 10 × 10^9/l, and the dose of erythropoietin was increased after 6 weeks if no response was observed.

Eight (38%) of 21 evaluable patients showed significant increases in hemoglobin. A complete response with a hemoglobin level above 115 g/l was obtained in 4 patients and another 4 transfusion-dependent patients became transfusion-free at a hemoglobin level above 100 g/l. One patient with a previous response and subsequent failure to erythropoietin alone improved in hemoglobin after the addition of granulocyte-CSF. Sixteen patients showed an increase in granulocyte count of $\geq 2 \times 10^9/l$. The percentage of bone marrow blasts increased in 4 patients, of whom 1 progressed to acute myelogenous leukemia. Responses were significantly more frequent in patients with less advanced pancytopenia and in patients with lower endogenous levels of serum-erythropoietin. Sixty percent of patients with ring sideroblasts in the bone marrow responded to treatment compared to 18% of those without ring sideroblasts ($p = 0.063$).

Treatment with granulocyte-CSF and erythropoietin resulted in a response frequency of 38%, which is higher than in any study of erythropoietin as mono-therapy. Patients with ring sideroblasts, who respond poorly to erythropoietin alone, showed a response rate of 60%. These findings, in combination with the case of granulocyte-CSF–induced second response to erythropoietin, are highly suggestive of a synergistic effect in vivo of granulocyte-CSF and erythropoietin in patients with myelodysplastic syndromes.

Introduction

The myelodysplastic syndromes (MDS) are chronic malignant bone marrow disorders characterized by ineffective hemopoiesis, progressive pancytopenia, and a risk for progression to acute myelogenous leukemia [1, 2]. Allogeneic bone marrow transplantation is at present the only possibility for a permanent cure but is, for several reasons, confined to a minority of the patients [3]. Other treatment alternatives aim at improving the clinical situation for the patient by reversing the peripheral cytopenia and inhibiting progression of the disease.

The number of treatment alternatives for MDS has increased during the last decade. The roles for high- and low-dose chemotherapy have been more clearly defined [4–6], and the effects of various differentiating inducing factors such as heme arginate [7] have been evaluated. None of these alternatives, however, has shown a positive effect in more than 30% of the cases. Recently, the development of several recombinant cytokines has made it possible to stimulate the usually ineffective myelodysplastic hemopoiesis. A majority of the cytokines tried as treatment for MDS exert their main effects on myelopoiesis. Granulocyte colony-stimulating factor (granulocyte-CSF) has been shown to increase the granulocyte count in a majority of granulocytopenic patients with MDS and has been given as maintenance treatment for up to 18 months [8–11]. This cytokine has few side effects and does not seem to increase the rate of leukemic transformation when compared to equivalent groups of untreated patients. Granulocyte-macrophage-CSF also has a favorable effect on the granulocyte count and has in one study been reported to reduce the frequency of severe infections [12, 13].

However, proliferation of myelodysplastic cells in vitro was stimulated to a greater extent by granulocyte-macrophage-CSF than by granulocyte-CSF [14]. In patients with MDS, the stimulatory effect on erythropoiesis of these cytokines seems to be limited, but in a small study of patients with aplastic anemia, 2 of 5 patients improved their hemoglobin levels after several months of treatment with granulocyte-CSF. Interleukin 3 has its main effect on myelopoiesis, but has also shown a positive effect on anemia in some patients with MDS [15].

For patients with MDS in chronic stable phase, anemia and the need for transfusions constitute the main clinical problems. Several reports on treatment with erythropoietin have shown that hemoglobin levels increase in approximately 20% of patients with MDS and anemia [16–19]. These studies have been too small to allow analyses of factors predictive for a response to treatment, but there has been a tendency towards a higher response rate in patients with lower endogenous levels of serum erythropoietin and in patients without ring sidero-blasts in the bone marrow.

In vitro, granulocyte-CSF alone has no direct stimulatory effect on the growth of erythroid colonies. In HIV-infected patients, treatment with granulocyte-CSF was found to increase the number of circulating burst-forming unit–erythroid (BFU-E), but the hemoglobin levels did not increase until the treatment with granulocyte-CSF was combined with erythropoietin [20, 21]. In another study, 2 patients with severe aplastic anemia treated with a combination of granulocyte-CSF and erythropoietin showed a trilinear response [22]. Studies on myelodysplastic erythropoiesis have shown that granulocyte-CSF synergizes with erythropoietin in stimulating the growth of BFU-E [23]. Furthermore, Hogge et al. [24] showed that the growth of BFU-E in long-term cultures of normal bone marrow was significantly increased when the feeder layer, by gene transfer, was made to produce granulocyte-CSF. This study also showed a higher proportion of primitive progenitors in S phase after granulocyte-CSF stimulation.

There is still no treatment alternative that is able to improve the hemoglobin levels in more than 30% of patients with MDS and anemia. The present study was designed to investigate the combined effects of two cytokines, granulocyte-CSF and erythropoietin, in such a group of patients.

Patients and Methods

Patients

Inclusion diagnoses were refractory anemia, refractory anemia with ring sidero-blasts, and refractory anemia with excess of blasts. Inclusion criterion were hemoglobin < 100 g/l + symptoms of anemia. Exclusion criteria were other active malignancy, uncontrolled hypertension, epilepsy, bleeding complications, and transfusion-dependent thrombocytopenia. The patients had not previously been treated with either of the two drugs and had not received chemotherapy during the previous 2 months.

Patient characteristics are shown in Table 1. A total of 22 consecutive patients from 8 Swedish and Norwegian hospitals were included in the study between November 1990 and September 1992. Five had refractory anemia, 4 refractory anemia, with ring sidero-blasts, and 13 refractory anemia with excess of blasts. The median age was 67 years (range 42–87), and 15 patients were male. Sixteen patients were transfusion dependent, and 6 had stable anemia. One patient with severe anemic symptoms was included with a hemoglobin of 105 g/l. The median granulocyte and platelet counts were 2.0 (range 0.1–5.0) and 188 (range 15–533), respectively. The median percentage of bone marrow blasts was 5.5 (range 2–17). Ten patients had ring sideroblasts in the bone marrow.

Another patient, a 32-year-old female with refractory anemia, was treated with granulocyte-CSF and erythropoietin but was not included in the study, as she previously had been treated with erythropoietin as monotherapy. In that study, she was transfusion-dependent (transfusion limit 70 g/l) at inclusion, but increased to a stable hemoglobin level of 80 g/l after 6 weeks of treatment with 5000 U of erythropoietin/day, s.c. This response ended after 3 months and could not be reinduced with 10,000 U of erythropoietin/day.

Treatment

A flow chart of the treatment schedule is shown in Figure 1. Granulocyte-CSF was given alone for 6 weeks and then in combination with erythropoietin for another 12 weeks. Both drugs were given s.c., once daily. There were 3 dose levels of granulocyte-CSF: 0.3, 1.0, and 3.0 mg/kg. Treatment was started at the lowest dose and increased every second week if the granulocyte count had not increased to between 6 and 10×10^9/l. After 6 weeks, erythropoietin was added at a dose of 60 U/kg. The erythropoietin dose was increased to 120 U/kg after 6 weeks, if hemoglobin had not increased with >15 g/l, and after 8 weeks, if hemoglobin then was <115 g/l.

A complete response in hemoglobin was defined as an increase to ≥ 115 g/l and a partial response as an increase with ≥ 15 g/l or, in transfusion-dependent patients, a stable hemoglobin level of >100 g/l without transfusions. A complete response in granulocyte count was defined as a level between 6 and 10×10^9/l and a partial response as an increase with $>2 \times 10^9$/l.

Tests

A bone marrow smear was taken before treatment, after 6 weeks in the study, and after the study period (weeks 1, 7, and 19). A bone marrow biopsy was taken at the first of these occasions. Before the patients were included in the study, all bone marrow samples were investigated by one pathologist and the subgroup of MDS was stated. Bone marrow smears were checked for the percentages of myeloblasts, ring sideroblasts, and erythro-poiesis. Bone marrow biopsies were used to estimate cellularity. Chromosomal analyses were performed before and, in most cases, after the study period. Peripheral blood values were followed weekly during the first 6 weeks and then every second week. Blood pressure, renal and liver function tests, and serum values for ferritin, erythropoietin, and

Table 1. Pretreatment variables

No.	Age/Sex	FAB	Dur	Blast%	Sid	Cytogenetics	S-EPO	S-GSF
1	66/F	RAEB	31	5	−	47,XX, +8 / 46,XX, 5q−	159	0
2	70/M	RAEB	4	7	−	46,XY	824	NT
3	73/M	RAEB	7	11	−	47,XY, +8	834	0.05
4	42/F	RA	16	3	−	46,XX, t (2;11), 5q−	1523	0
5	81/F	RAEB	28	10	+	NT	137	0.17
6	74/F	RA	26	4	+[a]	46,XX, 5q−	324	0.17
7	73/M	RAS	39	3	+	46,XY	1133	0
8	87/M	RAEB	5	8	+	46,XY	116	0
9	79/F	RA	73	4	−	46,XX, 5q−	265	0
10	59/M	RAEB	6	9	−	46,XY	5921	NT
11	79/M	RAEB	13	6	+	46,XY	3874	NT
12	56/M	RAEB	84	5	−	NT	136	0
13	51/M	RAEB	2	8	−	46,XY	35	0.80
14	53/M	RAEB	11	11	+	NT	243	0
15	79/M	RAS	3	3	+	46,XY, inv 9	NT	NT
16	56/M	RAEB	32	7	−	46,XY	103	0
17	83/M	RAS	2	2	+	46,XY	59	0
18	59/F	RA	3	2	−	46,XX	552	0
19	73/F	RAEB	2	13	−	NT	NT	NT
20	68/M	RAEB	8	17	−	47,XY, +8	NT	0.08
21	67/M	RA	40	4	+	46,XY,2q−, −6, 9q−, 12p+, 20q−, 22p+, +mar	85	0
22	58/M	RAS	51	3	+	46,XY	56	0

FAB, French-American-British classification of MDS; Dur, Duration of disease, in months, before start of treatment; Sid, Presence of ring sideroblasts in the bone marrow.

[a] This patient had ring sideroblasts but less than 15% of erythropoietic cells.

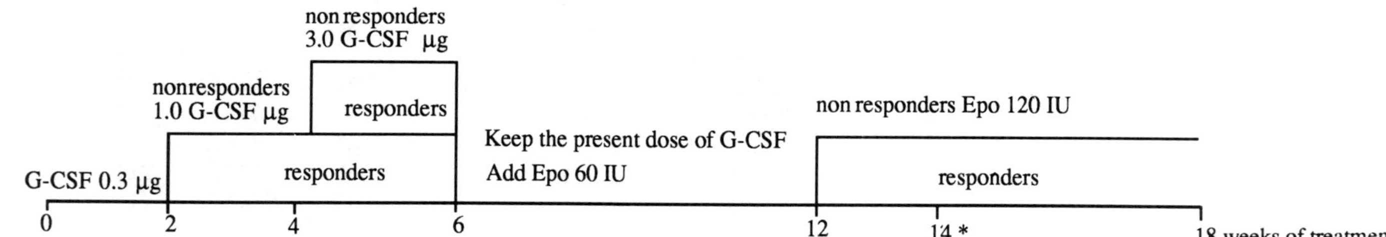

Fig. 1. Schedule of treatment and dose adjustments for one study. The dose of granulocyte-CSF was increased after the second and fourth week if the neutrophil count had not increased to 6–10 $\times$ 10^9/l. The dose of erythropoietin was increased if hemoglobin had not increased $\geq$15 g/l after the twelfth week or reached a level of $\geq$115 g/l after the fourteenth week.

granulocyte-CSF were taken before and after the study. Serum erythropoietin was analyzed with the radioimmunoassay method described by Wide et al. [25]. Serum granulocyte-CSF was analyzed with a commercial kit from R&D systems. Side effects were checked for continuously.

Statistical Analyses

Responders and nonresponders were compared using Student's t-test when the variables showed normal distribution and the Mann-Whitney U-test when they were skewed. Fisher's exact test was used for comparison of proportions.

Results

The results of treatment are shown in Table 2. Twenty-one patients were evaluable for a response to treatment. Eight patients (38%) responded with an increase in hemoglobin (Fig. 2). Four patients (3 with stable anemia and 1 with transfusion need) showed a complete response, reaching hemoglobin levels of 115–142 g/l. Partial responses were observed in 4 transfusion-dependent patients, who stabilized at hemoglobin levels above 100 g/l without transfusions. Three patients had a transfusion need exceeding 3 units of packed red blood cells/4 weeks. None of these responded to treatment, but one showed a 50% reduction of his transfusion need. An increase in granulocyte count to a level between 6 and 10 × 10^9/l was observed in 11 of 21 patients, and another 5 patients showed an increase of ≥2 × 10^9/l (Fig. 3). The 5 patients who did not fulfill the criteria for a partial response in granulocyte count all had pretreatment granulocyte counts <1 × 10^9/l. Three of these showed increases in granulocyte count during the first 6 weeks, which fell during the last part of the study. No significant effect on the platelet counts was observed (p = 0.85). The percentage of bone marrow blasts in the bone marrow before and after treatment is shown in Figure 4. Three patients showed a significant increase, and 1 of these progressed after 1 week to acute myelogenous leukemia (patient 12).

A chromosomal analysis was done in 18 of the 21 evaluable patients. Abnormal caryotype was found in 8 patients (Table 1). A follow-up analysis was made in 13 cases. Eleven of these showed unchanged chromosomal patterns after the end of the study. Patient 12, who also progressed to AML, developed a malignant clone, 46 XY, t(2q-; 18q +), and patient 20 showed an increase in the random loss of various chromosomes in combination with the previously found +8 clone. No significant changes in bone marrow morphology, liver and renal function tests, or blood pressure were observed.

Table 2. Results of treatment

No.	Result	Hemoglobin (g/l)		Granulocytes $\times 10^9$/l		Platelets $\times 10^9$/l		Blood transfusions at -18 to 18 weeks			Final doses G-CSF (μg/kg)	EPO (U/kg)
		pre	post	pre	post	pre	post	-18-0	0-9	9-18		
1	NR	80	80	1.4	5.1	190	284	8	6	4	3.0	120
2	NR	88	80	1.0	3.2	176	227	8	4	4	0.3	120
3	NR	86	85	2.0	6.6	100	325	4	2	4	3.0	120
4	NR	82	72	2.5	5.0	407	391	6	4	2	3.0	120
5	PR	104	105	1.5	10.2	148	175	4	4	0	1.0	120
6	PR	99	105	3.1	10.6	533	564	6	2	0	0.3	120
7	NR	73	81	2.4	7.2	396	388	8	4	2	1.0	120
8	CR	96	115	4.0	7.1	393	322	0	0	0	0.3	60
9	PR	92	101	3.5	8.0	322	382	6	0	0	1.0	120
10	NR	90	77	0.1	1.5	100	87	16	8	10	3.0	120
11	NR	87	87	0.8	0.3	89	70	7	2	6	0.3	120
12	NR	95	93	0.8	0.7	15	10	0	0	10[a]	3.0	120
13	CR	105	142	1.3	8.5	326	286	0	0	0	1.0	60
14	NR	82	62	0.4	2.0	185	121	36	4	13	1.0	120
15	PR	76	103	4.3	6.2	188	78	4	2	0	1.0	120
16	NR	87	73	0.1	0.2	40	23	0	0	2	3.0	60
17	CR	91	118	1.9	16.0	262	336	2	2	0	1.0	120
18	NR	67	64	2.2	5.2	138	62	0	4	3	0.3	120
20	NR	82	107	2.0	5.0	112	151	4	4	4	3.0	120
21	NR	61	78	5.0	15.1	232	62	15	12	12	1.0	120
22	CR	97	129	3.0	10.0	436	369	0	0	0	1.0	120

[a] Gastrointestinal bleeding.

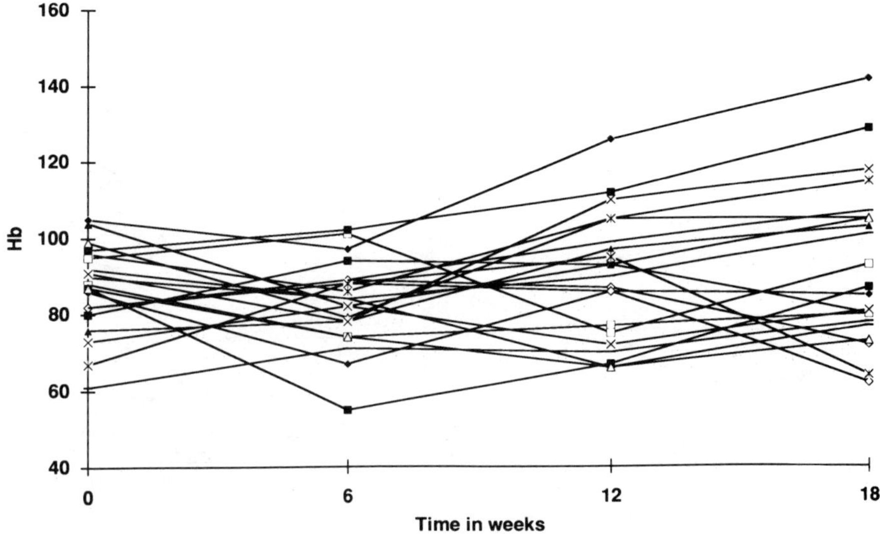

Fig. 2. Results of treatment with G-CSF and EPO on hemoglobin levels.

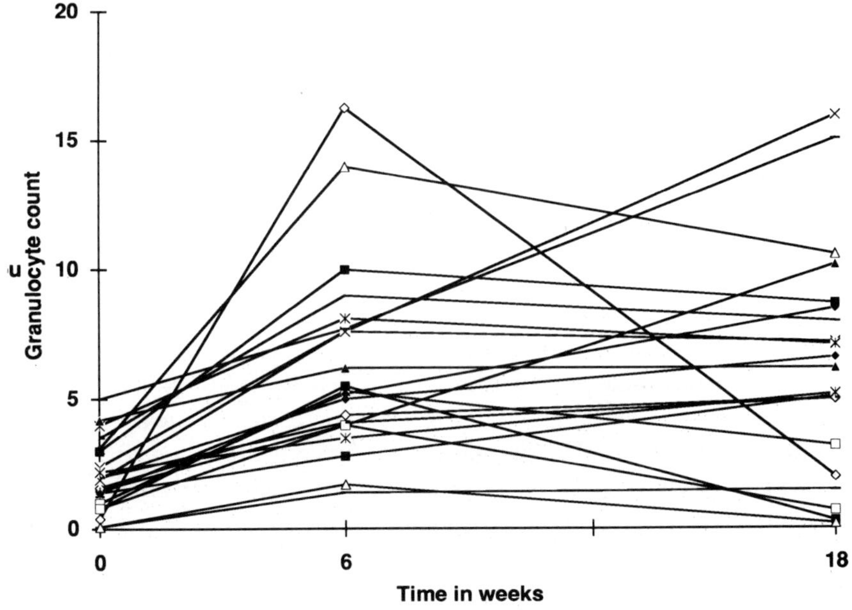

Fig. 3. Results of treatment with G-CSF and EPO on granulocyte counts.

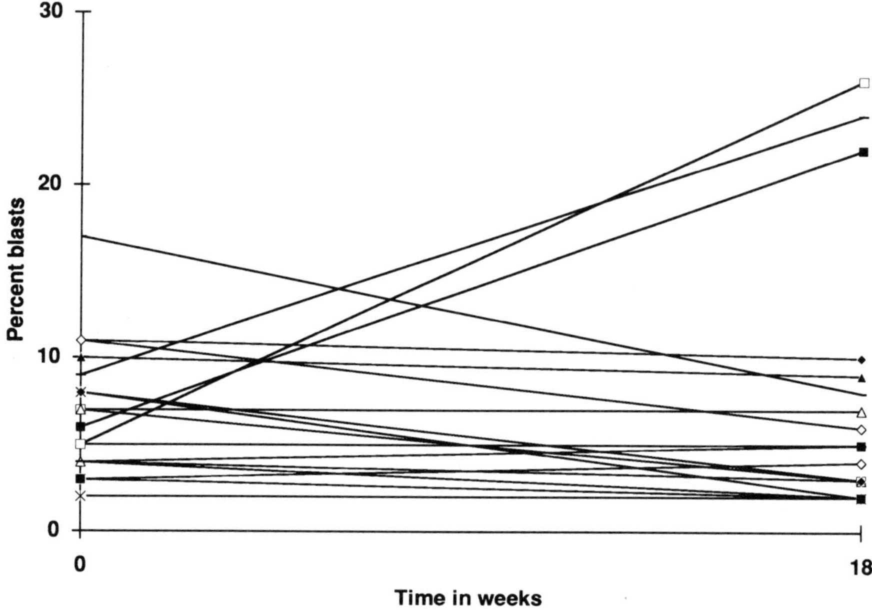

Fig. 4. Results of treatment with G-CSF and EPO on the percentage of bone marrow blasts.

Characteristics of Responders and Nonresponders

Table 3 shows pretreatment variables in patients with and without a response in hemoglobin. Hemoglobin levels and leukocyte, granulocyte, and platelet counts were significantly higher in the responding group. Three of 6 patients with stable hemoglobin levels and 5 of 15 with a need for transfusions responded to treatment. Responses were observed in 4 of 11 patients with normal karyotype and in 3 of 8 patients with chromosomal aberrations. None of the 3 patients with 2 or more clonal abnormalities were responders. Six of 10 patients with ring sideroblasts in the bone marrow and 2 of 11 without responded to treatment (p = 0.063). Bone marrow cellularity did not influence the response rate, but there was a tendency towards a higher percentage of bone marrow erythropoiesis in the responding group (p = 0.064). The responders had a median value for S-EPO of 116 U/L, compared to 824 U/l in the nonresponding group (p = 0.016). There was no difference in serum granulocyte-CSF between the two groups.

Table 3. Pretreatment variables in patients with and without a response
in hemoglobin

Variable	Responders	Nonresponders	p-Value
Hemoglobin, g/l[a]	95 ± 3.2	81.5 ± 2.6	0.005
Leukocyte count, × 10^9/l[a]	5.2 ± 0.6	2.9 ± 0.4	0.006
Granulocyte count, × 10^9/l[a]	2.8 ± 0.4	1.6 ± 0.4	0.043
Platelet count, × 10^9/l[a]	326 ± 45	167 ± 33	0.01
Age, y[a]	74 ± 5	64 ± 3	0.08
Duration of disease, months[a]	24	23	0.92
S-Ferritin, µg/l[a]	876 ± 229	1970 ± 881	0.38
Blasts in bone marrow, %[b]	4 (2–10)	6 (2–17)	0.36
Bone marrow cellularity, %[b]	70 (40–80)	80 (40–100)	0.24
Bone marrow erythropoiesis, %[b]	43 (18–50)	15 (5–71)	0.064
Serum erythropoietin, U/l[b]	116 (35–324)	824 (85–5921)	0.016
Serum G-CSF, ng/ml[b]	0 (0–0.8)	0 (0–0.8)	0.38
Stable hemoglobin, 6 pts	3	3	
Transfusion dependent, 15 pts[c]	5	10	0.41
Sideroblasts present, 10 pts	6	4	
Sideroblasts absent, 11 pts[c]	2	9	0.063
Karyotype, normal, 11 pts	4	7	
Karyotype, abnormal, 8 pts[c]	3	5	0.66

[a] Student's *t*-test, mean values ± SE.
[b] Mann-Whitney U-test, median values + range.
[c] Fisher's exact test.

Case Report

The patient who was treated outside the protocol had a transfusion need of 6
units/18 weeks and started at a hemoglobin level of 74 g/l. Treatment was
initiated with granulocyte-CSF, 30 µg/day and erythropoietin, 10,000 U/day.
The dose of granulocyte-CSF was increased to 90 µg/day after 2 weeks. Three
weeks after the start of treatment, the patient received her last transfusion at a
hemoglobin level of 70 g/l. The hemoglobin remained between 80 and 90 g/l for
3 months and then increased to >115 g/l, where it remained for 3 months. The
granulocyte count increased from 0.5 to 4.5 × 10^9/l.

Side Effects

All 22 patients were alive at the end of the study period, and 20 completed
the 18 weeks of treatment. All patients were evaluable for side effects. Patient 19

was withdrawn from the study and from the analysis of results after 18 days of treatment with granulocyte-CSF. At the start, this patient's platelet count was 9 $\times$ 10^9/l, the leukocyte count 1.6 $\times$ 10^9/l and the percentage of bone marrow blasts 13. After 18 days, the platelet count was 5 $\times$ 10^9/l, the leukocyte count 24.6 $\times$ 10^9/l, and the percentage of blasts 24. This patient developed confusion and was found to have a subdural hematoma. In patient number 15, treatment with granulocyte-CSF was withdrawn after 12 weeks because of erythema and itching, but EPO treatment continued as planned, and the patient was included in the analysis of results. Patient 12 was found to have acute myelogenous leukemia 1 week after the 19-week follow-up. Muscular pain and subfebrility after granulocyte-CSF injections were observed in 2 and 1 patient, respectively. These symptoms vanished after several weeks. Local irritation caused by the EPO injections occurred in 2 patients but could be easily overcome by diluting the erythropoietin.

Discussion

The results of this study are highly suggestive of an in vivo synergistic effect between granulocyte-CSF and erythropoietin in patients with myelodysplastic syndromes. This conclusion is supported both by the response rate itself and by the high proportion of responders in the group of patients with ring sideroblasts in the bone marrow. In the present study, 38% of the patients responded with an increase in hemoglobin levels, compared to treatment with erythropoietin alone, which has resulted in response rates between 0 and 27%. Our own erythropoietin study did not differ from the present study with regard to patient characteristics such as age or percentage of bone marrow blasts, and there were more cases with severe granulocytopenia and transfusion need in the present study. Thus, differences in patient selection have probably not positively influenced the response rate. Moreover, the synergistic hypothesis is supported by the case whose declining response to erythropoietin was first restored by the addition of granulocyte-CSF and after 3 months was further improved to a complete response. It is also in line with the case report of Bessho et al., which describes trilinear response to treatment with G-CSF and erythropoietin in 2 patients with severe aplastic anemia [22].

In several studies, patients with ring sideroblasts in the bone marrow have been reported to respond poorly to treatment with erythropoietin. The erythroid progenitors in sideroblastic anemia seem to lack the capacity to respond to erythropoietin, which acts on relatively mature erythropoietic cells. In our erythropoietin study [17], none of the 5 patients with ring sideroblasts responded to treatment. This should be compared with the present study, in which 6 of 10 sideroblasts patients showed significant responses. One mechanism behind this highly improved response rate could be that the combination has a direct synergistic effect on the erythroid precursor, but it is more likely that granulocyte-CSF increases the pool of multipotent progenitors and subsequently the amount of erythropoietin-responsive target cells. The latter explanation is supported by studies showing a stimulating effect of granulocyte-CSF on the number of primitive clonogenic progenitors [24, 26].

Greenberg et al. reported that while myelodysplastic bone marrow with low or absent spontaneous growth of BFU-E was not stimulated by the combination of granulocyte-CSF and erythropoietin, the same combination synergistically increased the growth in bone marrow with spontaneous intermediate or normal growth of BFU-E [23]. Patients with erythropoietic response to treatment with this combination had at least intermediate growth. This corresponds with our results showing that the responders had significantly higher pretreatment levels of hemoglobin.

The limited size of this study makes the analysis of differences between responders and nonresponders uncertain. It seems clear, however, that patients with less advanced cytopenia showed a higher response rate, probably due to less advanced damage to their multipotent progenitors. Pretreatment levels of serum erythropoietin were lower in the responding group and probably have a moderate predictive value for the response to treatment. It should be noted, however, that low erythropoietin values were also found in the nonresponding group: 1 of the 21 patients progressed to acute myelogenous leukemia. In a previously reported study of patients treated with low-dose cytosine arabinoside, 12% of patients with MDS and less than 20% of bone marrow blasts progressed to acute myelogenous leukemia within 18 weeks from start of treatment [6]. Thus, even if a proliferative effect in some of the cases cannot be excluded, there does not seem to be a generally increased risk of progression after treatment with granulocyte-CSF and erythropoietin.

There have been several reports on the synergistic effects upon myelodysplastic bone marrow in vitro of various combinations of cytostatic agents, inducers of differentiation, and cytokines [27]. However, previous studies have not been able to show a corresponding synergistic effect in patients treated with these combinations [28]. Granulocyte-CSF and erythropoietin synergistically stimulate erythropoiesis in vitro, and our results from treatment with this combination indicate that these drugs also have synergistic effects in vivo. This might introduce a new phase in the management of patients with myelodysplastic syndromes in which pretreatment in vitro and clinical analyses can facilitate individual therapeutic decisions.

References

1 Galton DAG: The myelodysplastic syndromes. Clin Lab Haematol 1984; 6:99–112.

2 Kerkhofs H, Hermans J, Haak H, Leeksma C: Utility of the FAB classification for myelodysplastic syndromes: Investigation of prognostic factors in 237 patients. Br J Haematol 1987; 65:73–81.

3 Appelbaum F, Storb R, Ramberg R, Shulman H, Buckner D, Clift R, Deeg J, Fefer A, Sanders J, Self S, Singer J, Stewart P, Sullivan K, Witherspoon R, Thomas D: Treatment of preleukemic syndromes with marrow transplantation. Blood 1987; 69:92–96.

4 Fenaux P, Luc Lai J, Jouet J, Bauters F: Aggressive chemotherapy in adult primary myelodysplastic syndromes. Blut 1988; 57: 297–302.

5 Cheson B, Simon R: Low-dose ara-C in acute nonlymphocytic leukemia and myelodysplastic syndromes: A review of 20 years experience. Semin Oncol 1987; 14:126–133.

6 Hellström-Lindberg E, Robèrt KH, Gahrton G, Forsblom AM, Lindberg G, Kock Y, Öst Å: A predictive model for the clinical response to low dose ara-C: A study of 102 patients with myelodysplastic syndromes or acute leukemia. Br J Haematol 1992; 81:503–511.

7 Volin L, Ruutu T, Knutila S, Tenhunen R: Heme arginate treatment for myelodysplastic syndromes. Leuk Res 1988; 12:423–431.

8 Negrin R, Haeuber D, Nagler A, Donlon T, Souza L, Greenberg P: Treatment of myelodysplastic syndromes with recombinant human granulocyte colony-stimulating factor. Ann Intern Med 1989; 110:976–984.

9 Negrin R, Haeuber D, Nagler A, Kobayashi Y, Sklar J, Donlon T, Vincent M, Greenberg P: Maintenance treatment of patients with myelodysplastic syndromes using recombinant human granulocyte colony-stimulating factor. Blood 1990; 76:36–43.

10 Greenberg P, Negrin R, Nagler A, Vincent M, Donlon T: Effects of prolonged treatment of myelodysplastic syndromes with recombinant human granulocyte colony-stimulating factor. Int J Cell Cloning 1990; 8 (Suppl 1):293–302.

11 Yoshida Y, Hirashima K, Asano S, Takaku F: A phase II trial of recombinant human granulocyte colony-stimulating factor in the myelodysplastic syndromes. Br J Haematol 1991; 78:378–384.

12 Vadhan-Raj S, Keating M, LeMaistre A, Hittelman W, McCredie K, Trujillo J, Broxmeyer H, Henney C, Gutterman J: Effects of recombinant human granulocyte-macrophage colony-stimulating factor in patients with myelodysplastic syndromes. N Engl J Med 1987; 317:1545–1552.

13 Shuster MW, Larson RA, Thompson JA, Coiffier B, Bennett JM, Israel RJ for the Shering-Plough/Sandoz MDS Study Group: Granulocyte-macrophage colony-

stimulating factor (GM-CSF) for myelodysplastic syndrome (MDS): Results of a multi-center randomized controlled trial. Blood 1990; 76:318a.

14   Ganser A, Lindemann, Seipelt G, Ottmann O, Herrmann F, Eder M, Frisch J, Schulz G, Mertelsmann R, Hoelzer D: Effects of recombinant human interleukin-3 in patients with myelodysplastic syndromes. Blood 1990; 76:455–462.

15   Nagler A, Binet C, Mackichan ML, Negrin R, Bangs C, Donlon T, Greenberg P: Impact of marrow cytogenetics and morphology on in vitro hematopoiesis in the myelodysplastic syndromes: Comparison between recombinant human granulocyte colony-stimulating factor (CSF) and granulocyte-monocyte-CSF. Blood 1990; 76:1299–1307.

16   Bessho M, Jinnai I, Matsuda A, Saito M, Hirashima K: Improvement of anaemia by recombinant erythropoietin in patients with myelodysplastic syndromes and aplastic anaemia. Int J Cell Clon 1990; 8:445–458.

17   Hellström E, Birgegård G, Lockner D, Wide L, Helmers C, Öst Å: Treatment of myelodysplastic syndromes with recombinant human erythropoietin. Eur J Haematol 1991; 47:355–360.

18   Bowen D, Culligan D, Jacobs A: The treatment of anaemia in the myelodysplastic syndromes with recombinant human erythropoietin. Br J Haematol 1991; 77:419–423.

19   Stein R, Abels R, Krantz S: Pharmacological doses of recombinant human erythropoietin in the treatment of myelodysplastic syndromes. Blood 1991; 78:1658–1663.

20   Miles SA, Mitsuyasu RT, Moreno J, Baldwin G, Alton K, Souza L, Glaspy J: Combined therapy with recombinant granulocytic colony-stimulating factor and erythropoietin decreases hemotological recovery from zidovudine. Blood 1991; 77:2109–2117.

21   Miles SA, Mitsuyasu RT, Lee K, Moreno J, Alton K, Egrie J, Souza L, Glaspy J: Recombinant granulocytic colony-stimulating factor increases circulating burst forming unit-erythron and red blood cell production in patients with severe human immunodeficiency virus infection. Blood 1990; 75:2137–2142.

22   Bessho M, Toyoda A, Itoh Y, Sakata T, Kawai N, Jinnai I, Saito M, Hirashima K: Trilineage recovery by combination therapy with recombinant human granulocytic colony-stimulating factor (rhG-CSF) and erythropoietin (rhEpo) in severe aplastic anaemia. Br J Haematol 1992; 80:409–411.

23   Greenberg P, Negrin R, Ginzton N: In vitro–in vivo correlations of erythroid responses to G-CSF plus erythropoietin (epo) in myelodysplastic syndromes (MDS). Exp Hematol 1992, 6, p 733, abstract no 112.

24   Hogge DE, Cashman JD, Humphries K, Eaves C: Differential and synergistic effects of human granulocyte-macrophage colony-stimulating factor and human granulocyte colony-stimulating factor on hematopoiesis in human long-term marrow cultures. Blood 1991; 77:493–499.

25   Wide L, Bengtsson C, Birgegård G: Circadian rhythm of human serum erythropoietin. Br J Haematol 1989; 72:85–90.

26   Ikebuchi K, Ihle JN, Hirai Y, Wong GG, Clark SC, Ogawa M: Synergistic factors for stem cell proliferation: Further studies of the target stem cells and the mechanism

of stimulation by interleukin 1, interleukin 6 and granulocyte colony-stimulating factor. Blood 1988; 72:2007–2014.

27 Francis G, Guimaraes J, Berney J, Wing M: Synergistic interaction between differentiation inducers and DNA synthesis inhibitors: A new approach to differentiation induction in myelodysplastic and acute leukemia. Leuk Res 1985; 9:573–581.

28 Hellström E, Robèrt KH, Samuelsson J, Lindemalm C, Grimfors G, Kimby E, Öberg G, Winqvist I, Billström R, Carneskog J, Dahlén M, Stockner M, Wislöff F, Dybedall I, Dahl IM, Öst Å for the Scandinavian Myelodysplasia Group (SMG): Treatment of myelodysplastic syndromes with retinoic acid and 1α-dihydroxyvitamin D3 in combination with low-dose ara-C is not superior to ara-C alone. Results from a randomized study. Eur J Haematol 1990; 45:255–261.

Eva Hellström-Lindberg, Division of Clinical Haematology and Oncology, Department of Medicine, Huddinge University Hospital, 141 86 Huddinge, Sweden

Discussion

to the Paper by E. Hellström-Lindberg et al.

Bowen (Cardiff): There were some patients here who initially on G-CSF increased their neutrophil count, which then fell when you started erythropoietin? Were they the patients who had a hemoglobin response as well?

Hellström-Lindberg: No, they were all patients with advanced cytopenia who did not respond to EPO. So all responders in hemoglobin had a good granulocyte response as well.

Miller (Baltimore): Do you look at myeloid or erythroid progenitor assays in your patients?

Hellström-Lindberg: Do you mean by bone marrow culture? No, we didn't, because this was a multicenter trail and we could not do that.

Wardrop (Cardiff): I am not quite clear how long the response persists in responding patients. Does this represent several months of good health or perhaps potentially longer than that?

Hellström-Lindberg: Well, we haven't done this study as a long-term study. But G-CSF patients have been treated for several years with a long-lasting good response. There are data on EPO treatment in MDS with persistent responses of up to 1.5 years. I think it is possible to maintain a long-term response. We don't know very much about that yet.

[Unidentified]: Do you distinguish patients responding from patients non-responding on the basis of their EPO levels?

Hellström-Lindberg: Well, as I said, it's just significant and I don't think you can draw any conclusions before you have a larger [patient population]. I don't think that a high EPO level should leave out patients from the trial, not so far.

Bowen: Do you look at the infection rates on G-CSF in those responders?

Hellström-Lindberg: These patients were basically outpatients and they didn't have any infections. As I said before, infection problems mostly occur in patients with advanced MDS, like MDS leukemia or MDS type 5.

Combined Use of Erythropoietin and Granulocyte–Macrophage–Colony-Stimulating Factor in Patients Undergoing Bone Marrow Transplantation

Preliminary Results of a Pilot Study

Manuel Abecasis, Maria José Passos

Bone Marrow Transplant Unit, Instituto Português de Oncologia,
Lisbon, Portugal

Introduction

Bone marrow transplantation (BMT), either allogeneic or autologous, is an effective treatment for a variety of hematological and neoplastic diseases. Many of the problems associated with BMT are related to the period of profound cytopenia that follows high-dose chemotherapy. Consequently, there has been great interest in the use of hemopoietic growth factors to stimulate early hemopoietic recovery and thus reduce morbidity.

The period of severe neutropenia following BMT can be substantially shortened by giving either granulocyte–macrophage–colony-stimulating factor (GM-CSF) or granulocyte colony-stimulating factor (G-CSF) [1]. The former stimulates an earlier progenitor than G-CSF, and recently it has also been shown that it possesses a moderate degree of megakaryocyte colony-stimulating activity by stimulating the proliferation of both burst-forming unit and colony-forming unit megakaryocyte [2].

Erythropoietin (EPO), a major hormone in erythropoiesis, has also been shown to be involved in the modulation of megakaryopoiesis in vitro [3] and thrombopoiesis in vivo [4]. EPO promotes megakaryocyte maturation in vitro, and in primate models a synergistically enhanced stimulation of hematopoiesis, including thrombopoiesis, was observed when GM-CSF and EPO were given in combination [5].

We first used such a combination to treat a patient with severe aplastic anemia who rejected 2 previous transplants and whose good graft functioning, with stable trilineage engraftment, was only achieved when GM-CSF and EPO were introduced after a third transplant [6].

We therefore decided to conduct a pilot study to evaluate the role of this combination of hemopoietic growth factors in patients submitted to autologous or allogeneic BMT for nonmyeloid diseases. The preliminary results of such a study, involving 7 patients, are reported here.

Patients and Methods

Between December 1991 and April 1992, 7 patients with nonmyeloid diseases submitted to autologous or allogeneic BMT were included in this study. Patients were nursed in single rooms equipped with HEPA-filtered air, and reserve isolation techniques were used. All had a central venous line placed on admission and were given a low bacterial content diet together with selective gut decontamination. Prophylactic acyclovir and i.v. were given to all patients. Intravenous antibiotics were given empirically when temperature was above 38°C and continued until either the neutrophil count was above 0.5 $\times 10^9$/l for 3 days or the fever had resolved. Random platelets were transfused to keep the platelet count above 20×10^9/l, and red blood cells were given to keep the hemoglobin above 7 g/dl or when symptomatic. All blood products were irradiated at 1500 rad.

Patients submitted to autologous BMT had their bone marrow harvested and refrigerated at 4°C before being given 48 h later, when the conditioning regimen consisting of melphalan 110 mg/m^2 and total body irradiation (3 fractions of 350 rad each) was terminated (Table 1). Patients submitted to allogeneic BMT received busulfan 4 mg/kg daily, then cyclophosphamide 60 mg/kg for 2 days. A patient with Fanconi's anemia was conditioned with cyclophosphamide 5 mg/kg for 4 days, antithymocyte globulin 30 mg/kg for 3 days, and total body irradiation (3 fractions of 200 rad each).

The dose of GM-CSF was 10 µg/kg daily given as a 4-h infusion for 15 days, starting on the day after BMT. The dose of EPO was 100 U/kg i.v. on alternate days, 3 days a week, for the first 4 weeks.

Patients were monitored with daily physical examinations and daily blood counts. Kidney and liver function tests and electrolyte measurements were performed 3 times a week. The results of the present study were compared with those of 2 groups of patients: group A, which included patients with myeloid malignancies transplanted during the same period of time, and group B, which included patients with nonmyeloid diseases trans-

Table 1. Conditioning regimen for autologous BMT

	Day		
	−2	−1	0
BM harvesting	×		
High-dose melphalan	×		
Total body irradiation	×	×	×
BM infusion			×

Table 2.   Patient characteristics

	Study group (n = 7)	Group A (n = 8)	Group B (n = 7)
Median age (range) in years	9 (2–29)	19 (6–36)	11 (1–21)
Male/female	3/4	5/3	4/3
Autologous/Allogeneic, BMT	3/4	1/7	0/7
Diagnosis			
ALL	5	0	5
AML	0	2	0
CML	0	5	0
NHL	1	0	1
Other	1	1	1
Conditioning			
Chemotherapy only	3	6	4
Chemotherapy and radiotherapy	4	2	3
GVHD prophylaxis			
Cyclosporine	3	1	3
Cyclosporine and methotrexate	1	6	4

ALL, acute lymphoblastic leukemia; AML, acute myeloblastic leukemia; CML, chronic myeloid leukemia; NHL, non-Hodgkins lymphoma; GVHD, graft-versus-host-disease.

planted the year before (Table 2). All clinical care policies were maintained unchanged throughout the studies and the period during which group B patients were transplanted.

Results

The median time for the neutrophil count to reach $0.5 \times 10^9/l$ was 14 days in the study group, 24 days in group A, and 17 days in group B. Patients in the study group had a platelet count $>25 \times 10^9/l$ after 18 days, as compared to 24 and 21 days in groups A and B, respectively. They required a median of 1 U of red cells as compared with 2 U for the patients in Group A and 1 U in group B (Table 3).

No adverse clinical events attributable to GM-CSF or EPO administration were observed. The patients did not differ in median values for the maximal serum creatinine and bilirubin concentrations, which were very similar in the three groups. The median number of days in isolation after BMT was 26 days in

Table 3. Findings after transplantation

	Study group (n = 7)	Group A (n = 8)	Group B (n = 7)
Number of days:			
to neutrophil >0.5 × 10^9/l	14	24	17
with neutrophils <0.5 × 10^9/l	12	20	15
to platelets >25 × 10^9/l	18	24	21
in isolation	26	30	26
of parenteral antibiotics	14	18	17

the study group and 30 and 26 days in groups A and B, respectively. Cessation of GM-CSF administration was followed by a rapid decrease in the absolute neutrophil count to almost the level of group B patients, with subsequent recovery in a manner comparable to this group.

Although the number of patients in this study is too small to allow for any significant comparisons, we found no major differences between the study group and group B, meaning that patients transplanted for nonmyeloid malignancies or diseases had a very similar hemopoietic recovery and similar needs in supportive treatment whether they were given GM-CSF plus EPO or not. Patients with myeloid malignancies had a slower recovery, although this may have been influenced by the short course of methotrexate given to 6 of them as prophylaxis against graft-versus-host disease.

Conclusions

The administration of GM-CSF plus EPO proved to be a safe and well-tolerated combination in this small group of patients and have a favorable effect on the recovery of neutrophils and platelets when compared to both groups of patients not receiving growth factors. These differences were more impressive when comparing the study groups with those patients transplanted for myeloid malignancies.

Alterations in the schedule of administration of GM-CSF have been recently suggested [7]. The administration of this factor first in the combination could increase the cell pool through an effect of priming and recruitment of progenitors. This would give EPO a larger number of cells to act on, which might prove to be a more effective way of combining these two growth factors.

Acknowledgments

We are grateful to Boehringer Mannheim and Sandoz/Schering Plough for providing us with EPO and with GM-CSF.

References

1 Mertelsmann R, Herman F, Hecht T, Schiller G: Hematopoietic growth factors in bone marrow transplantation. Bone Marrow Transplant 1990;6:73–77.
2 Gordon MS, Hoffman R: Growth factors affecting human thrombocytopoiesis: Potential agents for the treatment of thrombocytopenia. Blood 1992;80:302–307.
3 Dukes PP, Egrie JC, Strickland TW, Browne JK, Lin FK: Megakaryocyte colony stimulating activity of recombinant human erythropoietin, in Levine RF, Williams N, Levin J, Evatt BL (eds): Megakaryocyte Development and Function. New York, Alan R Liss, 1986, pp 105–115.
4 Shikama Y, Ishibashi T, Kimura H, Kawaguchi M, Uchida T, Maruyama Y: Transient effect of erythropoietin on thrombocytopoiesis in vivo in mice. Exp Hematol 1992:20:216–222.
5 Kanz L, Brugger W, Bross K, Mertelsmann R: Combination of cytokines: Current status and future prospects. Br J Haematol 1991;79(Suppl 1):96–104.
6 Abecasis M, Nolasco I, Gonçalves A, Rodrigues A, Coelho R: Successful third bone marrow transplantation for severe aplastic anemia. Possible in vivo synergism of GM-CSF and erythropoietin; in Freund, Link, Schmidt, Welte (eds): Cytokines in Hemopoiesis, Oncology and AIDS II. Berlin, Springer-Verlag, 1992; pp 565–567.
7 Lui kart S, MacDonald M, Herzan D, Modeas C, Goutsan M, Clamon G, Maurer H, Perry MC, Green MR: Ability of twice daily granulocyte-macrophage colony-stimulating factor (GM-CSF) to support those escalation of etoposide (VP-16) and carboplatin (CBDCA) in extensive small cell lung cancer (SCLC). Proc Am Soc Clin Oncol 1991;10:825a.

M. Abecasis, Bone Marrow Transplant Unit, Instituto Português Oncologia, Rua Professor Llma Basto, 1093 Lisbon CoDEX, Portugal

Discussion

to the Paper by M. Abecasis and M.J. Passos

Cazzola (Pavia): You have not shown any data on the reticulocyte count.

Passos: Yes, you studied, of course, the increase in the number of reticulocytes but we prefer not to present these results now, due to the small number of patients at this moment.

Cazzola: In a recent study on the use of rhEPO after allogeneic bone marrow transplantation, we were able to show that the median time to reach a reticulocyte count of 50×10^9 per liter was significantly shorter in treated patients than in historical controls.

Passos: The only thing we can say is that the number of transfusions utilized in these patients was less than the number of transfusions in the historical controls, although we cannot say that this difference is statistically significant.

Miller (Baltimore): We also looked at rhEPO in 18 patients after allogeneic bone marrow transplant. There was a decrease of the median time to a hematocrit of greater than 35 without transfusion from greater than 250 days down to 54 days in our patient population, as well as improving the time to reticulocyte count of greater than 2% corrected from 44 days to 17 days. These data suggested that we can stimulate erythropoiesis after bone marrow transplantation. There are quite a few studies going on in the U.S. looking at rhEPO in autologous transplantation. We are presently almost three-quarters of the way through a trial of recombinant human erythropoietin after autologous transplantation purged with 4HC, a drug like cytoxin. So I think there is going to be quite a lot of data coming out in the next 6 to 8 months looking at EPO after allogeneic and autologous bone marrow transplantation.

Oncology and Hematology

What is the clinical rationale for treating cancer patients with rhEPO?

Miller (Baltimore): I think, from my standpoint, the first reason to treat cancer patients with EPO is to avoid homologous blood transfusion. And the second reason, which is also very important, is to improve quality of life. This has often been ignored in patients with terminal diseases who are getting a lot of other therapies.

Adamson (New York): I am not sure I completely agree with that. There are some studies which have not been done. Would individuals with malignancy who are transfused to the target hematocrit level—as opposed to receiving EPO to achieve the target hematocrit level—be benefited equally in terms of quality of life from transfusions as compared to EPO therapy? I suspect that the outcome would be in favor of EPO therapy. We hematologists and oncologists need to be reminded that one of the benefits of EPO therapy in dialysis patients was the stimulation of protein synthesis which was accompanied by improved appetite, particularly in young patients. While there is a physiological and pharmacological rationale that one can make for using EPO therapy, the clinical rationale for treating elderly patients with malignancy, perhaps metastatic malignancy, and for which chemotherapy is only palliative, is not clear. I would argue that some selection is going to be necessary because of the costs involved in a large number of patients with malignancy. And that selection, at least in part, should be a selection on the basis of individuals who have been treated with intent to cure and those individuals who receive chemotherapy and can expect a prolonged survival.

Birgegård (Uppsala): I would like to make a case for the palliation of patients with terminal disease or with a short life expectancy. I think it's even more important in those patients to give them a good quality of life for the short time that they have left. In a curable disease you can tell the patient that he will have a short time of hardship and then later on he will be cured and his hemoglobin will be all right. What can you tell the dying cancer patient who has a year? So, I think I would take exactly the opposite standpoint if I had to choose, which at the moment I don't have to.

Adamson: Can I come back to Dr. Birgegård on that? Two points: One, the study has not been done, as I pointed out, to determine if palliation might be met equally well with transfusions as compared to EPO therapy. And second: One of the things that was brought out from the reporting of larger trials of patients with malignancy at the recent International Society of Hematology meeting in London is that those individuals who were least likely to respond to exogenous EPO therapy were those with poor performance status. These, unfortunately, very likely would fall into the category that you have just described.

Birgegård: On the other hand, people who try treatment with EPO in cancer patients repeatedly show that it works in most patients tried. One more thing: You yourself pointed out that we hematologists need to be reminded that there were other benefits than the increase in hemoglobin as you mentioned recently yourself. So why should we not try to give those benefits to these patients too?

Brunner (Bern): I have difficulties [in seeing] how EPO can really be shown in clinical trials to improve the quality of life in cancer patients who undergo palliative treatment, because these patients have many other problems and it is very difficult to distinguish between the improvement of quality of life induced by, let's say, EPO treatment or induced by chemotherapy or other supportive palliative care. We have great difficulties even to do quality-of-life studies in adjuvant chemotherapy in breast cancer to demonstrate how much patients benefit from these treatments effectively. And in palliative treatment, it seems to me extremely difficult to separate different factors. It is not only the anemia which bothers the patient; it is pain, it is loss of appetite, it is effects of both treatment and tumor progression. How do you want to distinguish all these factors? The quality-of-life studies before treatment and after treatment that you have done in your study, in my opinion, do not prove the specific effect of EPO because you have to look at the distribution of all other factors in the treated and in the control group which may not be equalized by randomization, such as tumor response rates, disease stages, performance status, age, etc. It seems to me that it is extremely difficult to do good quality-of-life studies to demonstrate that EPO-induced improvement of anemia is an independent factor of an improvement of quality of life.

Miller: I agree that quality of life is difficult to examine in cancer patients, but a lot of things that you are saying about patients with cancer is what people said five years ago about patients with uremia. As Dr. Eschbach said, many of the symptoms that people were associating with uremia really were associated with the anemia. I feel that some of the studies have supported that a patient with cancer who has a hematocrit of 25 or 30 will feel better when the hematocrit is raised to 36. Yes, we are not curing the disease, but I think you need to raise the point that quality of life in those patients is important and further studies need to be performed.

Goodnough (St. Louis): I would like to make a comment as both an oncologist and a blood banker. I feel that there are certain populations [for which] we should be able to reassure our patients that the blood supply is safe. One obvious example would be in trauma and non-elective surgery, and the second example would be in the palliative care of the terminal cancer patients whom you are not going to cure. These patients have too much else to worry about than the safety of the blood supply, and rather than to suggest an expensive medication for a series of subcutaneous injections, when even in that circumstance up to 30% of patients still will require blood transfusions, I just don't think it is worth the effort. In terms of their quality of life, simply reassure them that when they need red cells and platelet transfusions, they will be there for them.

Rank the order of oncologic indications which are most suitable for rhEPO.

Miller: From my standpoint, of the data that has been presented, I think one of the most interesting uses of EPO at this point is in cisplatin-induced anemia, especially cisplatin therapy such as was shown in the Austrian study of patients with osteosarcoma and Ewing sarcoma. The second place would be in intensive chemotherapy-induced anemia, such as seen with intensive therapy for breast cancer and/or intensive chemotherapy not containing cisplatin for sarcomas, etc. As a bone marrow transplanter I have to list BMT as the third indication, even though the data is very sketchy right now. My personal opinion is that over the next year or two we will get quite a lot more data about the role of EPO in bone marrow transplant. Fourth, I think the data that was reported today on myelodysplastic syndrome in combination with other growth factors is very interesting. Considering what the other therapeutic options are for myelodysplastic syndrome, I still think we should proceed at looking what EPO will do in this disease. And the fifth indication would be multiple myeloma, because different responses were seen in different studies.

Cazzola (Pavia): I will try to go back to the previous question first. I don't agree with Dr. Adamson in his view on the use of EPO in cancer patients. I believe that this should not be restricted only to patients with curable cancer. We have used EPO for the treatment of anemia in patients with prostatic carcinoma.

None of these patients had a curable disease but all of them had a long-lasting disease, and some of them were heavily transfusion-dependent: All patients responded to EPO by abolishing their transfusion requirements. Treatment was not only effective in terms of hemoglobin level but also in terms of quality of life; moreover, it was also cost-effective. Therefore, the decision to treat the anemia of cancer with EPO should be individualized for each patient, looking especially at quality of life.

With respect to the second question, I am sure that patients with malignant lymphoma who become anemic under first-line chemotherapy and have a curable disease should be treated with EPO to avoid transfusion. A substantial portion of patients with multiple myeloma may benefit from EPO. Finally, the data that Dr. Hellström-Lindberg has presented—that is, about a 40% response by combining EPO with G-CSF—are very interesting because myelodysplastic syndromes are poorly responsive disorders and are becoming more and more frequent. Thus, from the point of view of a hematologist, I would suggest that at least some subsets of patients with malignant lymphoma, multiple myeloma, and myelodysplastic syndromes could be treated with EPO.

Kubanek (Ulm): Are there any factors which you can predict will respond to EPO in patients with myelodysplastic syndrome?—because there is a small fraction of patients who do respond but I don't think we know who does respond.

Cazzola: We have discussed this point. We have not yet identified factors clearly predicting response. The impression is that patients at clinical onset are more likely to respond, possibly because they have normal residual stem cells responsive to EPO. Moreover, patients with blunted endogenous EPO production are more likely to respond, although there is no clear cut between responders and nonresponders (i.e., there is an overlap in terms of endogenous EPO production). At present, I think that these two factors may be considered predictors of response.

Is there any risk of worsening the underlying disease—e.g., in patients with multiple myeloma, non-Hodgkin lymphoma, or solid tumors—due to a stimulating effect of rhEPO on tumor cells?

Cazzola: To the best of my knowledge, there has been just one report indicating that a cell line derived from a patient with multiple myeloma expressed EPO receptors and responded in a proliferative way to EPO. We have tested the effects of EPO on a number of leukemic cell lines and solid tumor cell lines. The leukemic cell lines included also K562 and HEL, which do express

EPO receptors but at a low density (30 to 40 receptors per cell). None of these cell lines did respond to EPO by increasing the number of clonogenic cells or the percentage of cells in the S-phase of the cell cycle. This was true also for the K562 and the HEL cell lines. My feeling is that it is very unlikely to have a stimulatory effect on the basic disorder unless the malignant cells express, let us say, at least 1000 EPO receptors per cell. Any questions, comments, or opinions?

Miller: I think many people would avoid EPO in M6 leukemia because there have been some reports on tumor stimulation in that disease. Clinically, tumor stimulation has not been shown to be a problem.

Cazzola: I am not sure about that. In fact, we are using combinations of GM-CSF and chemotherapy to treat the patients with refractory anemia with an excess of blasts, or even those with acute myeloid leukemia in order to recruit clonogenic leukemia cells and kill them with chemotherapy. Maybe EPO could also be used—although I am not suggesting to use it—to treat M6 in combination with chemotherapy.

A. Huch (Zurich): What is the direct effect of improvement of the delivery of oxygen to the tumor itself by improvement of the hematocrit? Is there any indication that in some cases this improvement makes it worse?

Miller: I don't think there is any evidence that it makes it worse in the chemotherapy. However, this is an active research interest in radiation therapy, evaluating whether you can improve the response to radiation by providing more oxygen by an increased hematrocrit. I don't think anybody has looked at that in chemotherapy except from clinical experience that would suggest that there is not a worsening of the tumor.

What are possible synergisms between rhEPO and other cytokines in the treatment of malignant disorders (e.g., facilitation of intensified chemotherapy and bone marrow transplantation)?

Cazzola: Eva Hellström-Lindberg has presented nice data on this, obtained by using rhEPO in combination with G-CSF. EPO is ineffective in aplastic anemia, both in vitro and in vivo. But recent in vitro data suggest that the combination of stem cell factor and EPO may be effective in aplastic anemia. It is possible that the combination of stem cell factor and EPO will also be more effective than EPO alone in patients with myelodysplastic syndrome.

Kaltwasser (Frankfurt): I wonder if your last comment is correct, because of the enormous increase of endogenous EPO in aplastic anemia. I would doubt this comment in that way, that exogenous EPO could hardly overcome marrow aplasia. It would be a better idea to combine stem cell growth factors with the endogenous EPO in aplastic anemia, after, e.g., immunosuppressive treatment.

Cazzola: I partly agree with you, but there are four or five reports on patients with pure red cell aplasia and elevated endogenous EPO production who did respond to exogenous EPO. This is really strange, because this condition is very unlikely to respond for at least two reasons: lack of erythroid progenitors and high endogenous EPO. Nevertheless, the patients did respond. Your statement is okay, but often the clinical results are unpredictable.

Brunner: Are there any studies performed at present which looked at the combination of EPO and other cytokines in autologous bone marrow transplantation and after intensification of chemotherapy in non-Hodgkin lymphoma, Hodgkin disease, and breast cancer, where such intensive treatments are studied?

Miller: I think the data are being collected now. There are at least two studies in the U.S. looking at combination growth factors. I know there are studies elsewhere as well, but none of the studies have been reported. There may be some information from those who attended the meeting of the American Society of Hematology, but I do not know.

Cazzola: A clinical trial is being carried out in Italy to evaluate the effects of rhEPO and GM-CSF after autologous bone marrow transplantation; apparently there is no additional effect on erythropoiesis by using the two factors.

Based on current clinical experience, what recommendations are possible regarding dose, dose frequency, treatment duration, and treatment timing (before, together with, or after chemotherapy)?

Miller: That is a very hard question to answer at this point because the data are not anywhere near as advanced as the data in renal insufficiency. But I think it is good evidence that there is a minimum effective dose, and so I think that further studies should be performed using doses of at least 100 to 200 International Units per kilogram. In practice, most people use approximately between those doses and round up and down to the appropriate vial size.

The frequency: Most of the studies that have been randomized have been done with three-times-a-week based on the renal failure data, and so at this point most clinical experience has been done with three-times-a-week. In an absence of a study situation, I think that would be the most appropriate dose. In some of the myelodysplastic studies and the bone marrow transplant studies, daily dosing is being used; however, this is still being evaluated.

To the duration of treatment: We recommend treatment until they reach target hematocrit, which has been higher in cancer patients than in renal-failure patients. People have been using 38 as a target hematocrit. In a setting where the patient is continuing to receive either the chemotherapy or other immunosuppressive agents after bone marrow transplantation, it may be important to decrease but not stop the dose when they reach their target hematocrit, because there has been data in bone marrow transplantation that if you stop EPO the hematocrit can rapidly drop off and require either reinstitution or transfusion.

From the timing standpoint, there is no evidence of adverse experience when you use concurrent administration of EPO and chemotherapy, and therefore we recommend starting with EPO when the patient's hematrocit is decreasing. I think that in the absence of a study setting, it is important that you look at the rate of fall in the hematocrit and decide based on how fast the hematocrit is falling when you want to start. It would take—in the cancer patient, at least, in most of the studies—2 weeks between when you give EPO and see a significant reticulocyte and hematocrit response. So you need to guess where the patient is going to be in 2 weeks, if you are going to continue the chemotherapy.

Brunner: What is the exact timing? If you give chemotherapy you give it, usually, intermittently. When do you start EPO? Four days after the dose of chemotherapy, or later, or earlier? You are dealing with an expanding red-cell population if you give EPO, and if you give chemotherapy too close to EPO you may induce an increase of progenitor red-cell destruction. Therefore, timing may be important.

Miller: The studies in chemotherapy that have been done at this point have all been done with the EPO continuing irrespective of giving the chemotherapy, and it has not appeared to have any negative effects such as we have seen with the myeloid growth factor, such as 5FU and GM-CSF. At this point people have started with EPO when the patient gets anemic irrespective of the chemotherapy.

Cazzola: I would like to have the opinion of Dr. Bondurant at this point. If the major effect of EPO is the prevention of apoptosis, which are your suggestions on timing of EPO with respect to chemotherapy? Should we give EPO after or during chemotherapy?

Bondurant (Nashville): I do not really have an opinion on that based on the prevention of apoptosis by EPO. Our evidence does not suggest that the erythroid progenitor cells would be resistant to chemotherapeutic agents at any particular time or that their cycling status would matter. We have done some studies with methotrexate in vitro, but not with other agents. EPO does not offer significant protection to cells against the toxic action of methotrexate.

Does rhEPO treatment affect mortality and morbidity of cancer patients?

Miller: There is no evidence that EPO affects mortality at this point. Morbidity . . . I think some of those studies with regimen-specific treatment with EPO will help answer that question. From the large randomized trial, it is hard to really look at morbidity in the absence of looking at specific adverse events. However, at this point, I cannot say that we have shown that EPO affects the mortality or real morbidity.

Is iron substitution necessary (dosage, supplementation per os, or parenterally)?

Cazzola: My view is the following. If under EPO therapy serum iron falls below 60 micrograms per deciliter and/or transferrin saturation below 20%, we must administer iron. It is possible that in some patients oral iron is ineffective, even if given at full dosage (100 to 200 milligrams per day). Parenteral iron is required in these cases, which will include most patients with excessive cytokine production and reticuloendothelial iron block. In Europe, we can use iron saccharate, which is very effective and safe. It is a colloidal iron which is taken up by the reticuloendothelial cells. We haven't observed any adverse effect by using this iron in more than 200 patients with cancer. The only concern in patients with cancer is, some studies have suggested, that iron may stimulate malignant cell proliferation. So, from the point of view of the efficacy of EPO, iron supplementation is required in most patients. Future studies, however, should evaluate any possible effect of iron supplementation on malignant cell proliferation.

What is the cost-benefit to support rhEPO treatment in oncologic patients?

Miller: It is a very difficult question to answer at this point because formal cost–benefit analyses are not yet available. I think it depends on the cost of the transfusion of your patients and whether you want to look just at the cost of the blood and the time it takes to transfuse the blood or whether you need a factor in quality of life. So at this point there is very little data available. At my center, on a strictly cost–benefit ratio, where we have relatively expensive blood, I have a feeling that if a patient is requiring more than two units of blood a month, then a dose of EPO 100 to 200 units per kilogram three times a week is equivalent. But that is just at our center, and I think you have to look at each center separately. I heard that in some countries in Europe the blood is much less expensive. At our institution it is $800 per unit. Dr. Adamson, can you talk about that at all?

Adamson: No, I really don't have anything to add. The costs are going to vary country by country, and within the U.S. on a region-by-region basis, because the hospital gets a unit of red cells at one price, then the nurses' costs, the administrative costs, and other costs mushroom to the kind of figure that you have just given. So I think that the modeling that's going to have to be done around this will be very important. One of the things that Dr. Miller and I deal with in hematology and oncology patients, particularly in the U.S., is the inordinate concern about the safety of the blood supply. Many people are willing—whether it is right or not I will not argue—to assume added costs in order to avoid exposure to homologous blood. So it is going to be a very difficult cost–benefit analysis to be carried out at the present time.

Kubanek: I only would like to add this: It is very difficult to make a cost–benefit calculation, but I think $800 per unit of blood is much too high for our country, and we cannot calculate with this kind of price. It differs by a factor of four now in Germany. And I think this makes the calculation quite different. I think John Adamson pointed out that you add on cost, but you add on costs of EPO too, as we heard from Dr. Eschbach. So I think if you do calculations on cost–benefit, you have to do it right or you'd better not do them.

Lindsay (Ontario): As a simple nephrologist but also a taxpayer, I think this issue is very, very important. I am not going to get into the issue of cost–benefit, but can you give us some possible idea of the burden? What—in the U.S., for example—would be the number of people per year who are likely to get it? Give us some idea.

Miller: I am sorry; I don't have that data available. I can't even make a guess. I think it depends on, similar to the renal-failure patients, at what point you maintain the hematocrit. Do you want to keep your cancer patients on a hematocrit of 25 without transfusion? Do you want to keep them at 30? Do you think cancer patients do better with a hematocrit of 35? It's the same evaluation you need to do for the renal-failure patients. However, I think it is a little bit more difficult because of all of the other factors—the heterogeneity of the population is greater. But I agree that the cost–benefit is very important to look at.

The Anemia of Prematurity
Causes and Therapeutic Consequences

*Daniel S. Halpérin,[a] Martine Félix,[a] Pierre Wacker,[a] Gérald Lacourt,[b]
Jean-François Babel,[a] Marinette Wyss[a]*

[a]Hematology/Oncology Unit and [b]Division of Neonatology, Department
of Pediatrics, Hôpital Cantonal Universitaire, Geneva, Switzerland

Erythropoietin (EPO) is detectable in the human fetus as of the 19th week of
gestation [1]. During the last trimester, serum EPO concentration increases
simultaneously with cord blood hemoglobin level, and at term, it reaches values
2–4 times above those of nonanemic adults [1–4]. Postpartum, in response to the
newborn's exposure to an environment that is hyperoxic relative to the intra-
uterine milieu, red blood cell (RBC) production is down-regulated by a reduction
of endogenous EPO secretion. This "shut-off" phase usually lasts for 2–3
months during which the erythroid cell pool is modified from an initial state of
polycythemia to a state of slight oligocythemia, better known as the *physiological anemia of the newborn* [2, 5–8]. By the age of 8–12 weeks, nadir hemoglobin
concentration is usually reached and bone marrow erythroid hypoplasia is observed. At this point, spontaneous resumption of EPO production occurs, followed by active reticulocytosis and progressive normalization of the hemoglobin
concentration. Rarely does this physiological anemia cause clinical symptoms or
require any therapy in the term infant. In the preterm infant, however, this
hyporegenerative anemia is amplified by a variety of factors, the combination of
which leads to the *anemia of prematurity* (AP), a condition that is more often
symptomatic [6, 8]. These aggravating factors include the following: (a) a
reduced red cell mass at birth [9, 10], (b) extracellular volume expansion due to
rapid body growth [9, 11], (c) a short erythrocyte life span, which may be further
reduced in premature infants because of a particular sensitivity to oxidative
injury [9, 10, 12], (d) RBC losses due to blood sampling for laboratory monitoring [6, 9], (e) nutritional disorders associated with decreased protein and/or

caloric intake, since factors such as insulin-like growth factor-I (IGF-I) appear to have direct effects on fetal and early postnatal erythropoiesis [13], and EPO production itself may be dependent on body growth rate [14, 15], and (f) inappropriately low levels of circulating EPO in preterm infants, even in the face of pronounced anemia [16–22]. Serum EPO levels are lower in the first 2 months than at any other time in life. Only after the third month of postnatal age do they become comparable to those of nonanemic adults. The reasons for such a delay in the initiation of a functional erythropoietic regulation mechanism are unclear. In vitro, bone marrow as well as circulating erythroid progenitors from preterm infants are more numerous and equally sensitive to EPO as their adult counterparts [23–25]. These target cells should therefore be capable of proliferating and differentiating in vivo in the presence of adequate concentrations of EPO. On the other hand, animal studies have established that the site of EPO production in the fetus is the liver rather than the kidney [26] and that a greater degree of hypoxia may be needed to induce liver EPO release [27]. Thus, hypoxemia may be profound enough to elicit an appropriate secretion of EPO in utero, as is indicated by the high EPO levels measured in cord blood. Postnatally, however, the oxygen tension sensors, presumably located in the liver at this stage, may not be sensitive enough to detect the milder hypoxemia of anemic infants. This could account for the fact that preterm infants can respond to low central venous oxygen tension by increasing to some extent their EPO production, but in a very blunted way compared to older patients [16, 21, 22]. What stimulus underlies the liver-to-kidney switch is unknown. One might speculate that this event is developmentally determined, as serum EPO concentrations rise both with increasing gestation and postnatal ages.

It has been proposed that increased EPO production may not be necessary in preterm infants because their decreasing hemoglobin concentration should be compensated for by the rising production of adult hemoglobin, which has less affinity for oxygen than fetal hemoglobin [21, 28]. This, however, does not explain why both hematocrit and serum EPO concentration are simultaneously at their lowest levels in a lifetime. In addition, despite the progressive shift to the right of the hemoglobin dissociation curve, "oxygen availability" to the tissues decreases with postnatal age if it is calculated for a central venous oxygen tension of 20 mm Hg (a value that may be closer to reality in the most severely anemic patients than the 40 mm Hg traditionally used for determining "oxygen-unloading capacity") [5, 8, 22]. Moreover, clinical symptoms are commonly observed in the AP and include tachypnea, episodes of apnea/bradycardia, tachycardia, lethargy, and poor weight gain [8, 22, 29–32]. That these symptoms are related to decreased "oxygen availability" is suggested by their association with high blood lactate levels [32, 33] and by their resolution in some, but not all, studies after RBC transfusion [5, 22, 30–33]. Hence the clinical practice is to transfuse these patients if and when their anemia is considered symptomatic.

Since premature infants do not have complete immunological competence and are particularly vulnerable to blood-transmitted infections, the use of blood derivatives should be approached cautiously in these patients. Stringent blood donor selection criteria and optimal viral screening procedures cannot provide an absolute guarantee of safe blood products. Because EPO seems to be a major regulator of fetal and neonatal erythropoiesis, and since a temporary arrest of EPO-dependent erythropoietic activity characterizes the AP, the therapeutic use of recombinant human erythropoietin (rhEPO) in this situation may not only constitute a safer, but also a more physiological approach. We thus conducted a pilot study to verify the validity of this hypothesis.

Patients and Methods

Patients

The characteristics of 18 patients and 66 historical controls are shown in Table 1. Controls were matched with patients for gestational age, were clinically stable, had not been transfused beyond the second week of life, and had their blood counts checked weekly to monitor the progression of their anemia. All patients met the following eligibility criteria: gestational age was less than 34 weeks, they were 21–35 days old at entry into the study, venous hematocrit was less than 32% at 3 weeks or 30% at 4 weeks of age, they had no major symptoms related to their anemia (e.g., apnea/bradycardia

Table 1. Patient characteristics

	rhEPO patients (n = 18)	Historical controls (n = 66)
Mean gestational age (range), weeks	30.7 (28–33)	30.4 (26–34)
Mean birth weight (range), g	1350 (860–1800)	1320 (880–1830)
Mean age at initiation of rhEPO treatment (50), days	26.8 (3.9)	—
rhEPO regimen		
75 U/kg/week	3	—
150 U/kg/week	6	—
300 U/kg/week	5	—
600 U/kg/week	4 (patients 15-18)	—
Oral iron regimen		
2–5 mg/kg/day	14	66
7–8 mg/kg/day	4 (patients 15–18)	—

Modified from Halpérin DS et al., Eur J Pediatr 1992;151:661–667.

episodes), and their anemia was not caused by a hemolytic disease; they were not ventilated or dependent on an inspired fraction of oxygen higher than 25% or on total parenteral nutrition; none was so unstable clinically as to require blood tests totaling more than 7.5 ml/kg per week; they had no major congenital malformation, no renal, hepatic or hemostatic dysfunction, and were not hypertensive; they were not transfused in the 2 weeks preceding the study; and their parents gave informed consent in accordance with the ethics committee of our institution.

Therapy with rhEPO

The rhEPO supplied by Cilag A.G. (Switzerland) was recovered from supernatant of Chinese hamster ovary cells and conditioned as a buffered solution of 4000 or 2000 U/ml. After dilution with 0.9% saline, solutions of 400–2000 U/ml were obtained, which were more suitable for small infants. Starting at 21–33 days of life, rhEPO was given s.c. 3 times a week for 4 weeks at dosages of 75, 150, 300, or 600 U/kg per week (Table 1). Oral supplements of elemental iron were given throughout rhEPO therapy at a dose of 2–5 mg/kg/day (patients 1–14) or 7–8 mg/kg/day (patients 15–18). Vitamin E (5–20 mg/day) was given orally to all patients.

Laboratory and Clinical Monitoring

The following data were recorded before, during, and up to 3 months after therapy: vital signs, noninvasive blood pressure measurements, number and duration of apneic episodes, cutaneous reactions, and weight gain; cerebral ultrasonography; complete venous blood counts, including reticulocytes and smear examination; serum electrolytes, iron, transferrin, and ferritin; hepatic and renal function tests; and trough serum EPO levels by radioimmunoassay (courtesy of Dr. K. Rhyner, Zurich). Peripheral blood clonogenic cultures in methylcellulose were performed in 12 patients prior to and at completion of rhEPO therapy, with slight modifications of the method described by Iscove et al. [34]. The volume of blood sampled from each patient did not exceed 12 ml over the 4 weeks of therapy. Blood transfusions were ordered by an independent medical team according to clinical and hematological criteria routinely used in our neonatal unit.

Data Analysis

Comparisons between repeated observations in the historical controls and in the patients receiving rhEPO or comparisons between the two groups were made with paired or unpaired t, ANOVA, Mann-Whitney, Wilcoxon, and χ^2 tests as appropriate. Results are mean (SD) unless otherwise stated.

Results

Serum Erythropoietin Levels

The median baseline serum EPO level was 7.0 mU/ml (Table 2), i.e., the lower limit of normal for nonanemic adults. There was no correlation between these levels and the concomitant hematocrit. After 2 weeks of treatment, the

Table 2. Hematological values

	Weeks from beginning of rhEPO therapy[a]							
	0	1	2	3	4	5	8	14
Reticulocytes ($\times$ 10^9/l)								
Controls	69 (39)	96 (48)	85 (43)	97 (49)	127 (60)*	136 (66)	92 (38)	not available
rhEPO patients	71 (33)	133 (66)**	186 (87)***	200 (121)***	172 (73)*,**	107 (67)	174 (55)***,****	73 (51)
Hematocrit (%)								
Controls	33.6 (3.3)	32.3 (4.3)	30.8 (4.6)	29.5 (5)	28.8 (6)*	28.8 (6.2)	30.2 (3.9)	not available
rhEPO patients	26.2 (3.1)***	27.2 (3.6)***	26.8 (3.3)**	27.3 (4.6)	27.8 (4.7)	27.6 (4.4)	28.3 (4.4)	31.8 (2.7)
Serum erythropoietin (mU/ml)[b]								
Median	7.0	—	12.6*****	—	9.1	9.6	16.3******	9.9
Range	<0.5–14.5		2.3–90.7		<0.5–41.3	5.2–14.4	10.4–79.4	6.6–48.0

[a] Or corresponding postnatal age in controls.
[b] Data from rhEPO patients only.

*p $\leq$ 0.0001 week 0–4, ANOVA; **p $\leq$ 0.01 vs. historical controls, unpaired *t*-test; ***p $\leq$ 0.0005 vs. historical controls, unpaired *t*-test; ****p $\leq$ 0.01 vs. week 0, paired *t*-test; *****p = 0.02, signed-rank test; ******p = 0.008, signed-rank test.

median value of EPO reached 12.6 mU/ml (p = 0.02), and 4 weeks after rhEPO therapy it spontaneously rose to a median of 16.3 mU/ml (p = 0.008), which coincided with increased reticulocyte production.

Reticulocytes

A 2- to 10-fold increase in the absolute number of reticulocytes was observed in all but one of the patients (Table 2 and Fig. 1A) from a mean baseline count of 71 × 10^9/l (range 16–128) to 118, 133, 189, and 200 × 10^9/l on days 3, 7, 10, and 21, respectively (p ≤ 0.0001). Peak reticulocyte count occurred on average on day 21 (range 10–28) of rhEPO therapy, at least 2 weeks earlier than in historical controls, in which it was noted at 9 weeks of age. It was also higher than the peak count of controls [200 (121.1) × 10^9/l vs. 136 (66) × 10^9/l, p ≤ 0.05]. The magnitude of the reticulocyte count increase was directly related to the dose of rhEPO administered. Patients receiving the lowest dose achieved a 2-fold increase, whereas those on the highest dose had an approximate 5-fold increase (Fig. 1A). After discontinuation of therapy, the reticulocyte count returned to baseline values within 1 week, but increased again spontaneously up to a peak of 174 (55) × 10^9/l 3 weeks later. This second episode of reticulocytosis lasted for 2 weeks and coincided with a rise in serum EPO concentration, as shown in Table 2.

Hematocrit

Although the mean baseline hematocrit of rhEPO-treated patients was 2 SD below that of controls, at the end of treatment no significant difference remained between the 2 groups (Table 2 and Fig. 1B). This was not so much due to a rise of the hematocrit in rhEPO-treated patients, but rather to its continuous decline in historical controls until 8–9 weeks of postnatal age. Changes in hematocrit were not related to birth weight or gestational age, and only partly to the dose of rhEPO (r = 0.49, p ≤ 0.05). They were more significantly correlated with serum iron levels during therapy (Fig. 2A), and the 4 patients who received high-dose iron supplements had a mean hematocrit increase of 4.8 (3.5%), compared to a gain of 0.6 (3.1%) in the other patients (p ≤ 0.05).

Iron Metabolism

Serum iron, ferritin, and transferrin saturation values were normal in all patients before therapy. Within the 4 weeks of treatment, serum iron and transferrin saturation decreased by 49 and 58%, respectively, in patients on standard dose iron supplements, but were unchanged in patients on high-dose iron (Table 3). Serum ferritin decreased by 77% in both groups. By the end of

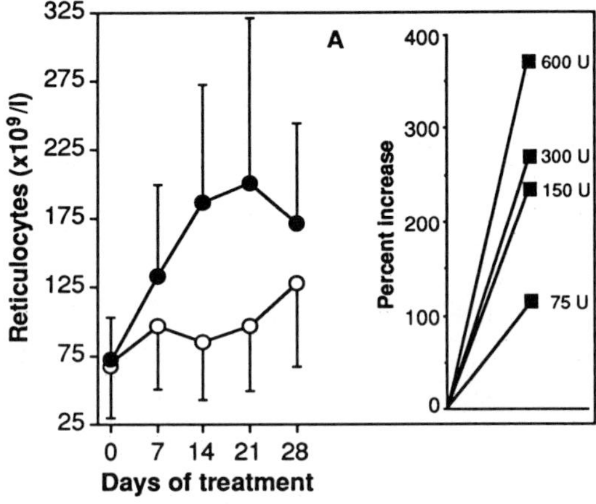

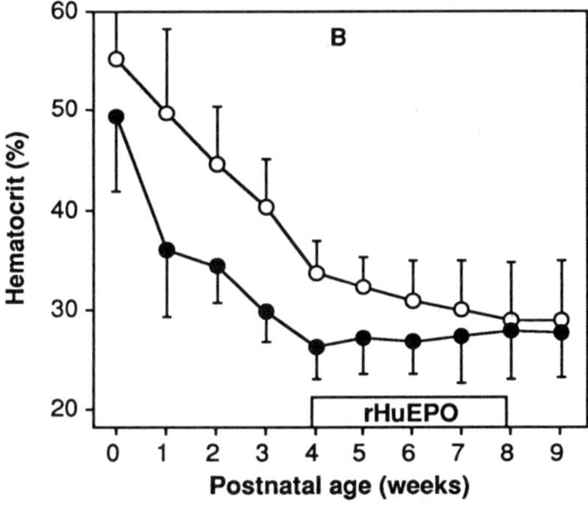

Fig. 1. Effects of rhEPO on (A) reticulocyte count and (B) hematocrit. ● = 18 patients treated with rhEPO and ○ = 66 historical controls. Values are means. Bars describe SD. Right insert in A shows maximal reticulocyte increase at different doses of rhEPO. For statistical significance of differences, see Table 2. (Modified from Halpérin DS et al., Eur J Pediatr 1992;151:661–667.)

therapy, 3 infants who had received rhEPO at 300 U/kg/per week and standard dose iron supplements were iron deficient as assessed biochemically and by RBC morphology. Regression analysis demonstrated a strong correlation between the dose of rhEPO and serum iron consumption in patients on standard dose iron (Fig. 2B). Patients on high-dose iron were able to maintain stable serum iron levels despite receiving the highest rhEPO dose.

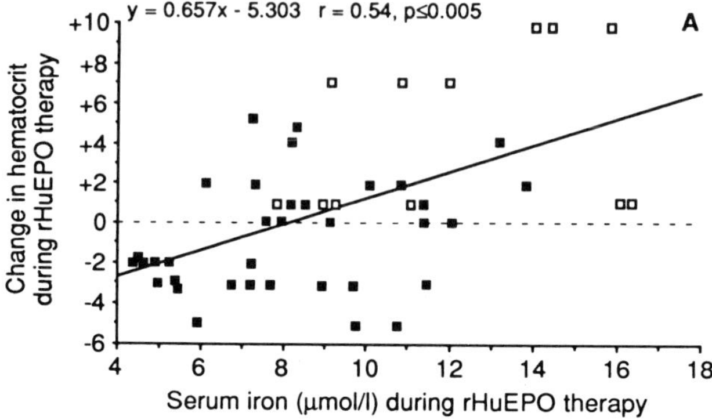

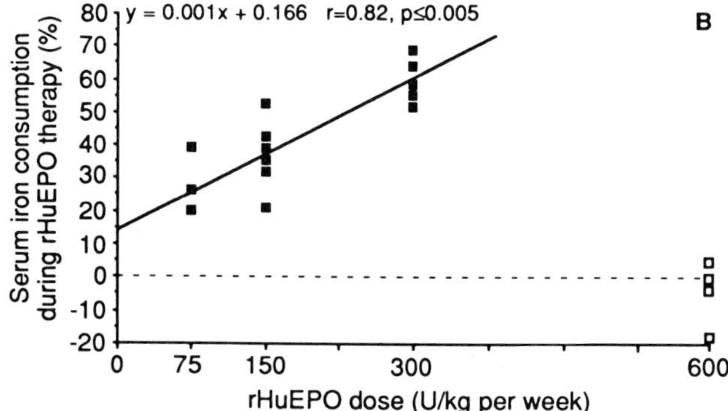

Fig. 2. Relation between serum iron concentration and hematocrit changes during (A) rhEPO therapy and (B) between rhEPO dose and serum iron consumption. ■ = 14 patients on standard dose oral iron (2–5 mg/kg/day) and ☐ = 4 patients on high-dose oral iron (7–8 mg/kg/day). (Modified from Halpérin DS et al., Eur J Pediatr 1992;151:661–667.)

Erythroid Progenitor Cells

The circulating erythroid progenitor cells (BFU-E) from 12 infants displayed normal proliferation and morphology in our clonogenic assay. Maximal growth was noted in the presence of 2 mU/ml of rhEPO, with 1340 (801) vs. 1239 (1635) colonies/ml blood before and after therapy, respectively. Identical sensitivity to rhEPO before and after treatment was demonstrated by dose-response studies where half-maximal proliferation was obtained at a rhEPO concentration of 0.27 mU/ml.

Table 3. Iron metabolism

	Days of rhEPO therapy			
	0	10	21	28
Serum iron (μmol/l)				
Patients on standard-dose oral iron[a]	13.9 (3.9)	9.3 (2.4)	8.2 (2.9)	7.1 (2.1)*
Patients on high-dose oral iron[b]	14.2 (2.7)	11.4 (3.1)	10.5 (2.8)	14.6 (2.0)
Transferrin saturation (%)				
Patients on standard-dose oral iron[a]	30.3 (17)	19.8 (7)	15.5 (5)	12.8 (5)**
Patients on high-dose oral iron[b]	24.0 (5)	17.8 (6)	16.0 (4)	25.0 (5)
Serum ferritin (μg/l)				
All patients	217 (138)	126 (99)	70 (51)	48 (26)*

[a] 2–5 mg/kg/day.
[b] 7–8 mg/kg/day.
*$p \leq 0.0001$, ANOVA day 0–28; **$p \leq 0.005$, ANOVA day 0–28.

Modified from Halpérin DS et al., Eur J Pediatr 1992;151:661–667.

Transfusions

Three of 18 patients required a RBC transfusion. They were among the most anemic infants, with baseline hematocrits of 21–23%. Two of them were unable to complete rhEPO therapy at 75 and 300 U/kg per week and were transfused after receiving one half of the scheduled injections. One infant was transfused after a full course of rhEPO at 300 U/kg/week because of iron deficiency that developed in the later part of therapy. As a crude comparison, in our neonatal unit approximately 30% of premature infants of similar gestational age require transfusion for symptomatic anemia beyond the second week of life.

Clinical and Biochemical Monitoring

Administration of rhEPO was well tolerated by all patients. Transient erythema at the site of injection was noted on a single occasion. Mean heart and respiratory rate remained unchanged throughout therapy. Blood pressure increased normally with postnatal age. Hypertension was not recorded in any patient. Weight gain was 12.2 (5.2) g/kg per day before therapy and 13.0 (4.2) g/kg at its completion (not significant). Results of hepatic and renal function tests remained normal in all patients. Cerebral ultrasonography scans that were normal at the outset remained normal during rhEPO treatment, and those that were abnormal showed either no progression or improvement during therapy.

Discussion

Eighteen anemic but clinically stable, preterm infants were treated at 3–4 weeks of postnatal age with s.c. rhEPO and oral iron using different dose regimens for both medications. Their hematocrit was at least 1 SD below the mean of 66 historical controls in whom spontaneous recovery from the AP had not been altered by RBC transfusions. They were thus at a higher risk of needing a transfusion in the following weeks. In this setting, our findings provide compelling evidence that rhEPO exerted significant effects on red blood cell production of premature infants.

The reticulocyte response was particularly remarkable, but since the patients were more anemic than the historical controls, their early reticulocytosis might have been spontaneous rather than rhEPO induced. Contradicting this hypothesis is the lack of any correlation between baseline hematocrit and reticulocyte counts or serum EPO levels in these patients. Also, patients with the highest baseline hematocrit reached their peak reticulocyte count as quickly, and in some cases more quickly, as those with the lowest hematocrit, and reticulocytosis was strikingly synchronous regardless of postnatal age at the time of therapy. Moreover, the magnitude of the reticulocyte count increase was dependent on the dose of rhEPO administered.

Treatment with rhEPO was accompanied by a dose-dependent reduction in serum iron concentration and transferrin saturation that contrasted with the stable values measured in untreated premature infants of similar postnatal age [35,36]. These changes constitute additional evidence that rhEPO stimulated the proliferation of the erythroid cell pool, thereby increasing the incorporation of circulating iron into maturing red cells, as shown in older patients [37,38]. Interestingly, the standard dose of oral iron (2–5 mg/kg/day) usually sufficient to prevent late iron-deficiency anemia in premature infants proved insufficient in some patients to sustain effective erythropoiesis during rhEPO therapy. Thus, iron deficiency was documented in 3 of 5 infants who had received rhEPO at a dose of 300 U/kg/week, and while overall stabilization of the hematocrit was achieved in patients treated with rhEPO as compared with historical controls, in some patients no or only a transient rise of hematocrit was observed. Serum iron levels were actually predictive of hematocrit changes during therapy. A decline of the hematocrit was likely to occur during rhEPO therapy in patients whose serum iron level on day

10 of treatment was <8 μmol/l (positive predictive value, 80%), but was improbable in those with a level ≥10 μmol/l (negative predictive value, 88%). On the other hand, larger doses of iron (7–8 mg/kg/day) combined with vitamin E to avoid the risk of iron-induced hemolysis [39] were well tolerated and sufficient to maintain stable serum iron levels even at the highest rhEPO dose administered.

Administration of rhEPO did not appear to suppress endogenous EPO production since serum EPO levels continuously increased during and after therapy, as is the case in untreated infants of similar postnatal age [2]. Neither did rhEPO, in agreement with other studies [40], deplete the pool of circulating erythroid progenitors or alter their sensitivity to EPO, as demonstrated in our clonogenic assays.

We conclude that rhEPO caused a dose-dependent increase of the reticulocyte count in infants with the AP and shortened the progression of their anemia. Its effects were limited in some patients by an abrupt fall in serum iron concentration that was not compensated by standard oral iron supplementation. Larger doses of iron preserved the levels of serum iron and optimized the hematological response to rhEPO. The impact of such effects on transfusion requirements of premature infants remains to be studied.

References

1   Thomas RM, Canning CE, Cotes PM, Linch DC, Rodeck CH, Rossiter CE, Huehns ER: Erythropoietin and cord blood haemoglobin in the regulation of human fetal erythropoiesis. Br J Obstet Gynaecol 1983;90:795–800.
2   Eckardt K-U, Hartmann W, Vetter U, Pohlandt F, Burghardt R, Kurtz A: Serum immunoreactive erythropoietin of children in health and disease. Eur J Pediatr 1990;149:459–464.
3   Hellebostad M, Hågå P, Cotes PM: Serum immunoreactive erythropoietin in healthy normal children. Br J Haematol 1988;70:247–250.
4   Meberg A: Haemoglobin concentrations and erythropoietin levels in appropriate and small for gestational age infants. Scand J Haematol 1980;24:162–168.
5   Holland BM, Jones JG, Wardrop CAJ: Lessons from the anemia of prematurity. Hematol Oncol Clin North Am 1987;1:355–366.
6   Shannon KM: Anemia of prematurity: Progress and prospects. Am J Pediatr Hematol Oncol 1990;12:14–20.
7   Stockmann III JA: Anemia of prematurity. Current concepts in the issue of when to transfuse. Pediatr Clin North Am 1986;33:111–128.
8   Wardrop CAJ, Holland BM, Veale KEA, Jones JG, Gray OP: Nonphysiological anaemia of prematurity. Arch Dis Child 1978;53:855–860.

9   Blanchette V, Zipursky A: Neonatal hematology, in Avery G (ed): Neonatology: Pathophysiology and Management of the Newborn. Philadelphia, JB Lippincott, 1987, pp 638–686.

10 Oski FA: The erythrocyte and its disorders, in Nathan DG, Oski FA (eds): Hematology of Infancy and Childhood. Philadelphia, W.B. Saunders, 1987, 3rd ed, pp 16–44.

11 Bratteby LE: Studies on erythrokinetics in infants. IX. Prediction of red cell volume from venous haematocrit in early infancy. Acta Paediatr Scand 1968;57:125–131.

12 Pearson HA: Life-span of the fetal red blood cell. J Pediatr 1967;70:166–171.

13 Kurtz A, Zapf J, Eckardt K-U, Clemons G, Froesch ER, Bauer C: Insulin-like growth factor I stimulates erythropoiesis in hypophysectomized rats. Proc Natl Acad Sci USA 1988;85:7825–7829.

14 Bozzini CE, Alippi RM, Barceló AC, Caro J: Correlation between erythropoietic activity and body growth rate in hypertransfused polycythemic growing rats as the result of an erythropoietin-dependent operating mechanism. Exp Hematol 1989;17:77–80.

15 Widness JA, Sanengen T, Hågå P, Clemons GK, Myhre K, Halvorsen S: Correlation of plasma erythropoiesis stimulating factor(s) and immunoreactive erythropoietin levels during rapid growth in the mouse. Acta Physiol Scand 1989;136:527–533.

16 Brown MS, Garcia JF, Phibbs RH, Dallman PR: Decreased response of plasma immunoreactive erythropoietin to "available oxygen" in anemia of prematurity. J Pediatr 1984;105:793–798.

17 Brown MS, Phibbs RH, Garcia JF, Dallman PR: Postnatal changes in erythropoietin levels in untransfused premature infants. J Pediatr 1983;103:612–617.

18 Dallman PR. Erythropoietin and the anemia of prematurity: J Pediatr 1984;105: 756–757.

19 Hågå P, Meberg A, Halvorsen S: Plasma erythropoietin concentrations during the early anemia of prematurity. Acta Paediatr Scand 1983;72:827–831.

20 Saito T, Urabe A, Uramoto K, Hashimoto Y, Takaku F: Serum erythropoietin titres in the anaemia of premature infants. Br J Haematol 1983;54:53–58.

21 Stockman III J, Garcia J, Oski FA: The anemia of prematurity: Factors governing the erythropoietin response. N Engl J Med 1977;296:647–650.

22 Stockman III JA, Graeber JE, Clark DA, McClellan K, Garcia JF, Kavey REW: Anemia of prematurity: Determinants of the erythropoietin response. J Pediatr 1984;105:786–792.

23 Shannon KM, Naylor GS, Torkildson JC, Clemons GK, Schaffner V, Goldman SL, Lewis K, Bryant P, Phibbs R: Circulating erythroid progenitors in the anemia of prematurity. N Engl J Med 1987;317:728–733.

24 Rhondeau SM, Christensen RD, Ross MP, Rothstein G, Simmons MA: Responsiveness to recombinant human erythropoietin of marrow erythroid progenitors from infants with the "anemia of prematurity." J Pediatr 1988;112:935–940.

25 Emmerson A, Westwood N, Rackham R, Stern C, Pearson T: Erythropoietin responsive progenitors in anaemia of prematurity. Arch Dis Child 1991;66:810–811.

26 Zanjani E, Ascensao J, McGlave P, Banisadre M, Ash R: Studies on the liver to kidney switch of erythropoietin production. J Clin Invest 1981;67:1183–1188.

27 Meberg A, Hågå P: Plasma erythropoietin levels in mice. Response to hypoxia at different ages. Scand J Clin Lab Invest 1981;41:231–235.

28 Delivoria-Papadopoulos M, Roncevic NP, Oski FA: Postnatal changes in oxygen transport of term, premature, and sick infants: The role of red cell 2,3-diphosphoglycerate and adult hemoglobin. Pediatr Res 1971;5:235–245.

29 Brown MS, Berman ER, Luckey D: Prediction of the need for transfusion during anemia of prematurity. J Pediatr 1990;116:773–778.

30 Joshi A, Gerhardt T, Shandloff P, Bancalari E: Blood transfusion effect on the respiratory pattern of preterm infants. Pediatrics 1987;80:79–84.

31 Keyes WG, Donohue PK, Spivak JL, Jones MD, Oski FA: Assessing the need for transfusion of premature infants and role of hematocrit, clinical signs, and erythropoietin level. Pediatrics 1989;84:412–417.

32 Ross MP, Christensen RD, Rothstein G, Koenig J, Simmons MA, Noble NA, Kimura RE: A randomized trial to develop criteria for administering erythrocyte transfusions to anemic preterm infants 1 to 3 months of age. J Perinatol 1989;9: 246–253.

33 Ohls RK, Christensen RD: Recombinant erythropoietin compared with erythrocyte transfusion in the treatment of anemia of prematurity. J Pediatr 1991;119:781–788.

34 Iscove N, Sieber F, Winterhalter K: Erythroid colony formation in cultures of mouse and human bone marrow: Analysis of the requirement for erythropoietin by gel filtration and affinity chromatography on agarose-concanavalin-A. J Cell Physiol 1974;83:309–320.

35 Hågå P: Plasma ferritin concentrations in preterm infants in cord blood and during the early anaemia of prematurity. Acta Paediatr Scand 1980;69:637–641.

36 Lundström U, Siimes MA, Dallman PR: At what age does iron supplementation become necessary in low-birth-weight infants? J Pediatr 1977;91:878–883.

37 Bianchetti M, Hämmerli I, Roduit C, Neuhaus T, Leumann E, Oetilker O: Epoetin alfa in anaemic children or adolescents on regular dialysis. Eur J Pediatr 1991;150:509–512.

38 Eschbach JW, Kelly MR, Haley NR, Abels RI, Adamson JW: Treatment of the anemia of progressive renal failure with recombinant human erythropoietin. N Engl J Med 1989;321:158–163.

39 Melhorn D, Gross S: Vitamin E-dependent anemia in the premature infant. I. Effects of large doses of medicinal iron. J Pediatr 1971;79:569–580.

40 Reed CDL, Fidler J, Oliver DO, Cotes PM, Pippard MJ, Winearls CG: Erythroid progenitor cell kinetics in chronic haemodialysis patients responding to treatment with recombinant human erythropoietin. Br J Haematol 1988;70:375–380.

Daniel S. Halpérin, Unité d'Onco-Hématologie Pédiatrique, Hôpital des Enfants, 30 Bd. de la Cluse, CH-1211 Geneva 4, Switzerland

Discussion

to the Paper by D.S. Halpérin et al.

Breyman (Zürich): Why did you chose a dosage of 2 to 5 milligrams? Why didn't you take a fixed dosage—let's say, of 5 milligrams per kilogram?

Halpérin: Well, usually iron is given in drops for these very tiny babies. So you round up the doses according to the weight of the child. We had a whole range of weights between 800 grams up to 1500 grams at the beginning of the study. So that makes clear why some patients received 2 and others up to 5 milligrams. It's the usual range in our neonatal unit.

Wardrop (Cardiff): The amount of blood received from the placenta at birth by the preterm baby is important in influencing the respiratory-disease outcome, and it governs the hematological outcome. What is the practice in your unit, and did you find any link between cord-clamping practice—i.e., the amount of blood that the baby can get from the placenta—and the outcome, or has this not been studied yet?

Halpérin: We did not properly study the question. I think it's a very important issue. In our maternity unit, there is no real policy, to say the truth. Some obstetricians will clamp early and others late. Therefore we did not really address this question. But I think it may be a very useful point to study in further studies.

Wardrop: Could I ask a small supplementary question? Some of the babies obviously must have responded more effectively than others. Did you get any clues from your retrospective analysis of what seemed to be associated with a good response and what with bad response? Did infection inhibit response?

Halpérin: We did not have infectious episodes in any of these 18 babies when they were on EPO. So I have no answer available for that particular point. We have spoken at length about the problem of functional or even clinical iron deficiency. This study was not aiming at all at addressing the issue of whether or not EPO could decrease the number of transfusions given to these babies. This was not a proper methodological setting for that. However, we had three babies out of 18 who needed a transfusion. This is less than what was expected; usually around 30% of our preterm infants need a transfusion for late anemia of prematurity. So we had about 50% of that usual rate. Now, it is interesting to note that in two of these babies transfusion was required because treatment was interrupted after 2 weeks. These two babies were those who had the lowest hematocrit at start, and therefore the length of time that is necessary for the hematocrit to come up with EPO was too short and it continued to decline until they became symptomatic. The third one that was transfused was a patient that initially responded well in terms of reticulocyte count but unfortunately developed quite clearly clinical iron-deficiency anemia. Therefore, despite his very good initial reticulocyte response, there was absolutely no increase in hemoglobin—and actually a decrease, which rendered the transfusion necessary in this case.

Klinkmann (Rostock): Based on your data, would you dare to speculate that the prophylactic application of EPO for these cases would be around the corner?

Halpérin: It is a speculation, as you say yourself. Our study was a "rescue" study; babies were selected by the fact that they were anemic. And they were 4 weeks of age. Now, other studies, like that of Dr. Wardrop and Obladen, address that question of true prophylaxis, giving these patients EPO in the very first few days of life. The initial life of these patients is difficult, as you know; they need sometimes very intensive care. A lot of blood has to be drawn for blood cultures and so on; therefore the amount you push in through erythropoietin and draw back from phlebotomies may render the prophylactic approach inefficient. But this is a speculation.

Obladen (Berlin): Have you standardized for serum protein content or for amino acid administration, which both may be highly variable in preterm infants?

Halpérin: You mean in diet?

Obladen: Have you brought the serum protein concentration into a defined range, because obviously the infant needs some amount of protein to make red cells and not only iron and erythropoietin. And the protein content and the ability to produce protein is highly variable in preterm infants.

Halpérin: We have data on serum protein levels throughout the study period but did not look for a correlation with response to treatment. What was more or less standardized was the amount of calories that these children were given, which implies that the intake in terms of protein was also more or less standardized. But this is not exact science.

Is There a Need for Erythropoietin Treatment During and After Pregnancy?

Renate Huch

Department of Obstetrics, University Hospital Zürich, Zürich, Switzerland

Introduction

Is there a need for erythropoietin (EPO) treatment during and after pregnancy? Yes, because of the high prevalence of maternal anemia in pregnancy and postpartum; yes, because of the adverse effects of maternal anemia on the fetus; and yes, because increased physical strength and rapid correction of hemoglobin levels represent such advantages for mothers in terms of reducing puerperal complications and facilitating breast feeding and care of the newborn child. These opinions need to be backed by facts. It should be stated at the outset that we have relatively extensive experience with EPO treatment in the postpartum period, but that our experience with its use during pregnancy is still in the early stages.

Hematological Deviations During Pregnancy

Characteristic deviations in hemoglobin and hematocrit values occur during pregnancy compared to normal values in nonpregnant women [1, 2]. They begin to be detectable around the 10th week of gestation. Although red cell mass increases markedly during pregnancy—up to 800 ml is regarded as physiological—there is a proportionately greater increase in plasma volume, resulting in a relative decrease in circulating erythrocyte, hemoglobin, and hematocrit levels. Individual variation is considerable, and nadirs are reached between weeks 20 and 30 of gestation, with a slight increase at term. The proportionately greater expansion in plasma volume in pregnancy thus results in much disputed terms such as "dilutional anemia" or "physiological anemia of pregnancy." Since the

*Epoietin alfa kindly supplied by Cilag AG, CH.

erythrocyte lifespan remains virtually unchanged during pregnancy, the increase in erythrocyte volume is the result of increased marrow activity. Hemoglobin concentration, mean corpuscular volume, and hemoglobin content are virtually unchanged.

The increase in erythrocytes in pregnancy runs parallel with increasing levels of erythropoietin [3–5]. This increase is not stimulated by the normal circumstances triggering endogenous erythropoietin production, namely hypoxemia or anemia, since hyperventilation provides the pregnant woman with high oxygen pressure and saturation values [6], and since, as just said, the red cell mass increases markedly in pregnancy. The stimulus to erythropoietic activity in pregnancy is most probably to be found in the changed hormonal status, the best correlation being seen with placental HPL [4].

Iron Balance During Pregnancy

These changes are accompanied, during normal pregnancy, by negativization of the iron balance, sometimes with virtually total depletion of iron stores [1, 7]. Daily iron requirements are estimated as between 3 and 7 mg due to daily losses, on the one hand, and an increased requirement for hemopoiesis and fetal growth, on the other hand. These requirements cannot be met by nutritional sources alone, even given the increased rate of food absorption in pregnancy and assuming an optimum diet. Maternal iron stores are therefore mobilized. If these are already inadequate at the beginning of pregnancy, then latent iron deficiency becomes manifest. At the end of pregnancy, iron deficiency is prelatent in 40% of women, latent in 20–30%, and manifest in 20–30% [8].

Iron deficiency is the cause of approximately 95% of pregnancy anemias. It can be remedied to some extent by early iron replacement therapy, but clinically this has not become standard practice, at least in terms of routine prescribing. In addition, diagnosis of iron deficiency poses some problems in pregnancy as does treatment late in pregnancy.

WHO [9] sets the cutoff between the normal "dilutional anemia" of pregnancy and true anemia at 11 g/dl, and at 1 g/dl lower postpartum, to account for blood loss at and after delivery. The prevalence of anemia according to this definition is high—from 20 to 40% depending on the study population. Early treatment of iron deficiency tends to be associated with lower prevalence [10]. Approximately 3% of all pregnant women have values below 10 g/dl. A recent Australian study in 15,000 pregnancies showed that 3.7% of all pregnant women at term had values <9.2 g/dl [11]. It is undisputed that early iron replacement increases hemoglobin levels. However, compliance leaves much to be desired in pregnant patients, and the diagnosis of iron deficiency in pregnancy is more difficult. The treatment of anemia in late pregnancy can present problems. The pros and cons of prophylactic iron are subject to considerable controversy. Hemminky and Starfield, in a review of the major studies, came to the conclusion that prophylactic iron gave no detectable advantages in terms of birth weight, duration of gestation, or morbidity of mother or child [12].

Major Problems with Anemia During and After Pregnancy

Table 1 shows maternal and fetal problems that have been reported as associated with anemia. A prime example in the mother is an increased infection rate, particularly of the urinary tract. Dysmaturity and prematurity may affect the fetus. In addition to oxygen deprivation due to decreased maternal oxygen content and oxygen delivery, the pathogenesis of these problems may lie in iron and folate deficiency either per se or as factors often associated with anemia. An increase in premature labor with low ferritin values as an expression of severe iron deficiency anemia has been observed [13]. Perinatal mortality rates below 9.2 g/dl are double those in populations with values over 9.2 g/dl [11].

Only in the last 10 years has attention begun to focus on the potentially negative consequences of raised hemoglobin and hematocrit values. Garn et al.

Table 1. Major problems with anemia during and after pregnancy (WHO 1972)

Anemia in pregnancy (hemoglobin < 11g/dl)	Anemia postpartum (hemoglobin < 10g/dl)
Maternal problems	Maternal problems
Infections (pyelonephritis)	Fatigue
Shock with acute blood loss	Weakness
Premature labor contractions	Headache
Placental insufficiency	Tachycardia
Pregnancy-induced hypertension	Nursing problems
Fetal risks	Puerperal fever
Prematurity	Prolonged hospitalization
Growth retardation	
Increased mortality	

[From Refs. 8, 11, 13, and 14.]

[15], in a systematic analysis of 50,000 pregnancies, were the first to show the risks for pregnancy outcome of low *and* high values. A rise in hemoglobin or hematocrit should be seen as expressing failed or suboptimal plasma expansion, with adverse effects on blood rheology and the microcirculation, and hence on oxygen transport. Thus, in obstetrics there is not *one* critical hemoglobin or hematocrit value, but *two* such values. They define an optimal hemoglobin and hematocrit range encompassing the highest percentage of favorable pregnancy outcomes. The relevant studies define this optimal range with relative unanimity: the lower limit is 9–10 g/dl, and the upper limit 13.0–13.2 g/dl.

Postpartum the situation is aggravated by blood loss at and after delivery. According to a recent analysis, postpartum blood loss over 500 ml is still a problem in modern obstetrics [14] and is possibly on the increase. It appears to be associated in particular with the practices of induction of labor, epidural analgesia, acceptance of a prolonged second stage, and adoption of the sitting-up position for the second stage. A recent report from the American College of Obstetrics and Gynecology estimates that 5 out of 100 patients lose over 1000 ml of blood [16]. There is a general tendency to underestimate blood loss on visual assessment [17]. It has been reported that a blood loss of 500 ml at delivery will usually result in a 1-g reduction in hemoglobin [18]. For these reasons, there is a high prevalence of postpartum anemia, defined by WHO as a hemoglobin below 10 g/dl. Data on the prevalence of postpartum anemia in women with singleton pregnancies and vaginal delivery range between 4 and 10%. Approximately 10% of women have a value below 8 g/dl. The consequences, as well as prolonging hospital stay and reducing the mother's ability to cope, include breast feeding difficulties and a raised incidence of puerperal complications (Fig. 1).

Blood Transfusions in Pre- and Postpartum Anemia

The high prevalence of pre- and postpartum anemia is also reflected in the long unchallenged practice of treating severe anemia with red cell transfusions. The analysis in Figure 1 comes from our own hospital and shows the incidence during the 1980s to be of the usual order of magnitude for obstetrics. With the exception of very severe anemia, the well-known reservations on the part of both doctors and patients have drastically cut the number of blood transfusions.

rhEPO Treatment in Postpartum Anemia

An additional factor contributing to this reduction has been the availability of recombinant erythropoietin. A case such as the one shown in Figure 2 with a

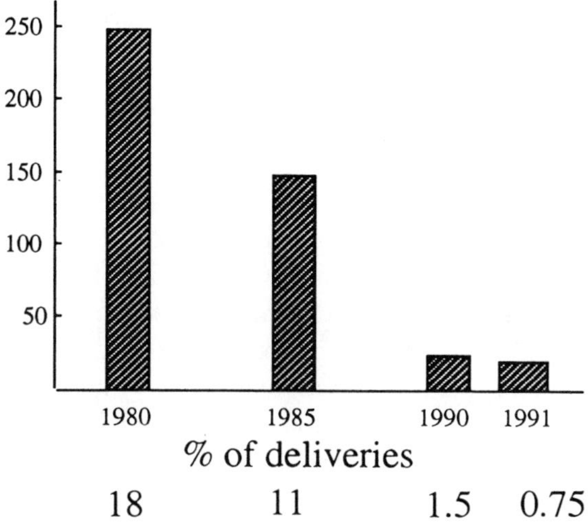

Fig. 1. Number of patients undergoing red blood cell transfusion (Department of Obstetrics, University Hospital Zurich, 1980–1991). [Data from Ref. 22.]

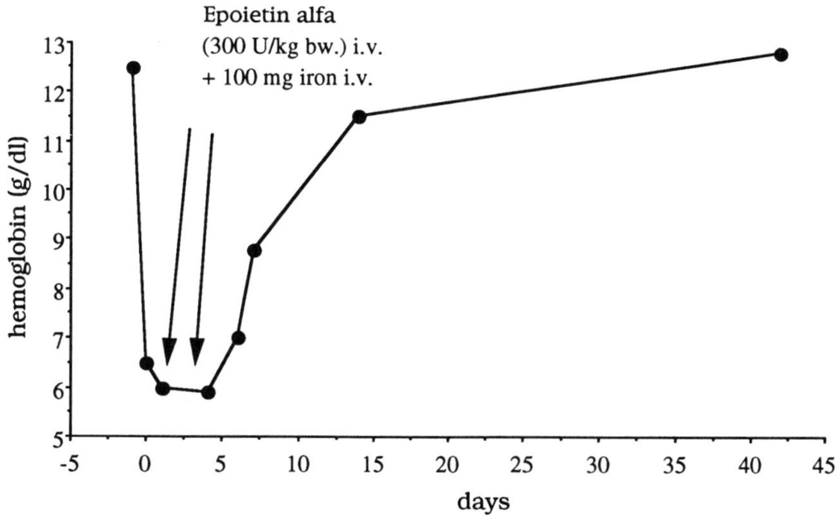

Fig. 2. Hemoglobin concentrations in a patient postpartum. Extensive blood loss at delivery resulted in a decrease in hemoglobin from 12.5 to 5.9 g/dl when treatment with EPO was started as indicated. [From Ref. 23.]

hemoglobin just under 6 g/dl due to severe postpartum hemorrhage would previously have been a candidate for transfusion. Two i.v. injections of EPO and iron restored the situation to normal in just 10 days.

In our first pilot study—when we were still giving EPO in repeated doses over 5 days postpartum, combined with oral iron—we showed rapid reversal of anemia within 5 days on EPO compared with oral iron alone [19]. We then confirmed this result in a randomized controlled study in 37 postpartum patients with hemoglobin values below 10 g/dl, treated either with 20,000 U EPO and iron or with iron alone [20]. Like those researching other applications, we have found that the efficacy of EPO depends on an adequate availability of iron, and we are currently conducting a systematic study to determine the optimal combination of i.v. or s.c. EPO with i.v. iron. During the puerperium, recombinant human erythropoietin can be considered an effective new treatment for anemia. The cost for postpartum use is about the same as that for 1–2 whole blood units. The advantages are obvious: quicker recovery and no negative side effects.

Evidence is still lacking for us to be equally affirmative as yet regarding treatment during pregnancy. The available experimental data and clinical observation show that an essential precondition is already in place: the human placental membranes form a barrier to the transfer of EPO (21). Fetuses of anemic mothers develop compensatory polycythemia. Co-treatment of the fetus with EPO would not be desirable.

We are just beginning our exploration of this field and have assembled 5 cases to date. EPO seems to be just as effective during pregnancy as during the postpartum period. This is a more than adequate justification in our view for systematically investigating the use of EPO in pregnancy.

References

1   Göltner E: Korpuskuläre Elemente des Blutes; in Friedberg V, Rathgen GH (eds): Physiologie der Schwangerschaft. Stuttgart, Georg Thieme Verlag, 1980; pp 44–67.
2   Hytten F, Chamberlain G: Clinical Physiology in Obstetrics. London, Blackwell Scientific Publications, 1980.
3   Beguin Y, Lipscei G, Oris R, Thoumsin H, Fillet G: Serum immunoreactive erythropoietin during pregnancy and in the early postpartum. Br J Haematol 1990;76:545–549.
4   Cotes PM, Canning CE: Changes in serum immunoreactive erythropoietin during the menstrual cycle and normal pregnancy. Br J Obstet Gynaecol 1983;90:304–311.
5   Widness JA, Clemons GK, Garcia JF, Schwartz R: Plasma immunoreactive erythropoietin in normal women studied sequentially during and after pregnancy. Am J Obstet Gynecol 1984;149:646–650.
6   Huch R: Maternal hyperventilation and the fetus. J Perinat Med 1986;14:3–17.

7 Pritchard J, Scott D: Iron demands in pregnancy; in Halberg L, Harwerth H, Vanottie A (eds): Iron Deficiency Pathogenesis, Clinical Aspects, Therapy. New York; Academic Press, 1970; pp 250–260.

8 Göltner E: Die Bedeutung der Anämien in Gynäkologie und Geburtshilfe. Med Welt 1981;32:1413–1415.

9 World Health Organisation: Nutritional Anaemias. Technical Report Series 1972; p 503.

10 Letsky E: The haematological system; in Hytten F, Chamberlain G (eds): Clinical Physiology in Obstetrics. London, Blackwell Scientific Publications, 1980; pp 43–78.

11 Ratten GJ, Beischer NA: The significance of anaemia in an obstetric population in Australia. J Obstet Gynaecol Br Commonw 1972;79:228–237.

12 Hemminki E, Starfield B: Routine administration of iron and vitamins during pregnancy: Review of controlled clinical trials. Br J Obstet Gynaecol 1978;85: 404–410.

13 Goepel E, Ulmer HU, Neth RD: Premature labor contractions and the value of serum ferritin during pregnancy. Gynecol Obstet Invest 1988;26:265–273.

14 Gilbert L, Porter W, Brown VA: Postpartum haemorrhage—a continuing problem. Br J Obstet Gynecol 1987;94:67–71.

15 Garn SM, Ridella SA, Petzold AS, Falkner F: Maternal hematologic levels and pregnancy outcomes. Semin Perinatol 1981;5:155–162.

16 American College of Obstetricians and Gynecologists: Diagnose und Behandlung postpartaler Blutungen. "ACOG Technical Bulletin" NR.143/1990. Geburtshilfe Frauenheilkd 1991;9:53–57.

17 Duthie SJ, Ghosh A, Ng A, Ho PC: Intra-operative blood loss during elective lower segment caesarean section. Br J Obstet Gynaecol 1992;99:364–367.

18 Hiss RG: Evaluation of the anemic patient; in Laros RK (ed): Blood Disorders in Pregnancy. Philadelphia, Lea & Febiger, 1986, pp 1–18.

19 Danko J, Huch R, Huch A: Epoetin alfa for treatment of postpartum anaemia. Lancet 1990;335:737–738.

20 Huch A, Eichhorn K-H, Danko J, Lauener P-A, Huch R: Recombinant human erythropoietin in the treatment of postpartum anemia. Obstet Gynecol 1992;80: 127–131.

21 Eichhorn K-H, Bauer C, Eckardt K-U, Huch A, Huch R: Lack of associations between fetal and maternal erythropoietin at birth. Eur J Obstet Gynecol Reprod Biol 1993;50(1).

22 Breymann C, Zimmermann R, Huch R, Huch A: Rekombinantes Erythropoietin (rHuEPO) in Kombination mit parenteraler Eisengabe zur Behandlung der schweren postpartalen Anämie. Perinatal Medizin 1991;3:147.

23 Breymann C, Richter C, Huch R, Huch A: Erythropoietin nach schwerer postpartaler Anämie. Poster bei der Jahresversammlung der Schweizerischen Gesellschaft für Gynäkologie und Geburtshilfe (SGGG) und der Schweizerischen Gesellschaft für Medizinische Genetik (SGMG). Montreux, June 18–20, 1992.

Renate Huch, Departement für Frauenheilkunde, Klinik für Geburtshilfe, Frauenklinikstrasse 10, CH-8901 Zurich, Switzerland

Discussion

to the Paper by R. Huch

Simoes (Lisbon): I did not understand whether you have utilized erythropoietin during pregnancy. It seems that you have utilized it in a small number of patients.

Huch: We have limited experience, as we only recently started to use erythropoietin in a pilot fashion during pregnancy. We are just in the process of conducting a systematic study during pregnancy. It will be a prospective, randomized, and controlled study. Anemic patients will be either treated with intravenous iron alone or with EPO and iron (provided iron deficiency is the underlying cause). Such a study during pregnancy only became realistic after enough experimental evidence was at hand that EPO does not cross the placenta.

Kokot (Katowice): Do you have some experience with EPO treatment in pregnant women with a functioning kidney transplant?

Huch: No, we have not.

Risks of Homologous Blood Transfusion

Bernhard Kubanek

DRK-Blutspendezentrale Ulm und Abteilung Transfusionsmedizin der Universität Ulm, Ulm, Germany

The homologous blood transfusion is, like most effective therapeutic measures, not without risk. Because there are alternative potentially beneficial strategies for patients undergoing elective surgery, the adverse effects of homologous blood transfusion must be defined as clearly as possible to enable us to estimate the risk/benefit ratio for the individual patient. Blood is donated from individual donors, a fact that defines the main risks of homologous transfusion: (a) the transmission of bloodborne infection, and (b) the alloimmunization and immunomodulation caused by immunological recognition of self and not self.

The key measures of preventing bloodborne infections include selection of safe donors, screening of donations, which identifies most donations made by infectious persons, and removal of leukocytes to prevent the transmission of cellbound viruses like CMV and, in addition, remove nonself antigens. Pooled plasma products are always viral inactivated. Viral-inactivated fresh frozen plasma is available and clinically evaluated in Germany. The strict indications for homologous transfusion and the use of alternative measures as autologous transfusion and intraoperative blood salvage, if indicated, reduce the individual risk.

Since there are regional variations in the prevalence of the relevant infections, and the epidemiology of infections is a dynamic time-dependent process, risk estimates can only be made for geographically defined donor populations from recently estimated prevalences. Most of the estimates discussed in this article are restricted to north and mid-European donor populations.

In Table 1, infectious agents transmitted by blood and tests for them are shown, to which every donation is subjected. Furthermore, the year of introduction of the test is indicated, since it may determine the degree of selection for the repeat donor population.

Table 1.   Infectious agents transmitted by blood

Infectious agent	Screening	Implemented in Germany since:
Hepatitis B virus (HBV)	HBs-Ag	1972
Hepatitis non-A–non-B (= HCV)	ALT ANTI-HCV	1958 1990
Hepatitis A (HVA)	Not tested	
HIV-1	Anti-HIV1	1985
HIV-2	Anti-HIV2	1989
CMV	Anti-CMV	Only for patients at risk
EBV	Not tested	
Treponema pallidum	Hemagglutination test	1971
Malaria	Anamnestic exclusion	1968
Bacteria	Anamnestic exclusion and on random sampling	

Fatal disease from bacterial contamination is rare, with an estimated risk of one in a million units [1]. However, it is the only infectious complication that can be expected in an even higher frequency in autologous transfusions. Syphilis transmitted by transfusion is now virtually nonexistent. Asymptomatic infection with herpesvirus CMV and EBV is so common in healthy adults that it can almost be viewed as normal flora. CMV transmission of the blood product can be prevented by testing or treatment of blood products for susceptible patients. The following information will be limited to the risks for transmitting HIV and hepatitis B and HCV by blood.

The confirmed prevalences of the seromarkers of the donations in Baden-Württemberg for 1991/92 are listed in Table 2. The prevalences are broken up for first-time donors and repeat donors. Notable is the greater than 10-fold difference between first-time and repeat donors for hepatitis B, HIV, and lues, which is an indication for the ongoing selection process. The overall rate of seromarkers is closer to the rate of the repeat donors, since 90% of all donations are given by them. Similar data have been published recently for the Netherlands and Great Britain [2].

Table 2.   Rate of seromarkers in blood donors in Baden-Württemberg (1991/92)

Test	Positive rate %	Positive rate in first-time donors (%)	Positive rate in repeat donors (%)
GPT > 35	3.1	3.1	3.1
Anti-HCV	0.53	0.33[a]	0.55[a]
	0.51	0.48[b]	0.52[b]
HBsAg	0.041	0.32	0.01
HIV-1-Ab	<0.002	0.006	0.001
HIV-2-Ab	0	0	0
Lues-Ab	0.01	0.1	0.005

[a] Anti-HCV 1. generation (C-100-3).
[b] Anti-HCV 2. generation (C-100-3, c33c, c22-3).

Figure 1 shows the HIV prevalences collected in the multicenter study of the German Red Cross Blood Banks separately for Berlin as a region, with a higher prevalence for HIV infection and the Red Cross Blood Centers that recruit donors from more rural areas. The study began testing for HIV-1 antibodies in 1985 [3].

The data show a quick decrease of HIV prevalence in the first year and, from there on steady, very low prevalences of 1–2 confirmed positive anti–HIV-positives per 100,000 donations. The initial prevalences in Berlin were about 20 times higher. However, in Berlin the current rate for HIV infection among active blood donors has decreased to 3–5 confirmed positives per 100,000, whereas the anticipated rate of HIV-infected persons in the general population probably has not changed. This indicates the strong selection that has occurred since 1985 in the donor population, as elsewhere [2].

The very low prevalences for HIV and HBV in the donor population shown in Table 2 indicate that it is virtually impossible to conduct transmission studies in mid-Europe on a logistically meaningful scale. Therefore, estimates of transfusion risk can only be attempted from current prevalences and the window period as well as the sensitivity of the screening tests. (The window period is the time from infection until the detection of a specific marker for infection.) The window period of HIV is approximately 45 days. We estimated the risk of transmitting HIV from an infected donor who is seronegative to be on the order of 1:300,000 to 1:3 million per unit in our donor population [3]. HIV transmitted by transfusion became an extremely rare event.

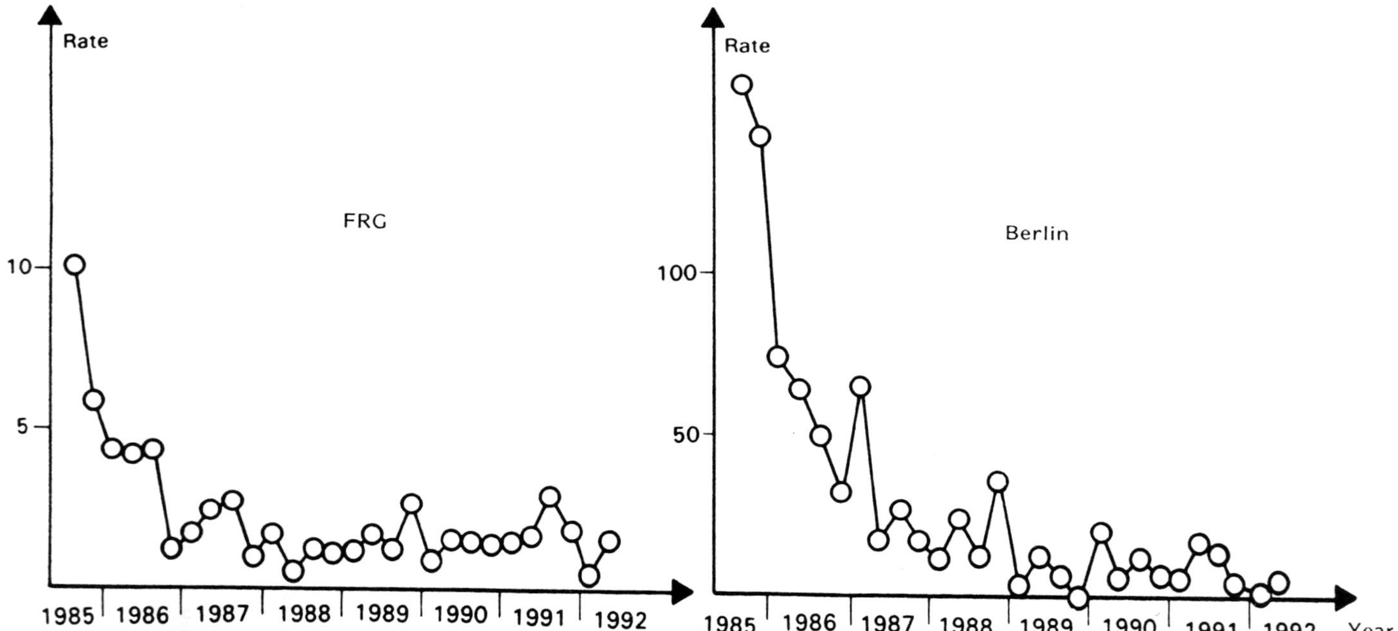

Fig. 1. HIV antibody prevalences per 100,000 donations reported quarterly in blood donors from Red Cross blood banks in Germany (FRG) and Berlin.

Non-A–non-B posttransfusion hepatitis (PTH) continued to be a significant problem until very recently, although it recently decreased as a consequence of stricter donor selection. Non-A–non-B PTH in mid- and northern Europe has a lower incidence than reported in United States or south European studies. In 1989 a new virus, the hepatitis C virus (HCV), was identified by molecular techniques for a clinically well-described disease—non-A–non-B posttransfusion hepatitis. HCV is an RNA virus that appears to be related to the pesti- and flaviviruses [4]. The protein C-100-3 derived from HCV clones was soon developed to detect antibodies to HCV in the serum by an enzyme-linked immunoabsorbent assay (ELISA). Routine screening of donors was begun in June 1990. It soon became obvious that the C-100-3 ELISA had sufficient sensitivity, but the specifity in the context of low seroprevalence population was questionable. A second-generation ELISA and a RIBA have been made more accurate by the addition of two further antigens from the structural region.

In order to obtain information regarding the prevalence of viral carriers in our donor population, donations that were repeatedly reactive were additionally tested with RIBA-2 and a nested HCV-RNA PCR [5]. It is apparent that 80% of the ELISA-reactive donors are false positive since they showed no reactivity in the RIBA-2 assay and were negative by PCR. The "true seroprevalence" based on RIBA positivity is 0.1%, i.e., 1 in 1000, 5 times lower than the "crude" 0.47% seroprevalence based just on the reactive ELISA. The association of positivity in the RIBA assay and PCR implies that these donors are viremic and potentially infectious. The data reported on donors from the United Kingdom and the Netherlands are very similar [2] (Table 3).

The clinical features and the natural history of the PTH-C were recently better defined by specific HCV diagnostics on previously conducted prospective studies [6, 7]. The mean interval between transfusion and anti-HCV conversion is 15 weeks. Approximately 25% develop clinical manifest hepatitis with jaundice. Fifty percent of patients with PTH-C show biochemical coincidence of chronic disease and histologically chronic persistent or chronic active hepatitis. About 10% develop cirrhosis after years. There are reports of liver failure and death. However, the actual frequency of symptomatic liver disease is not clear. A large retrospective case control study of PTH-C [8] and a study of hepatitis C in renal patients [9] did not find extensive morbidity and little excess mortality even years after the diagnosis of PTH-C.

The important question of how much testing for surrogate markers and HCV reduces the incidence of PTH-C was asked in two studies (Table 3). Donahue et al. [10] studied this question in a cohort of patients undergoing cardiac surgery

Table 3.   Prevalences of anti-HCV and HCV-RNA in mid- and north European blood donors

Population	Prevalence of anti-HCV	EIA-pos		RIBA-2 pos.		PCR		Prevalence of HCV
		n	%	n	%	n	%	
Donors Netherlands	0.5%	37	(100)	8	(22)	7	(19)	0.1%
Donors Ulm	0.47%	72	(100)	12	(17)	14	(19)	0.1%
Donors England	0.61%	65	(100)	5	(7)	6	(10)	0.06%

who were stratified in three groups according to the period in which certain screening methods were used on the blood they received: (a) 1985–1986, (b) October 1986 to November 1990, when additional screening for ALT and anti-HBc was introduced, and (c) from May 1991, when blood was screened for antibodies to HCV. The introduction of surrogate markers reduced the PTH-C significantly by 50%. This cannot be attributed just to testing but is probably a consequence of donor selection for HIV. The implementation of anti-HCV testing has further reduced the risk substantially for the transmission of PTH-C to less than 1 in 3000 units. A study by the Japanese Red Cross [11] shows a reduction of the same order of magnitude. A study by Contreras et al [12] was undertaken to assess the incidence of PTH-C in London and has shown a very low incidence of PTH-C even before the implementation of anti-HCV testing.

Transmission of the hepatitis B virus by transfusion is rare because of the mandatory screening of blood donors since 1972 with a rather sensitive ELISA (0.5 ng/ml). In addition, donor selection reduced the risk further, which is currently estimated at less than 1:50,000 per unit [13]. The risk of transmission of HCV is estimated at less that 1:5000 taking into account the prevalence of 1 in 1000, the 80% reduction of transmission by anti-HCV testing [10], and the rather long window period of several months. However, it can be expected that an improvement in the tests may shorten the window period and therefore lower the risk of PTH-C (Table 4).

The risks of transfusion of homologous blood other than transmission of disease are mainly immunologically mediated. Adverse effects like volume overload or poor transfusion practice are not dealt with since they are not specific for homologous transfusions but also occur with autologous transfusions.

Alloimmunization against antigens on blood cells, its etiology, and its clinical significance are better understood than immunomodulation. Non-autologous antigens on erythrocytes, leukocytes, and platelets are recognized as

Table 4.   Estimated risk of infection for HIV, HBV, and HCV of screened blood in Baden-Württemberg

Virus	Prevalence	Estimated risk per unit
HIV	2/100,000	1:500,000–1:1 million
HBV	40/100,000	1:50,000
HCV	100/100,000[a]	<1:5000

[a] RIBA-2 reactive donations.

nonself by the immune system, and, as a consequence, clinically significant alloantibodies can be produced.

Hemolytic reactions due to preformed antibodies are rare, but if they occur they can have disastrous consequences for the patient. Due to heavily regulated and improved compatibility testing, fatal hemolytic transfusion reactions are rarely (<15%) caused by serological errors [1]. Most fatal transfusion reactions are caused by clerical and managerial errors, although blood transfusion is one of the most regulated procedures in medicine. Most errors occur when "blood is given to the wrong person" in the intensive care unit or in the operation site. These risks are expected to occur with at least equal frequency in autologous transfusions.

Clinically significant antibodies against RBC are detected with a frequency of 1% of transfused hospitalized patients. In chronically transfused patients, up to 10% RBC alloantibodies can occur [14]. They rarely cause transfusion reactions when proper compatibility testing is applied, but render further transfusion therapy more difficult. Delayed hemolytic transfusion reactions are usually due to alloantibodies to RBC antigens formed after transfusion or during pregnancy.

Febrile transfusion reactions are caused by antibodies to HLA determinants on leukocytes. They can cause very unpleasant reactions with fever and are clinically important for chronically transfused thrombocytopenic patients because of the immune destruction of transfused platelets. HLA immunization can be avoided by removal of leukocytes from blood components by filters.

In the last 15 years evidence has accumulated that homologous blood transfusions may induce changes in the reactivity of the immune system of recipients which may have clinical significance. The suppression of the immune system has been studied extensively in patients undergoing kidney allografting who have benefited by pretransplant blood transfusions [15]. This effect could clearly be related to the transfused leukocytes. This observation led to speculations as to whether blood transfusions impair immune surveillance of cancer and thereby enhance the regrowth of cancer [16].

Although animal studies and several retrospective studies suggest a detrimental effect of homologous blood transfusion on the prognoses of patients, particularly with colorectal carcinoma, methodological difficulties in the interpretation of these studies do not allow a firm conclusion.

In a recent large, not yet published randomized prospective study on 474 patients operated on for colon carcinoma, no difference was observed between disease-free survival of patients receiving autologous transfusion and patients receiving homologous transfusion. There was also no difference in the occurrence of postoperative infection (R.L. Marquet, personal communication). In a similar prospective randomized study (Heiss et al., personal communication), no significant difference of recurrence of cancer was observed, but there were significant increases in peri- and postoperative infections.

Initial clinical observations suggest that autologous transfusions are associated with a decreased risk in postoperative bacterial infection as compared to homologous blood transfusion in patients undergoing orthopedic surgery [17]. In one of these studies [18], this observation could only be confirmed in a subset of patients receiving homologous whole blood, whereas there was no difference between autologous and homologous recipients of packed RBC. A recent report by Jensen and coworkers [19] suggests that WBC-reduced transfusions abrogate the deleterious effect of allogeneic transfusion on enhancing postoperative infections. The evidence from the data so far published (mainly retrospective) in which ill-defined homologous blood products were transfused is suggestive of an increased risk for postoperative infection but is not enough to draw firm conclusions. The issue can only be solved by well-designed prospective studies.

Conclusions

The transmission of infectious disease by transfusion is a real but often overestimated risk. The recognition of HIV risk has improved the safety of the mid-European blood supply, e.g., by stricter donor selection and viral inactivation. The transmission of HCV has been markedly reduced by anti-HCV testing.

Transfusion-associated death by hemolytic reactions is rare, but is mainly caused by managerial and clerical errors. The immunomodulation by homologous blood is not well understood. Individual risk can be reduced by strict indication for homologous blood and by the use of alternative methods such as autologous transfusions and intraoperative blood salvage.

References

1 Sazama K: Reports of 355 transfusion-associated deaths. Transfusion 1990;30:583–590.

2 Reesink HW, Nydegger UE: Blood donor screening or "over-screening": How far to go in avoiding transmission of infectious agents? Vox Sang 1992;63:59–69.

3 Glück D, Vornwald A, Gossrau E, Kubanek B: HIV prevalence in blood donors in urban and in rural areas of the FRG. Blut 1990;60:304–307.

4 Kuo G, Choo Q-L, Alter HJ, et al.: An assay for circulating antibodies to a major etiologic virus of human non-A, non-B hepatitis. Science 1989;244:362–364.

5 Da Silva Cardoso M, Koerner K, Epple S, Kubanek B: Prevalence of HCV-RNA-positive blood donors and correlation to ELISA and RIBA status. Ann Hematol 1993;66:147–151.

6 Aach RD, Stevens CE, Hollinger FB, et al.: Hepatitis C virus infection in post-transfusion hepatitis. N Engl J Med 1991;325:1325–1329.

7 Esteban JI, González A, Hernández JM, et al.: Evaluation of antibodies to hepatitis C virus in a study of transfusion-associated hepatitis. N Engl J Med 1990;323:1107–1112.

8 Seeff LB, National Heart, Lung, and Blood Institute Hepatitis Study Group: Mortality of non-A, non-B transfusion-associated hepatitis (NANB TAH) in the U.S. 18 years after infection (abstract). Hepatology 1991;14:90A.

9 Roth D, Fernandez JA, Babischkin S, et al.: Detection of hepatitis C virus infection among cadaver organ donors: Evidence for low transmission of disease. Ann Intern Med 1992;117:470–475.

10 Donahue JJ, Munoz A, Ness PM, et al.: The declining risk of post-transfusion hepatitis C virus infection. N Engl J Med 1992;327:369–373.

11 Japanese Red Cross Non-A, Non-B Hepatitis Research Group: Effect of screening for hepatitis C virus antibody and hepatitis B virus core antibody on incidence of post-transfusion hepatitis. Lancet 1991;II:1040–1041.

12 Contreras M, Barbara JAJ, Anderson CC, et al.: Low incidence of non-A, non-B post-transfusion hepatitis in London confirmed by hepatitis C virus serology. Lancet 1991;337:753–757.

13 Public Health Service Inter-Agency Guidelines for Screening Donors of Blood, Plasma, Organs, Tissues, and Semen for Evidence of Hepatitis B and Hepatitis C. MMWR 1991;40(RR-4).

14 Walker RH, Lin D-T, Hartrick MB: Alloimmunization following blood transfusion. Arch Pathol Lab Med 1989;113:254–261.

15 Opelz G, Terasaki PI: Poor kidney-transplant survival in recipients with frozen blood transfusions or no transfusions. Lancet;1974:2:696–698.

16 Van Aken WG: Does perioperative blood transfusion promote tumor growth? Transfusion Med Rev 1989;3:243–252.

17 Triulzi DJ, Vanek K, Ryan DH, Blumberg N: A clinical and immunologic study of blood transfusion and postoperative bacterial infection in spinal surgery. Transfusion 1992;32:517–524.

18 Fernandez MC, Gottlieb M, Menitove JE: Blood transfusion and post-operative infection in orthopedic patients. Transfusion 1992;32:318–322.

19   Jensen LS, Anderson AJ, Christiansen PM, et al.: Postoperative infection and natural
     killer cell function following blood transfusion in patients undergoing elective
     colorectal surgery. Br J Surg 1992;79:513–516.

Bernhard Kubanek, DRK-Blutspendezentrale Ulm and Abteilung Transfusionsmedizin der Universität Ulm, Helmholtzstrasse 10, 89081 Ulm, Germany

Discussion

to the Paper by B. Kubanek

Winearls (Oxford): Can you distinguish between seroconversion in these studies and true infection, because the two are very different in terms of clinical consequence?

Kubanek: I think we probably can be on the HCV because we got PCRs there, and it was very interesting how the PCRs overlapped with the anti-HCV. So I feel that most of these donors which were labeled as anti-HCV positive are infectious too. We have other data which I have not shown; we have taken up the donors into high-risk donors with elevated ALTs and they had in 60% anti-HCV and in 80% positive PCR. At the current state of knowledge, we feel most of RIBA-positive donors and patients are infectious.

Joven (Reus): Just to comment that I think your view of the homologous transfusion is too optimistic. I suppose, depending on which one is the invited speaker, the conclusion would be different and you would not be so peaceful after such a talk. But just handling your data, at least several patients in Germany are at risk every year to contract AIDS from a transfusion. And even more, your conclusions on the colonic carcinoma on 400 patients—I think they cannot be conclusive in the same way as other studies cannot be conclusive yet. However, if homologous transfusion can be avoided, this always will be an advantage to our patients.

Kubanek: I agree wholeheartedly that homologous blood transfusion should be avoided when possible. I did not say that you do not get HIV infection from transfusion; I only said that there is a very low prevalence in our donor population and a very low risk. We have done a look-back study and came up with the same numbers (a risk 1:Mio). And I estimate the risk for all transfused patients of Germany on the order of about five infected patients. I think this is the first large randomized and prospective study, and there is another randomized study which I did not cite, from Germany, which also could not show that there was an enhancement of cancer growth. All the other studies which showed that were retrospective studies with a lot of problems if you analyze them. In most of the studies, whole blood was given and it was not distinguished between whole blood and red blood cells, and red blood cells with leukocytes and without leukocytes, and I think this data is inconclusive.

The Rationale for Use of Recombinant Human Erythropoietin to Facilitate Autologous Blood Collection Before Elective Surgery

Lawrence Tim Goodnough

Division of Laboratory Medicine, Washington University School of Medicine, and Transfusion Services, Barnes Hospital, St. Louis, Mo., USA

Introduction

Interest in blood conservation interventions has been stimulated by recent issues related to blood safety and blood inventory [1]. For transfusion settings such as elective surgery, preoperative autologous blood donation represents an alternative to allogeneic blood transfusion and has become a standard of practice in elective orthopaedic surgery [2]. To ensure minimal exposure to allogeneic blood, aggressive autologous blood procurement coupled with innovative blood conservation interventions such as recombinant human erythropoietin (rhEPO) is necessary in this setting. The evidence to support the use of EPO therapy to facilitate autologous blood procurement is reviewed in this article.

Underording Leads to Undercollection of Autologous Blood

Candidates for autologous blood donation include any patient scheduled for an elective procedure with a request for blood type and cross-match, indicating a minimum 10% likelihood of requiring blood transfusion using a maximum surgical blood ordering schedule [3]. A recent study uses this approach to determine the number of autologous blood units that should be requested for surgery and found that 9% of all patients undergoing elective surgery were transfused with allogeneic blood [4]. For patients undergoing procedures that routinely have significant blood loss and require considerable transfusion support, however, this approach would result in, at best, the avoidance of allogeneic blood in 10% of patients; in practice, unexpected bleeding or blood needs results in considerably more autologous donor patients who require allogeneic blood. As shown in Table 1, 17% of all orthopaedic patients and 20% of patients undergoing hip arthroplasty in one study were transfused with allogeneic blood despite enrollment in an autologous blood program [5]. Thus, underordering of autologous blood units contributes, in part, to subsequent allogeneic blood exposure in elective orthopedic surgery.

Autologous blood-ordering practices designed to minimize allogeneic blood exposure should be based on audited transfusion requirements in patients who did not have autologous blood available. Table 2 summarizes the number of autologous blood units required for a selected group of orthopedic procedures to ensure a 95% likelihood of avoiding additional allogeneic blood unit transfusions. For example, in a study of 3 tertiary care and 3 community hospitals, Toy et al. [6] found that 4 and 6 autologous blood units would be necessary for primary and revision total hip arthroplastys, respectively. At our institution, 8 units would be required for bilateral hip replacement and 3 and 6 units for unilateral and bilateral knee replacement, respectively.

Undercollection of Autologous Blood Leads to Allogeneic Blood Exposure

The American Association of Blood Bank Standards allow autologous blood donation every 72 hours until 72 hours before the procedure, as long as the patient's hematocrit is greater than or equal to 33%. Patients are routinely given oral iron supplementation during this period [7]. Since liquid blood can be stored for up to 6 weeks, in theory as many as a dozen autologous blood units might be procured. Donation success (i.e., donating the number of units re-

Table 1. Homologous blood transfusion in elective orthopedic surgery[a] [5]

Procedure (n)	Blood units transfused						
	1	2	3	4	5	6	
Hip (152)	0	1	5	9	11	4	
Knee (89)	0	1	1	6	3	3	
Spine (150)	0	0	4	7	7	6	
Misc. (39)	0	1	0	2	1	0	
Total (430)	0 +	3 +	10 +	24 +	22 +	13	= 72 (16.7%)

[a] In patients who predonated autologous blood, 7/1/85 to 6/30/88.

Table 2. Number of autologous blood units required to avoid allogeneic blood with 95% certainty [10]

	Six Hospitals[a]	One Hospital[b]
Total hip arthroplasty		
Primary	5	4
Revision	6	6
Bilateral		8
Total knee arthroplasty		
Unilateral		3
Bilateral		6

[a] Ref. 6.
[b] Ref. 10.

quested) becomes limited, however, by either iron-restricted erythropoiesis or erythropoietin-modulated erythropoietic response to serial phlebotomy, or both. Early analysis of our hospital-based program revealed that 23 (40%) of 58 patients asked to donate ≥4 units were unable to do so [8], subsequently confirmed by McVay et al. [9] in a regional blood center's experience in which 123 (33%) of 368 patients asked to donate ≥4 units were unsuccessful. The likelihood of donation success is correlated with the presence of anemia at initial donation. At our hospital-based program, 53 (82%) of 65 nonanemic (HCT >39%) patients successfully donated ≥4 units, compared to only 11 (33%) of 34 patients who were anemic at first donation [10]. Ninety percent of our autologous donors presenting with anemia were female. Similarly, at a regional blood center 233 (87%) of 268 nonanemic (Hgb ≥12.5 g/l) patients successfully donated ≥4 autologous units, compared to only 12 (33%) of 36 patients with anemia at first donation.

Subsequent studies of patients in this setting have shown that endogenous erythropoietin levels during the preoperative storage interval do not increase above the normal range for this assay [11], irrespective of iron status [12], indicating that the erythropoietin-modulated erythropoietic response to serial phlebotomy is inadequate. In addition, initial iron status of the patient is important in determining whether the patient will successfully donate autologous blood [12], particularly in premenopausal females [13].

Not only do autologous blood donors have difficulty in predonating 4 or more units before surgery, but the oxygen-carrying capacity of sequential autologous units donated is significantly less than allogeneic units. A previous study found that 26% of all autologous units donated were below a 95% confidence interval for the red cell volume content (200 ± 19 ml, M ± SD) of allogeneic blood units [14].

For these reasons, requests for more autologous blood units and the inability to successfully donate the number requested result in an increased likelihood of subsequent exposure to allogeneic blood. As shown in Table 3, the likelihood of allogeneic transfusion is greatest in anemic patients who were asked to donate ≥4 units, in which 7 (41%) of 17 patients subsequently received allogeneic blood [10].

Erythropoietin Therapy Facilitates Autologous Red Cell Collection

These results suggested that treatment with rhEPO would prevent the development of anemia in these patients and increase the volume of autologous blood that could be collected before surgery. This was confirmed in a randomized, double-blind, placebo-controlled multicenter study to determine whether erythropoietin therapy could facilitate preoperative autologous donation [15]. Patients receiving erythropoietin twice weekly (600 U/kg i.v.) donated 41% greater red blood cell volume when compared to placebo-treated patients (Fig. 1). An

Table 3. Relationship between number of autologous units requested and presence of anemia at initial donation on subsequent exposure to allogeneic blood

No. autologous units requested	Anemic[a]	Not anemic
≤ 3 Units		
No. patients	17	89
No. received	5	10
Allogeneic blood	29%	11%
≤ 4 Units		
No. patients	17	39
No. received	7	8
Allogeneic blood	41%	21%
All patients	34	128
No. received	12	18
Allogeneic blood	35%	14%

[a] Hematocrit ≤ 39% at first donation.

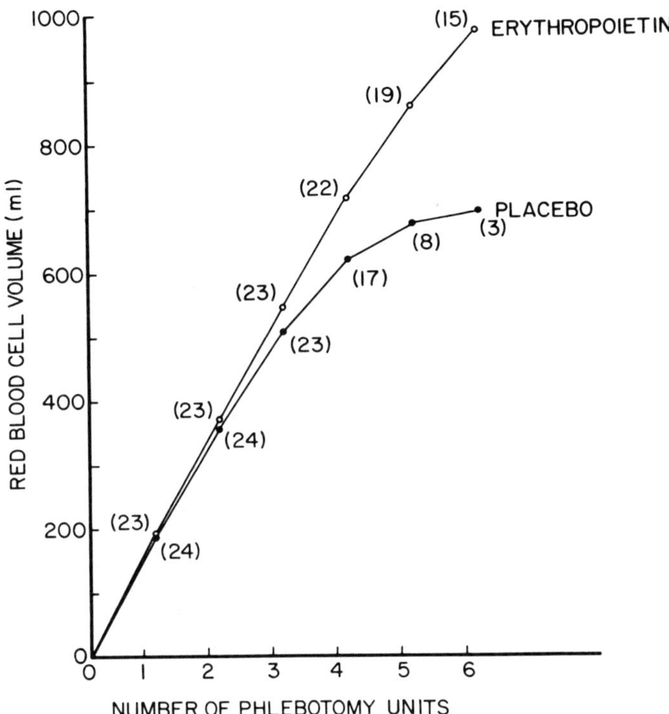

Fig. 1. Cumulative red blood cell volume procured per patient. Number of patients at each donation is indicated in parentheses. Mean cumulative interval in days for each visit: 3.5 for visit 2; 7.2 for visit 3; 10.6 for visit 4; 14.2 for visit 5; 17.6 for visit 6. [From Ref. 15.]

analysis of hematocrit changes in these patients suggested that the equivalent of approximately 4 units of blood could be generated in this setting [16] to provide efficacy for elimination of homologous blood transfusion.

Further analysis of preoperative red blood cell production (taking into account both in vivo and ex vivo [stored] red blood cell volumes) indicated that patients who underwent aggressive autologous blood phlebotomy had a significant (28%) expansion of red blood cell volume preoperatively (Fig. 2), along with accelerated erythropoiesis at the time of surgery [17]. However, the increase (48%) in the patients treated with erythropoietin was significantly higher. The major difference in red blood cell production between the placebo and erythropoietin groups occurred early in the collection period; by the time of surgery, there may have been enough of an endogenous erythropoietin effect in

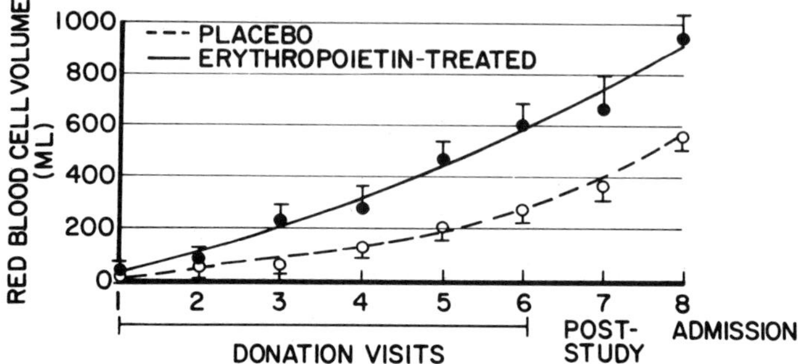

Fig. 2. Red blood cell volume preoperatively during autologous blood donation in 24 placebo- and 23 erythropoietin-treated patients. Data points represent calculated total volume of RBC (both in vivo and ex vivo) at donation visits 1 through 6, poststudy visit, and hospital admission. The length of time to expand RBCs by 200 ml (equivalent to 1 unit of allogeneic blood [14]) can be derived for any preoperative interval. From Ref. 17.

the placebo patients to have diminished the differences between groups [18]. This result was undoubtedly dependent on the fact that the phlebotomy program was an aggressive one involving the attempted removal of 2 units of blood per week. Not all patients can tolerate such a schedule [19]. For some, the limiting factor may be the loss of oxygen-carrying capacity involved in reaching hematocrits in the 30% range, such as patients undergoing coronary artery bypass graft surgery [20]. Since the increased erythropoiesis can be attributed to the drug rather than to the aggressive phlebotomy program in erythropoietin-treated patients, a more modest autologous blood-procurement program coupled with administration of erythropoietin may well be preferable [19, 21] in patients unsuited for aggressive autologous phlebotomy. Our analysis of preoperative red blood cell production in erythropoietin-treated patients indicates that the autologous blood equivalent of nearly 5 units of homologous blood could be generated in this setting [17] to provide efficacy for a 50% reduced exposure to allogeneic blood transfusion. Clinical trials to demonstrate this are currently underway in elective orthopedic and coronary artery bypass surgery [16].

This analysis indicates that for surgical procedures associated with significant blood loss requiring large transfusion needs (e.g. ≥4 blood units), an aggressive autologous blood phlebotomy program is necessary in order to minimize homologous blood exposure. The value of erythropoietin in this setting would be to not only facilitate autologous blood procurement, but to prevent the anemia associated with blood donation in individuals who may have medical risks and poor tolerance for anemia and/or aggressive phlebotomy [17–19, 21].

Based on the above analysis of the prevalence of anemia at first autologous blood donation, along with the prevalence of allogeneic blood transfusion, the number of orthopedic patients undergoing initial hip replacement annually who could benefit from EPO therapy can be derived. As illustrated in Table 4, EPO therapy would benefit 4800 patients annually in the United States, assuming a 50% reduction in allogeneic exposure in patients receiving EPO. This represents only 3.5% of all patients, but 20% of all anemic patients who receive treatment.

Some issues remain in need of definition for the use of erythropoietin therapy in the surgical setting. Prudent use of this agent suggests that erythropoietin therapy should be linked to ongoing blood losses (either autologous blood donation or perisurgical bleeding) in order to avoid potential complication related to polycythemia and hyperviscosity in patients at risk [22]. The use of this agent to correct preoperative anemia should be coupled with autologous blood procurement when the hematocrit exceeds 33% not only because of safety concerns but also to enhance the effectiveness of this therapy in reducing perisurgical homologous blood transfusions; most blood transfusion support in coronary artery bypass surgery, for example, is given on the day of operation and could be best avoided if autologous blood were available preoperatively [23]. The ultimate goal of erythropoietin therapy should be to reduce the need for homologous blood transfusion; erythropoietin should be used only in clinical settings in which this has been shown to occur. Clinical trials that use homologous blood exposure as outcome are currently in progress in a variety of settings to demonstrate this.

Finally, questions of optimal dose, route, and interval of administration for erythropoietin therapy have yet to be established and are the object of study in ongoing clinical trials [24]. Based on the estimate of 2 additional allogenic unit red cell volume equivalents produced by the patients treated with EPO compared to placebo (Fig. 2), acquisition costs of approximately $150 for two units [25] would represent cost savings compared to approximately $2500 in drug therapy

Table 4. Annual number of 135,000 orthopedic patients undergoing hip replacement surgery annually who could benefit from EPO therapy

25% of 135,000	=	24,000 anemic donors
40% of 24,000	=	9,600 would receive HB w/o EPO
20% of 24,000	=	4,800 would receive HB with EPO

Benefit: 4800 (3.5%) of all patients
(20%) of 24,000 treated patients

costs (at 600 U/kg i.v. for 6 doses in a 70-kg patient, totally 252,000 units at $0.01 per unit) [26]. This cost benefit imbalance must be addressed with issues related to drug dose, route of administration, drug charges, and iron supplementation in order to fulfill the promise of erythropoietin as a new tool in blood conservation as an alternative to allogeneic blood in elective surgery [1].

References

1 Goodnough LT, Shuck J: Blood transfusion in elective surgery: review of risks, options, and informed consent. Am J Surg 1990;159:602–609.
2 Goodnough LT, Shaffron D, Marcus RE: Impact of preoperative autologous blood donation in elective orthopaedic surgery. Vox Sang 1990;59:65–69.
3 Mintz PD, Nordine RB, Henry SB, Webb WR: Expected hemotherapy in elective surgery. NY State J Med 1976;76:532–537.
4 Renner SW, Howanitz PJ, Bachner P: Preoperative autologous blood donation in 612 hospitals. Arch Pathol Lab Med 1992;116:613–619.
5 Goodnough LT: Erythropoietic hormone: A review, in Johnson RG (ed): Blood Loss: Its Prevention and Replacement in Spine Surgery, Spine: State of the Art Reviews. Philadelphia, Hanley and Belfus, Inc., 1991, pp 109–118.
6 Toy PTCY, Kaplan EB, McVay PA, Lee SJ, Strauss RG, Stehling LC: Blood loss and replacement in total hip arthroplasty: a multicenter study. Transfusion 1992;32:63–67.
7 Wasman J, Goodnough LT: Effect of autologous blood donation for elective surgery on physician transfusion behavior: A matched, controlled study. JAMA 1987;258:3135–3137.
8 Goodnough LT, Wasman J, Corlucci K, Chernosky A: Limitations to donating adequate autologous blood prior to elective orthopaedic surgery. Arch Surg 1969;124:494–496.
9 McVay PA, Hoag MS, Lee SJ, Toy PTCY: Factors associated with successful autologous blood donation for elective surgery. Am J Clin Path 1992;97:304–308.
10 Goodnough LT, Vizmeg K, Sobecks R, Schwarz A, Soegiarso W: Prevalence and classification of anemia in elective orthopaedic surgery patients: Implications for blood conservation programs. Vox Sang 1992;63:90–95.
11 Kickler TS, Spivak JL: Effect of repeated whole blood donations on serum immunoreactive erythropoietin levels in autologous donors. JAMA 1988;260:65–67.
12 Goodnough LT, Brittenham G: Limitations of the erythropoietic response to serial phlebotomy: Implications for autologous blood donor programs. J Lab Clin Med 1990;115:28–35.
13 Goodnough LT, Price TH, Rudnick S: Iron-restricted erythropoiesis as a limitation to autologous blood donation in the erythropoietin-stimulated bone marrow. J Lab Clin Med 1991;188:289–296.
14 Goodnough LT, Bravo J, Hsueh J, Keating L, Brittenham GM: Red blood cell volume in autologous and homologous blood units: Implications for risk/benefit

assessment for autologous blood "crossover" and directed blood transfusion. Transfusion 1989;29:821–822.

15 Goodnough LT, Rudnick S, Price TH, et al.: Increased collection of autologous blood properatively with recombinant human erythropoietin therapy. N Engl J Med 1989;321:1163–1167.

16 Goodnough LT: Erythropoietin as a pharmacologic alternative to homologous blood transfusion in the surgical patient. Transfusion Med Rev 1990;4:288–296.

17 Goodnough LT, Price TH, Rudnick S, Soegiarso RW: Preoperative red cell production in patients undergoing aggressive autologous blood phlebotomy with and without erythropoietin therapy. Transfusion 1992;32:441–445.

18 Kempen PM: Repeated blood donations and erythropoietin levels (letter). JAMA 1989;261:1443.

19 Bell K, Gillon J: Erythropoietin and preoperative autologous blood donation (letter). N Engl J Med 1990;322:1157–1159.

20 Goodnough LT, Johnston MFM, Toy PTYC, et al.: The variability of transfusion practice in coronary artery bypass graft surgery. JAMA 1991;265:86–90.

21 Goodnough LT, Marcus RE: Homologous blood transfusion needs in elective orthopaedic surgery: Potential role of erythropoietin therapy (reply to letter). N Engl J Med 1990;322:1158–1159.

22 Raine AEG: Hypertension, blood viscosity, and cardiovascular morbidity in renal failure: Implications for erythropoietin therapy. Lancet 1988;1:97–99.

23 Goodnough LT, Soegiarso RW: Surgical blood lost, the "transfusion trigger," and blood transfusions in coronary artery bypass graft surgery: Implications for blood conservation strategies. Surg, Obstet, Gyn (in press).

24 Goodnough LT, Geha AS: A new era in blood conservation. Ann Thor Surg 1991;151:703–704.

25 Forbes JM, Anderson MD, Anderson GF, et al.: Blood transfusion costs. A multicenter study. Transfusion 1991;31:319–323.

26 Doolittle RF: Biotechnology—the enormous cost of success. N Engl J Med 1991;324:1360–1361.

Lawrence Tim Goodnough, MD, Division of Laboratory Medicine, Washington University Medical Center, 660 South Euclid Avenue, St. Louis, MO 63110 (USA)

Discussion

to the Paper by Goodnough et al.

Wardrop (Cardiff): I enjoyed your presentation very much but, like flying in commercial aircraft, homologous blood transfusion is almost totally safe. Are you saying that there are no adverse events potentially when your system gets widespread in the U. S.?

Goodnough: Well, I hoped to convince you that almost totally safe is inherently unsafe, and we could have had this conversation in 1981 too, and I think that many people had that feeling. To me the issue of blood conservation and issues related to blood safety are timeless. I am thankful that there has been arithmetic success and the blood supply is safer than ever, but I do not agree with the philosophy that we should no longer be prudent about transfusion practice, that we should no longer take the time and expense and effort to develop conservation strategies.

Winearls (Oxford): Do you still recommend 600 units per kilogram i.v. twice weekly?

Goodnough: Well, I did not have time to show you the dose-response data, but I believe that you can tailor this to the individual patient. There is a tight linear correlation between the amount of erythropoietin you give on a per-week basis and the milliter-per-kilogram production. So for a 70-kilogram patient in whom you would like to have 700 milliters for blood conservation, you can calculate that it would be 250 units per kilogram intravenously in six divided doses. I do not believe it has to be 600 units per kilogram; I believe it to be dependent on the weight of the patient and how much blood the surgeon is asking for you to supply with them as conservation equivalents. To answer your question, 300 units per kilogram intravenously, and if you give it subcutaneously I believe the pharmacokinetics would show us that you probably could get by with lower doses than that, and if we address issues of relative iron deficiency and come up with that or iron supplement alternatives I think that would also improve the cost–benefit relationship.

Blanchard (Boston): It is my understanding that the major risk of transfusion for an acute bad outcome is receiving a wrong unit of blood. Do you have any evidence that this is more or less likely in the autologous setting?

Goodnough: That is a good question, and I think that it is probably the same—that the risk of an acute hemolytic transfusion reaction because of a blood-administrated error or a bacterial sepsis result would be the same for autologous as it would be for allogenic.

Preoperative Autologous Blood Donation with rhEPO Therapy in Patients Scheduled for Cardiac Surgery: Preliminary Results of a Dose-Response Finding Multicenter Trial

H. G. Güse,[a] *K. Wens,*[a] *W. Behr,*[b] *K. Doukas,*[b] *W. Franke,*[c]
D. Messinger,[c] *P. Scigalla*[c]

[a]Abteilung für Anästhesie und Intensivmedizin, Zentralkrankenhaus Links der Weser Bremen; [b]Abteilung für Transfusionsmedizin, Zentralklinikum Augsburg; [c]Boehringer Mannheim GmbH, Germany

Many publications have dealt with the necessity of reducing the use of homologous blood. One way of achieving this is by deposit of the patient's own blood prior to elective surgery [1]. However, more than 30% of our patients are unable to donate the amount of blood required because they develop anemia after autologous blood donation and because of the lack of time to compensate for this anemia. Animal studies and several well-controlled trials in humans have shown the efficacy of rhEPO as adjuvant therapy to accelerate the recovery of red cell counts following autologous blood donation [2–6]. The dose–response relationship and the subgroups of patients that might benefit most from this therapy still need to be determined more precisely. In addition, the suitability and compatibility of rhEPO administration in patients undergoing cardiac surgery also need to be evaluated.

We therefore initiated a randomized, multicenter, placebo-controlled, double-blind clinical study to assess the efficacy of rhEPO at four dose levels in patients undergoing autologous blood donation prior to elective cardiac surgery.

Study Design

Prior to enrollment, the study was approved by the institutional review board of each participating institution (Table 1). Informed consent was obtained from each patient enrolled in the study. The participating 212 patients scheduled for cardiac surgery were

Table 1.   Trial centers

---

1.   W. Behr and E. Struck (Augsburg)
2.   H. G. Güse (Bremen)
3.   R. Hetzer (Berlin)
4.   S. Massonet-Castel (Paris)
5.   J. Melo (Lisbon)
6.   M. Schmoeckel and B. Reichart (Munich)

---

randomly assigned to one of five equivalent groups to be treated with twice-weekly doses of 800, 400, 200, or 100 U/kg rhEPO given intravenously, or to receive placebo. Patients were scheduled to attend a total of 16 times, as follows.

Visit 1	Enrollment, primary and anamnestic investigation, check of inclusion and exclusion criteria
Visits 2–9	Donation visits (4 weeks)
Visit 10	Admission to hospital
Visit 11	Surgery
Visits 12–15	Postoperative phase (2 weeks)
Visit 16	Follow-up visit 12 weeks after surgery

If clinical and laboratory parameters permitted, autologous blood was collected depending on the patient's body weight (40–60 kg: 400 ml; 60–80 kg: 450 ml; >80 kg: 500 ml) prior to dosing at each donation visit.

The following parameters were monitored:

Blood pressure, hemoglobin, hematocrit—each visit
Reticulocytes, erythrocytes, platelets, iron, ferritin, transferrin, and creatine kinase—visits 1, 2, 4, 6, 8, 10, 15, and 16
Creatinine, sGPT, sodium, potassium, and differential blood count at visits 1, 10, 15, and 16.

Donation was postponed if a patient's hemoglobin value was less than 12 g/dl and if the current clinical condition did not allow donation. Furthermore, the treatment could be discontinued if a patient wished to withdraw from the study. Each patient was requested to take 100 mg iron sulfate three times a day during the preoperative period.

Patient Eligibility

All patients aged between 18 and 75 years scheduled to undergo elective cardiac surgery and who had a hemoglobin value of more than 12.0 g/dl (females) or 12.5 g/dl (males) were eligible for enrollment.

Patients were ineligible if they had severe aortic stenosis or a moderate degree of aortic stenosis associated with coronary heart disease; unstable angina; main-stem stenosis; current i.v. therapy with nitrates or heparin; lytic therapy; planned double operation (e.g., bypass surgery plus valve replacement); severe lung disease; extremely irregular body-mass index; severe hypertension (diastolic blood pressure >90 mmHg); a history of infections or severe disease of any other organ system, including bleeding/coagulation disorders; cerebral insufficiency; seizures; malignancy; or were pregnant or lactating. Patients were further excluded if they were taking more than two antihypertensive drugs or any cytotoxic immunosuppressant agent or if they had a deficiency of folic acid or vitamin B_{12}.

Objectives

Our primary objective was to determine the relationship between the red cell volume collected and the doses of rhEPO administered. Our secondary objectives were to observe hematological changes and iron metabolism, and to investigate the clinical tolerance of rhEPO and the influence of rhEPO on safety laboratory parameters.

Enrollment of 212 patients was completed on June 30, 1992. To date we have been able to assess the data of 117 patients with complete follow-up until October 1, 1992, all of whom were from centers 1, 2, and 6. Of these patients 107 actually underwent surgery. We report below on 117 patients with respect to safety and 107 patients with respect to efficacy.

Statistical Analysis

A patient was considered evaluable for efficacy if he or she received the assigned study medication at the first seven donation visits. This was the precondition for obtaining an accurate description of the dose-response relationship. The final dose was given after the last autologous blood donation and therefore had no influence on the primary variable.

In addition to the primary variable—the donated red cell volume—the net red cell volume was calculated:

Net red cell volume [ml] = donated red cell volume [ml] − blood volume [ml] × (baseline hct [%] − hct before surgery [%])/100

The donated and net red cell volumes were analyzed using one-sided Wilcoxon's rank sum test adjusted for sex. To guarantee the experimentwise error rate of 0.05 in a strong sense, the four pairwise comparisons of rhEPO dose versus placebo were ordered a priori from the highest to the lowest dosage and tested in a confirmatory manner in this sequence. The procedure stopped at the first nonsignificant test ($p > 0.05$) [7].

Adverse events were recorded throughout the entire study period applying the following definition:

An adverse event is any undesired, noxious, or pathological change in a patient or subject as indicated by signs, symptoms, and/or laboratory changes that occurs in association with the use of a drug or placebo whether or not considered drug-related.

Results

Patient Characteristics

The clinical characteristics of the 107 patients shown in Table 2 are fairly evenly distributed over the five groups. A markedly higher proportion of male patients were enrolled in the study up to this stage of investigation. A separate analysis according to sex was therefore not performed.

Hematocrit Changes During Donation Phase

Autologous blood donation resulted in a marked decrease in hematocrit in all treatment groups (Figure 1). The mean decrease was most pronounced in the placebo group (6.8%). The 800 U group showed the smallest decrease (3.2%).

Donated Red Cell Volume

As shown in Figure 2, the cumulative red cell volume donated was large in all groups but was enhanced significantly by administration of 400 or 800 U/kg of rhEPO. The red cell volume was determined by multiplying the amount of whole blood donated (ml) by the actual hematocrit (%). The actual gain in red

Table 2. Patient characteristics

		Treatment group—U/kg (n)				
		Placebo (22)	100 (22)	200 (24)	400 (19)	800 (20)
Sex (%)						
Male		77.3	72.7	79.2	73.7	75.0
Female		22.7	27.3	20.8	26.3	25.0
Age (yr)	$\overline{X}$	55.1	59.8	60.5	50.2	58.9
Body weight (kg)	$\overline{X}$	74.3	71.5	73.6	73.4	72.9
Type of surgery (%)						
Valve op.		31.8	18.1	41.6	21.1	30.0
CABG		68.2	81.9	58.4	78.9	70.0
Hb (g/dl)	$\overline{X}$	14.4	14.2	14.2	14.7	14.3
	± SD	±1.1	±0.9	±1.3	±0.9	±1.0
Hct (%)	$\overline{X}$	42.3	41.7	41.8	42.9	41.7
	± SD	±3.4	±2.8	±3.8	±2.8	±3.1

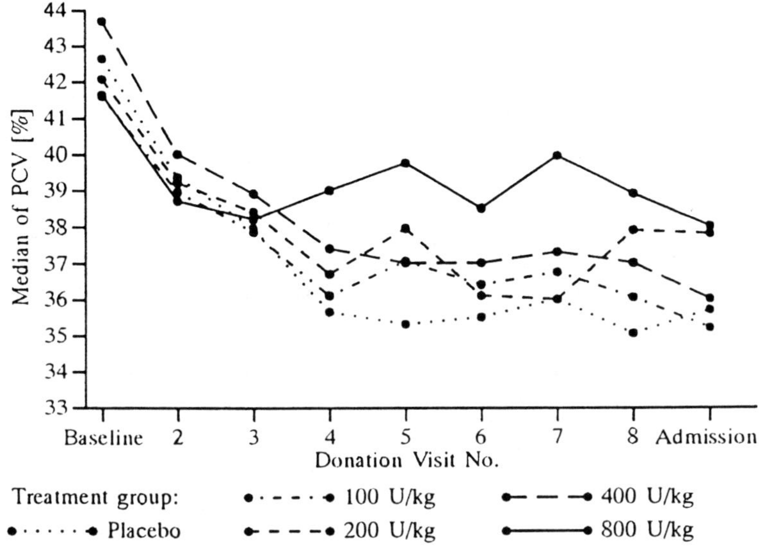

Fig. 1. PCV: Course of the median during preoperative treatment phase.

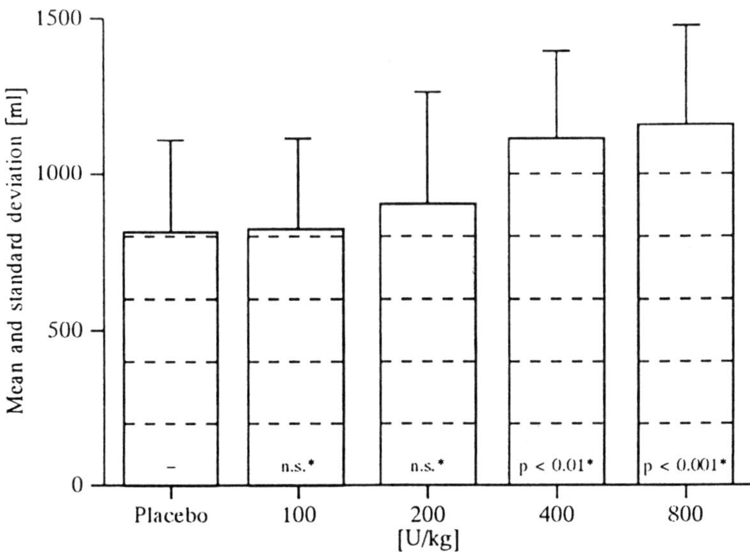

Fig. 2. Donated red cell volume.

cell volume at the end of the donation phase is a function of the sum of the individually donated red cell volume and the change of the body's red cell volume calculated from the patient's estimated total blood volume and the change in hematocrit (net red cell volume).

This is analogous to the mathematical assumption of re-establishing the baseline hematocrit in each patient at the end of the donation phase and allows calculation of the real mean/median surplus gain of red cells in each treatment group (Figure 3). Compared with placebo, the mean net red cell volume per donor was 11% higher in the 100 U group, 39% higher in the 200 U group, 65% higher in the 400 U group, and 100% higher in the 800 U group. This mathematical maneuver was used to take into account the varying degrees of hematocrit decrease in the donation phase. This parameter describes the red cell volume additionally obtained exclusively as a result of increased erythropoiesis in the donation phase. The occurrence of this net effect demonstrated the marked dose-dependent increase in the red cell volume obtained due to administration of rhEPO in the donation phase. Furthermore, there was already a significant therapeutic effect of rhEPO administration at 200 U compared to placebo. The gain in packed red cells caused by each doubling of the dose was similar.

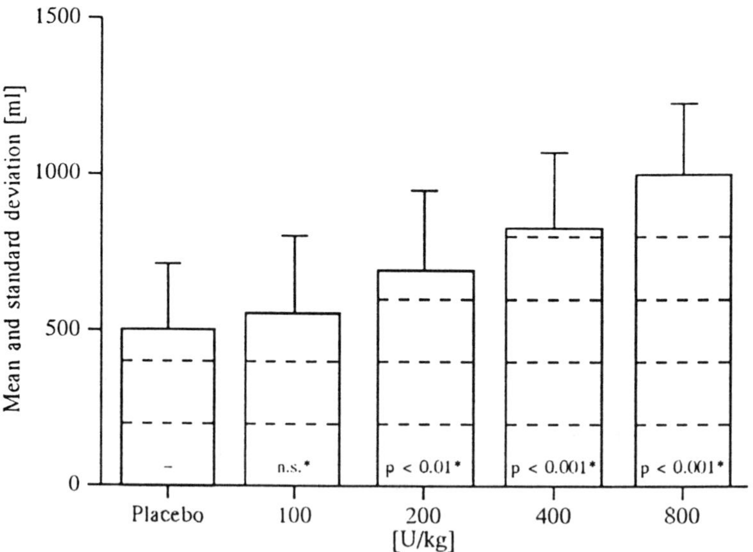

Fig. 3. Net red cell volume.

Iron Metabolism

The parameters of iron metabolism—ferritin levels and transferrin saturation (Table 3)—reflected the marked depletion of endogenous iron reserves due to autologous blood donation in all treatment groups. Oral iron substitution during the treatment phase was not sufficient to compensate for the iron loss caused by autologous blood donation.

Homologous Transfusion Requirements

Due to the large volume of autologous blood collected in all groups during the donation phase, 92 patients (86%) received no homologous transfusions. The number of homologous transfusions is an inconsistent parameter for the assessment of the efficacy of any autologous blood donation program because guidelines and specific clinical circumstances necessitating homologous transfusions were not defined identically by the individual centers. Fifteen of the 107 patients evaluated up to now received 37 U of homologous blood. Patients with homologous transfusions were evenly distributed among the five groups (three: placebo; four: 100 U; three: 200 U; two: 400 U; and three: 800 U).

Course of Hematological Parameters in the Postoperative Phase

During the first 3 days of the postoperative recovery phase, hematocrit values behaved inconsistently. The placebo group and the 100 and 200 U groups showed the lowest values, whereas the 400 U group and the 800 U group showed

Table 3. Iron metabolism: change in donation phase from baseline to admission (median values)

| | Treatment group—U/kg | | | | |
	Placebo	100	200	400	800
Ferritin (ng/ml)					
Baseline	85	202	91	89	115
Change	-29	-96	-53	-62	-79
Rel. change (%)	-43	-59	-53	-62	-69
Transferrin saturation (%)					
Baseline	21.9	26.6	25.4	27.6	25.9
Change	-6.1	-10.9	-13.4	-14.8	-17.7
Rel. change (%)	-31	-48	-53	-65	-60

a stable recovery of hematocrit values. At the time of discharge, only the 800 U group had reached its baseline value (Figure 4).

Platelets

During the donation phase, the platelet counts increased within the normal range in all treatment groups. The increase was more pronounced in the rhEPO groups, but the difference in increase compared to the placebo group was small and did not appear to be dose-dependent (Table 4).

At discharge, however, there was a nearly twofold rise in platelet counts compared to baseline in all groups due to the postoperative thrombocytosis. This is a well-known phenomenon, particularly in patients after open-heart surgery.

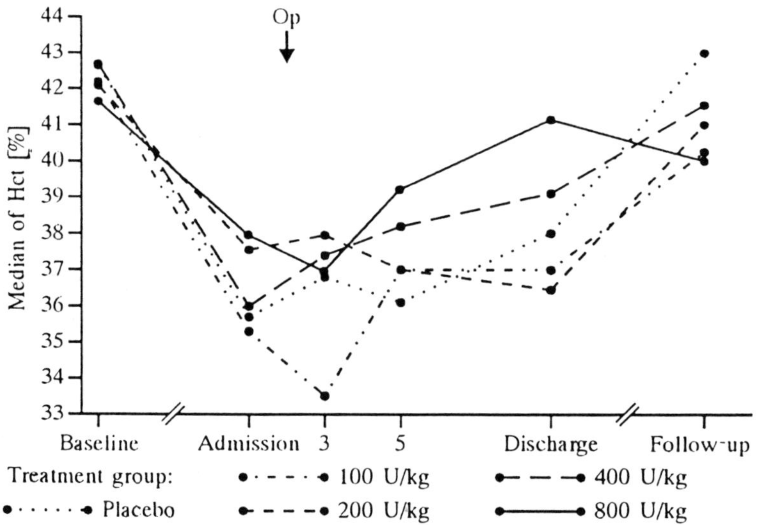

Fig. 4. Postoperative hematocrit (median).

Table 4. Platelets (10^9 gl, median values)

| | Treatment group—U/kg | | | | |
	Placebo	100	200	400	800
Baseline	224	253	220	239	233
Admission	236	283	244	253	260
Discharge	370	417	360	403	396
Follow up	235	256	224	229	239

Blood Pressure and Safety Laboratory Parameters

Assessments of all other clinical or laboratory parameters did not reveal any significant differences compared to the placebo group. There was a slight decrease in systolic and diastolic blood pressure during the donation phase in all groups. There was no higher incidence in hypertensive events in the rhEPO groups compared to placebo.

Adverse Events

During the entire study period, all adverse events were documented irrespective of whether they were considered drug-related. Adverse events were evenly distributed and occurred in all treatment groups with a frequency similar to that in the placebo group. The most frequent preoperative adverse events (Table 5) were angina pectoris (24 cases), dizziness (11 cases), upper respiratory tract infections (nine cases), headache (seven cases), and syncope (six cases). Serious adverse events were documented in seven cases preoperatively (Table 6). There was no significant difference in the frequency of adverse events between the study groups, apart from two patients in the 200 U group who suffered myocardial infarction (Table 5).

Table 5. Number of patients with adverse events in preoperative phase (multiple AEs per patient possible)

	Treatment group—U/kg					
	Placebo	100	200	400	800	Total
No. of patients included	24	23	25	22	23	117
No. of patients with AEs	15	15	13	13	10	66
Angina pectoris	5	5	5	5	4	24
Arrythmia	1	—	1	1	—	3
Dizziness	4	1	—	2	4	11
Upper respiratory tract infection	1	4	3	1	0	9
Flu syndrome	—	—	1	1	2	4
Headache	1	2	2	2	—	7
Heart failure	1	—	—	—	—	1
Hypertension	—	1	—	—	—	1
Hypotension	1	1	1	—	—	3
Syncope	3	—	2	—	1	6
Myocardial infarction	—	—	2	—	—	2
Leukocytosis	—	1	—	—	—	1
Allergic reaction	1	—	—	1	—	2
Pruritus	1	1	—	—	—	2
Rash	—	—	—	1	—	1
Ulcer	—	1	—	1	—	2

Table 6. Number of patients with serious adverse events (intra- and postoperative)

	Treatment group—U/kg					
	Placebo	100	200	400	800	Total
Patients with op.	22	22	23	20	20	107
Patients with serious AEs	4	3	7	4	6	24
Angina pectoris	1	—	1	1	1	4
Arrhythmia	—	—	1	1[a]	—	2
Convulsion	—	—	1	—	—	1
Embolus	1	—	—	—	1	2
Heart failure	2[a]	—	1	—	—	3
Hemorrhage	—	—	2	—	3	5
Myocardial infarction	—	1 + 1[a]	—	1[a]	1	4
Thrombosis	—	—	—	—	1	1
Sepsis	—	—	—	1[a]	—	1
Other	2	1	7	1	5	16

[a]Death.

The number of fatal outcomes was rather high: eight of the 117 patients presented here died. Six of these fatal events occurred during or after surgery. (We must add, however, that there were no further fatal events in the 95 patients who are still to be evaluated.) Two of the fatal events occurred in the placebo group, one in the 100 U group, and three in the 400 U group. There were no fatal events in the 800 U group.

Two patients (2/117 = 1.7% or 2/212 = 0.9%) in the 200 U group suffered myocardial infarction at the end of the donation phase. The first of these was hospitalized on schedule for the elective bypass operation after having completed the donation phase. On the evening after hospitalization the patient suffered an anterior wall infarction. He underwent CABG under emergency conditions and died 10 days later of septicemia. The second patient was admitted to hospital on schedule after an uncomplicated donation phase and suffered myocardial infarction on the second night after admission. A bypass operation was not considered advisable, and after 3 weeks' inpatient treatment the patient was discharged as asymptomatic. Three days after discharge the patient died of sudden cardiac arrest at home. These two fatal outcomes might have been associated with the procedure of donation; however, there is no significant difference between the 0.8–2.5% lethality rate in patients waiting for cardiac surgery at the respective centers without any autologous donation and the group reported on here. Patients suffering from coronary heart disease are constantly at risk of infarction, and we cannot determine whether the events happened by chance or were influenced by autologous blood donation. A causal relationship with rhEPO therapy was not assumed.

Regarding the cases of postoperative fatal outcome, we must state that the mean intra- and postoperative lethality rates in patients not enrolled in this study at the respective centers were comparable or even higher than in the study group.

Discussion

These preliminary results demonstrate the dose-dependent efficacy of pharmacological doses of rhEPO with respect to the collection of autologous blood. A statistically significant and clinically relevant effect can be seen starting from doses of 200 U/kg twice a week. These data confirm the findings of studies on patients scheduled for elective orthopedic surgery [1–3].

Whereas nearly all these studies used a fixed dose of rhEPO, we formed four groups with different rhEPO doses in order to establish a dose-response relationship. Administration of rhEPO may be useful in patients undergoing open-heart surgery because of the expected high blood loss. Normally patients remain on a waiting list for several weeks, providing sufficient time for routine preoperative autologous blood donation. Nevertheless, a considerable percentage of the patients scheduled for elective cardiac surgery cannot be included in an autologous blood donation program because of low baseline hematocrit values. Our preliminary results indicate that these subgroups of patients, in particular, could benefit most from drug enhancement of erythropoiesis by rhEPO. We found that the patients' response to rhEPO therapy was similar to that of orthopedic patients [1–3], although the frequency of adverse events was much higher in our population. We attribute this to the risk of their underlying disease. Adverse events were not more prevalent in the rhEPO groups compared to the placebo group; nor was there a difference when the study patients were compared to those not enrolled in the study or not participating in a blood donation program. During the trial we found no signs of either dangerous hemoconcentration or any obvious adverse dose-dependent increase in platelet counts. It is especially important for cardiovascular patients that there was no evidence of side effects such as hypertensive episodes.

Our data confirm the results of other studies that found that rhEPO treatment does not cause hypertension in patients with non-renal anemia [3]. The autologous blood donation scheme used in our study resulted in a marked depletion of iron stores in all study groups. The oral iron substitution during the treatment phase was not sufficient to compensate for the iron loss caused by autologous blood donation. Considering the dose-dependent increase in red cells, the depletion of iron stores does not appear to be a limiting factor for the stimulation of erythropoiesis by rhEPO in the investigated dose range and duration of treatment. Further evaluation should reveal the extent to which our results were influenced by subgroups of patients becoming iron-deficient. Finally, we hope to be able to develop a therapeutic schedule that takes into account patients' baseline values and their expected transfusion needs.

References

1   Lorentz A, Schipplick M, Gmehlin U, Osswald PM, Winter M: Präoperative Eigenblutspende mit Flüssiglagerung bei künstlichem Gelenkersatz. Anaesthesist 1989;38:480–489.

2   Goodnough TL, Rudnick S, Price TH, Ballas SK, et al.: Increased preoperative collection of autologous blood with recombinant human erythropoietin therapy. N Engl J Med 1989;321:1163–1168.

3   Graf H, Watzinger U, Ludvik B, Wagner A, Höcker P, Zweymüller KK: Recombinant human erythropoietin as adjuvant treatment for autologous blood donation. Br Med J 1990;300:1627–1628.

4   von Bormann B, Weidler B, Friedrich M, von Andrian-Werburg H: Rekombiniertes Erythropoietin während autologer Blutspenden. Anaesthesist 1991;40:386–390.

5   Levine EA, Rosen AL, Gould SA, Sehgal LR, Egrie JC, Browne JK, Sehgal HL, Moss GS: Recombinant human erythropoietin and autologous blood donation. Surgery 1988;104:365–369.

6   Levine EA: Increasing autologous blood donation with recombinant human erythropoietin. In: Gurland HJ, Moran J, Samtleben W, Scigalla P, Wieczorek L, eds. Erythropoietin in Renal and Non-Renal Anemias. Contributions to Nephrology, Vol 88. Basel: Karger, 1991:327–333.

7   Hothorn L, Lehmacher W: A simple testing procedure "control versus treatment" for one-sided ordered alternatives with application in toxicology. Biomet J 1991; 33(2):179–189.

H.G. Güse, Abteilung für Anästhesie und Intensivmedizin, Zentralkrankenhaus Links der Weser Bremen, Senator Wessling-Str. 1, 28277 Bremen 61, Germany

Discussion

to the Paper by H. G. Güse et al.

Kubanek (Ulm): Could the increase in platelets be due to an iron deficiency that patients developed and not due to erythropoietin?

Güse: Well, I mentioned that in the postoperative period of cardiac surgery we can routinely recognize a remarkable increase of platelets. In our trial we cannot [distinguish] if this increase is influenced by erythropoietin additionally. But I think this phase must be under further close observation. As well, we cannot realize if the increase in platelet count is due to any development of iron level.

Adamson (New York): Perhaps you might help me and Dr. Kubanek. I believe the slide shows that the peak in platelet count was plotted some number of days after the surgery. That rise in platelet count was probably surgically dependent and not EPO-dependent.

Güse: Of course, you are right. We counted platelets only for one time approximately 10 days after surgery. So we take neither data on the development of platelet counts nor on the special impact of erythropoietin. But in general you are right; in fact there is a postsurgical increase of platelets.

Blackburn (Leeds): Could you have predicted which patients would have responded badly to the donation of the blood? The two patients that actually died as a result of the venisection, were they especially unstable in terms of their cardiovascular system or was it out of the blue?

Güse: Several studies showed that there is only a bad predictability [as to] which patient would develop any complications during predonation. Patients with a bad cardiac performance had not been enrolled. I want to point out that there is only a coincidence of time between predonation and the two severe adverse events with fatal outcome. Everyone knows that a certain percentage of patients get myocardial infarction even without any treatment. So we do not know exactly if these events are due to our management or if they happened by chance.

Blackburn: It is a serious problem. If you go to an ethical committee trying to get a ratification to run a large trial, [do you] say that you have got a 2% mortality that could be attributable to your technique, or would you say that's not the case when you are going to an ethics committee?

Güse: If I understand your question correctly, you mentioned our striking rate of fatal outcomes. Regarding this fact, I must admit that we caught a period of very high mortality rate which was not comparable to any other periods of the past and which was due to a lot of surgical problems. Of course, we are obliged to discuss the results of our study together with our ethical committee and they have to decide on further procedures. But I want to repeat once more: If you want to get a correct statement, you must compare our results with a group without any treatment.

Dose-Response Relationship of rhEPO in Preoperative Autologous Blood Donation in Patients Scheduled for Elective Orthopedic Surgery

P. M. Osswald,[a] A. Osmers,[a] A. Lorentz,[a] W. Franke,[b] D. Messinger,[b] P. Scigalla,[b] P. Haux[c]

[a]Institut für Anästhesiologie und Operative Intensivmedizin, Fakultät für klinische Medizin Mannheim der Universität Heidelberg; [b]Boehringer Mannheim GmbH; [c]Institut für Klinische Chemie, Fakultät für klinische Medizin Mannheim der Universität Heidelberg, Germany

Homologous transfusions in surgical patients continue to involve such risks as intolerance reactions, sensitization, and transmission of infections. In the past, this led to the increased use of autologous transfusion. Even with intensive use of these autologous methods in elective orthopedic surgery, however, the need for homologous blood transfusions and the attendant risks can never be completely eliminated. In the search for ways to increase the effectiveness of autologous blood collection programs, different preoperative autologous blood donation schedules, combinations of different autologous methods, modified iron substitution regimens, and the administration of erythropoietin have been tried, with varying degrees of success [1–4]. Prompted by the proven effectiveness of recombinant human erythropoietin (rhEPO) in the treatment of renal anemia [5,6], various investigators have succeeded in demonstrating that rhEPO is in principle capable of stimulating erythropoiesis during autologous blood donation and thereby increasing the amount of autologous blood that can be collected [7,8]. The purpose of our study was to evaluate different dosages of rhEPO for their effectiveness in increasing autologous blood deposit compared to a placebo control group. The selected dosages were essentially based on those used in a study by Goodnough, who observed a clinically relevant increase in donated red cell volume in his patients at a weekly dosage of 2 × 600 U/kg BW i.v. [7]. The prominent concern of our study was to examine the dose-response relationship between pharmacological dosages of rhEPO and the amount of donated red cell volume (RCV). Further aspects of interest were the pre- and postoperative course of hematological variables, the possibility of reducing homologous transfusion requirements, the impact of donation and treatment on iron metabolism, and the tolerance of rhEPO therapy.

Materials and Methods

Study Procedure

One hundred fifty-six patients who were scheduled for an elective orthopedic procedure with an anticipated blood loss of >1000 ml and who were to participate in the autologous donation program (for inclusion and exclusion criteria, see Table 1) were enrolled at eight centers (Table 2). Following informed consent, the patients were randomized into one of five dose groups (100, 200, 400, or 800 U/kg, or placebo, twice weekly i.v.). The study medication was administered on a double-blind basis. The patients could donate autologous blood twice weekly over a 4-week period. In accordance with autologous blood donation guidelines, patients with a hematocrit value ≥ 34 vol % (or Hb $\geq$ 11.5 g/dl) gave 500 ml blood; donation volumes that diverged from this amount

Table 1. Patient eligibility

Inclusion criteria
    Elective orthopedic surgery
    Anticipated blood loss > 1000 ml
    Hb > 12.0 g/dl (female)
    Hb > 14.0 g/dl (male)

Exclusion criteria (Patients unsuited as autologous blood donors were
    excluded from participation in the study)
    Overt cardiovascular diseases (e.g., heart failure, unstable angina pectoris,
      uncontrolled hypertension)
    Pronounced obstructive or restrictive lung diseases
    Cerebral sclerosis
    Convulsive seizures and epilepsy
    Coagulation disorders
    Hepatic diseases (SGPT above 80 units/L)
    Renal diseases (creatinine > 2 mg/dl)
    Bleeding (e.g., gastrointestional bleeding)
    Pregnancy, lactation, or inadequate contraception
    Diseases of the hemopoietic system
    Malignant neoplasms
    Immunosuppressive or cytostatic therapy
    Acute infections or inflammations
    Iron deficiency, folic acid, or vitamin B_{12} deficiency despite substitution

Table 2. Trial centers

1. W. Buzello (Cologne)
2. H. Gombotz (Graz)
3. H. J. Heidel (Bad Düben)
4. I. Linde (Hanover)
5. H. H. Mehrkens (Ulm)
6. P. M. Osswald (Mannheim)
7. G. F. Riedler (Lucerne)
8. W. Schleinzer (Hamburg)

were documented. Blood was collected in plastic bags containing CPDA 1, PAGGS, or SAG-mannitol stabilizer and stored at 4 to 6°C as whole blood or fractionated. At each donation visit, rhEPO or placebo was given intravenously irrespective of whether the patient could donate. Hematological variables (erythrocytes, erythrocyte indices, reticulocytes, platelets) and parameters of iron metabolism (ferritin, transferrin saturation, serum iron, erythrocyte porphyrins) were determined once weekly; blood pressure was monitored regularly. All patients were scheduled to take a daily oral iron supplement of 200–300 mg Fe^{2+}. The patients underwent surgery at the earliest on the fourth day and at the latest on the eighth day after the last donation visit. After the operation, the patients were followed up until the fourteenth postoperative day, which was succeeded by a further postoperative follow-up phase of 10 weeks. The study protocol was submitted to the ethical review committee and approved.

Statistical Analysis

The calculated sample size was based on the assumptions that a difference of one additionally donated unit of blood (about 180 ml red cell volume) is to be regarded as clinically relevant and that the standard deviation of the primary variable is also 180 ml (significance level = 0.05; power = 0.9, one-sided hypothesis). A patient was considered evaluable for efficacy if he received the assigned study medication on the first seven donation visits. This was the precondition for obtaining an accurate description of the dose-response relationship. The final dose was given after the last autologous blood donation and therefore had no influence on the primary variable.

In addition to the primary variable—the donated red cell volume RCV_D—the following parameters were calculated:

$ERCR_B$	BV (ml) $\times$ (Hct_B − 34 vol %)/100
$ERCR_F$	BV (ml) $\times$ (Hct_F − 34 vol %)/100
RCV_N	RCV_D (ml) − $ERCR_B$ + $ERCR_F$
RCV_C	RCV_D (ml) + $ERCR_F$
$ERCR_B$	Endogenous red cell reserve at baseline
$ERCR_F$	Endogenous red cell reserve before surgery
RCV_N	Net red cell volume
BV	Blood volume
RCV_C	Corrected red cell volume before surgery

| Hct_B | Hematocrit at baseline |
| Hct_F | Hematocrit before surgery |

The primary variable RCV_D was analyzed using one-sided Wilcoxon's rank sum test adjusted for sex. To guarantee the experimentwise error rate of 0.05 in a strong sense, the four pairwise comparisons of rhEPO dose versus placebo were ordered a priori from the highest to the lowest dosage and tested in a confirmatory manner in this sequence [9]. The procedure stopped at the first nonsignificant test ($p > 0.05$). RCV_N was analyzed descriptively in an analogous manner. Analyses of covariance were also performed to describe the influence of $ERCR_B$ and Hct_B on RCV_D and RCV_C. Investigator-treatment interactions were examined by means of ANOVAs.

Adverse events were recorded throughout the entire study period applying the following definition:

> An adverse event is any undesired, noxious, or pathological change in a patient or subject as indicated by signs, symptoms, and/or laboratory changes that occurs in association with the use of a drug or placebo whether or not considered drug-related.

Results

Patients

One hundred fifty-six patients were enrolled at eight centers between December 1990 and June 1992. Two patients dropped out before beginning the treatment phase. Twenty other patients stopped participation after beginning treatment: 12 due to adverse events and eight patients for other reasons. Of the 134 patients who completed the treatment phase, 127 received study medication seven or eight times and could be evaluated for efficacy. The general patient data and the blood volumes calculated according to Nadler et al. [10] are listed in Table 3. The patient groups were comparable at baseline. Because of the rather higher percentage of men in the placebo group, the blood volume in this group was slightly greater than the blood volume in the four rhEPO groups. Mean patient age was in accordance with the underlying disease. Ninety percent of the patients were undergoing total hip replacement or revision arthroplasty.

Autologous Blood Donation

The total donated red cell volume was calculated for each patient from the volume and hematocrit of the individual donations. The patients in the placebo group donated 839 ± 320 ml (mean ± SD). The corresponding donation volumes in the rhEPO groups were as follows: 100 U rhEPO group: 958 ± 311 ml; 200 U rhEPO group: 880 ± 276 ml; 400 U rhEPO group: 1020 ± 361 ml; and 800 U rhEPO group: 1058 ± 277 ml (Figure 1). The larger donation volume

Table 3. Patient characteristics

		Treatment group—U/kg (n)				
		Placebo (28)	100 (25)	200 (24)	400 (26)	800 (24)
Sex (%)						
Male		50	44	41.7	42.3	41.7
Female		50	56	58.3	57.7	58.3
Age (yr)	$\overline{X}$	63.0	68.9	66.8	65.5	66.6
	± SD	±8.3	±5.1	±6.6	±9.1	±5.9
Calculated blood	$\overline{X}$	4.70	4.41	4.30	4.39	4.41
volume (L)	± SD	±0.84	±0.70	±0.83	±0.85	±0.68
Weight (kg)	$\overline{X}$	79.8	72.4	70.9	72.6	73.9
Hb (g/dl)	$\overline{X}$	14.1	14.3	14.0	14.0	14.2
	± SD	±1.1	±1.3	±1.0	±1.1	±0.9
Hct (%)	$\overline{X}$	42.5	42.8	41.7	41.7	42.3
	± SD	±3.6	±3.8	±3.1	±3.3	±3.2

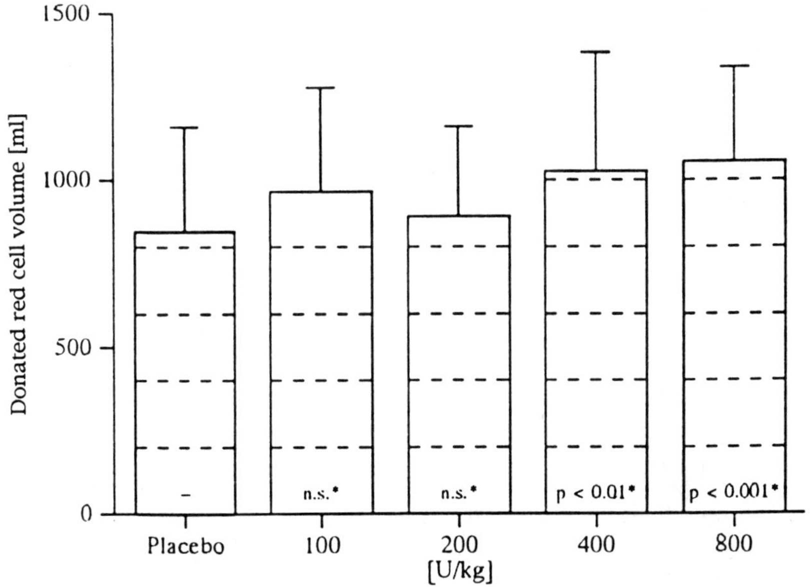

Fig. 1. Donated red cell volume (mean and standard deviation).

in the patient groups with 400 and 800 U rhEPO was statistically significant compared to placebo.

Reticulocytes showed a marked dose-dependent increase in all treatment groups during the donation phase. The highest values were reached at donation visit 5 or 7. Compared to baseline, this was an increase by 125% in the placebo group, 186% in the 100 U group, 173% in the 200 U group, 317% in the 400 U group, and 323% in the 800 U group (Figure 2).

The course of hematocrit in the donation phase showed a drastic decrease of about 6–7 vol % in all five treatment groups between baseline and donation visit 3 (Figure 3). Hematocrit subsequently recovered to some extent in the two high-dose groups, whereas the values of the placebo group and the two low-dose groups continued to fall or remained unchanged at a low level. At the end of the donation phase, the median decrease in the two low-dose groups and placebo group was 5.5 to 7.5 vol %, whereas in the two high-dose groups the decrease (2.8 and 3.5 vol %) was statistically significantly smaller than in the placebo group, despite the greater donation volume.

Effective Erythropoiesis

To demonstrate exclusively the effect of increased erythropoiesis in the donation phase, the varying degrees of decrease of hematocrit in the donation phase must be taken into account when comparing the donation volumes. The net

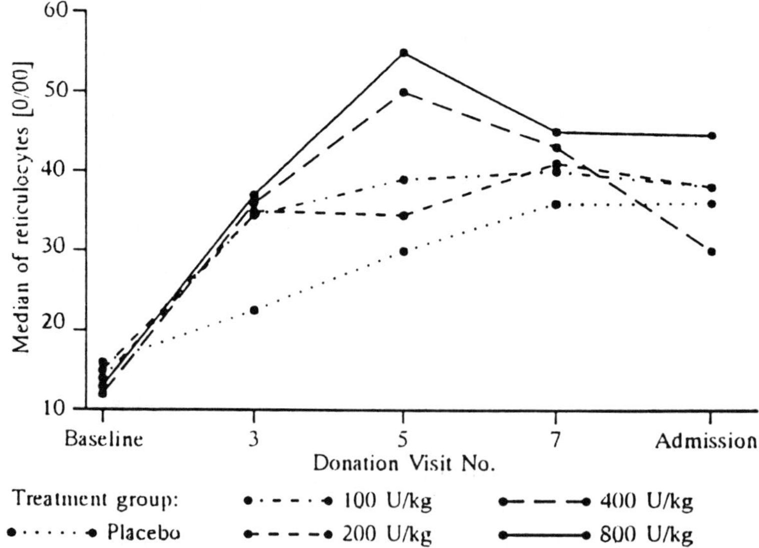

Fig. 2. Reticulocytes: course of the median during preoperative treatment phase.

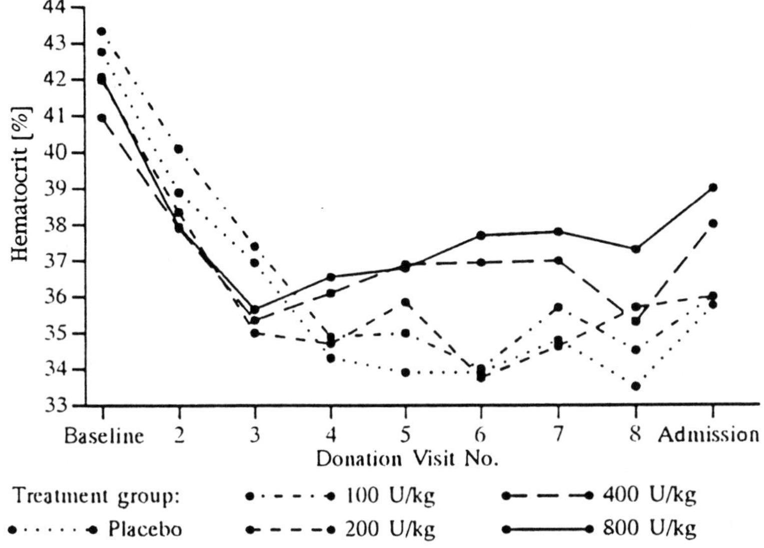

Fig. 3. Hematocrit: course of the median during preoperative treatment phase (median).

red cell volume RCV_N is the donated red cell volume RCV_D minus the endogenous red cell volume reduced due to the fall in hematocrit ($ERCR_B$ minus $ERCR_F$). The difference in RCV_N between the rhEPO groups and the placebo group defines the red cell volume additionally produced exclusively as a result of rhEPO treatment. Compared to the net red cell volume of 529 ml obtained in the placebo group of the total population, in the 800 U group a 79.6% higher (950 ml) volume was obtained, and in the 400 U group a 61.4% higher (854 ml) volume was obtained (Figure 4). The gain in the two low-dose groups was 25.3 and 18.3%. All differences were statistically significant compared to placebo. The percentage gains were higher in the women than in the men (400 U group: 80.4 versus 56.4%; 800 U group: 105.9 versus 70.4%), whereas the absolute gains in the men were slightly above those of the women (368 ml versus 326 ml in the 400 U group; 460 ml versus 426 ml in the 800 U group).

The ability of a patient to donate a given amount of autologous blood is highly dependent on his $ERCR_B$ at the start of the donation phase, i.e., the amount of red blood cells representing the difference between the baseline hematocrit before the donation phase and the donation criterion of 34 vol %.

The regression lines of analysis of covariance show that a 100 ml higher $ERCR_B$ leads to a mean increase in donation volume RCV_D of just under 100 ml in both men and women (Figure 4).

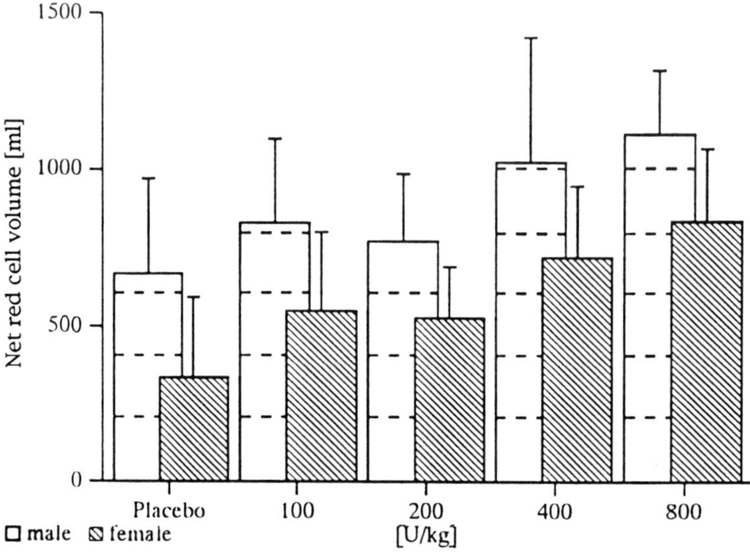

Fig. 4.   Net red cell volume (RCV_N) stratified by sex (mean and standard deviation).

Blood Loss and Transfusions

Blood loss was comparable in the individual treatment groups with the exception of the 100 U group, in which the total blood loss was slightly lower. In the placebo group, on average a higher proportion of the autologous blood units were retransfused than in the rhEPO groups (87% versus 68–78%), probably due to the smaller donated amount. A mean 2.6 units were transfused in the 100 U group, whereas this figure was 3.3 U in the other groups. Only nine of the 123 patients evaluable for efficacy who underwent surgery (7.3%) required in total 21 units of homologous blood (Table 4).

Postoperatively, the two high-rhEPO-dose groups showed less pronounced decreases in hematocrit compared to the other treatment groups. Whereas the placebo group exhibited a median maximum fall in hematocrit to 30 vol % 5 days after surgery, the comparative values for the 400 and 800 U groups were 5 and 4 vol % higher, respectively. An excessive postoperative increase in the haematocrit value was not observed in the rhEPO groups.

One additional patient in the placebo group who was not evaluable for efficacy received 7 units of homologous blood after surgery.

Iron Metabolism

The serum ferritin values and transferrin saturation decreased sharply in all groups during the donation phase (Table 5). The ferritin decreases in the rhEPO-

Table 4. Blood loss and blood transfusions (only patients with surgery)

		Placebo (28)	100 (25)	200 (23)	400 (25)	800 (22)
Blood loss (ml) (intra- and	$\overline{X}$	2157	1831	1958	2080	2175
postoperative)	± SD	±1312	±783	±817	±1010	±1737
Autologous transfusions (U)	$\overline{X}$	3.3	2.6	3.3	3.3	3.3
	± SD	±1.02	±1.50	±1.23	±1.54	±1.69
Homologous transfusions						
No. of patients		2	1	2	2	2
Sum of units		5	5	2	6	3

Table 5. Iron metabolism: change in donation phase from baseline to admission (median values)

	Placebo	100	200	400	800
Ferritin (ng/ml)					
Baseline	159	149	149	102	151
Change	−69	−88	−91	−56	−86
Rel. change (%)	−42	−58	−65	−64	−61
Transferrin saturation (%)					
Baseline	23.9	24.8	23.0	21.8	23.8
Change	−8.7	−9.0	−9.3	−9.8	−8.1
Rel. change (%)	−32	−36	−46	−49	−30
Erythrocyte porphyrins (μg/dl)					
Baseline	42.8	38.0	40.3	36.5	49.0
Change	13.5	16.5	33.1	42.0	63.0
Rel. change (%)	33	51	81	98	139

treated groups were 58% (100 U), 65% (200 U), 64% (400 U), and 61% (800 U) of the baseline value and thus much more pronounced than in the placebo group, in which the ferritin values decreased by 42%. Transferrin saturation underwent a median preoperative decrease to levels around or below 15% in all groups. Erythrocyte porphyrins exhibited a marked dose-dependent increase in the donation phase. An increase of 33% was observed in the placebo group, whereas in the two high-dose groups the median increases were 98 and 139%. Both differences are statistically significant compared to placebo. Postoperative normalization of the iron metabolism variables indicated that iron stores were rapidly replenished.

Blood Pressure

The changes in systolic and diastolic blood pressure values revealed no differences between the individual treatment groups. Median blood pressure values decreased slightly during the donation phase.

Platelets

During the autologous blood donation phase, the platelet count increased slightly within normal limits in all treatment groups. The non-dose-dependent increase was smallest in the placebo group with a median $35 \times 10^9/L$ and most pronounced in the 200 U group with $62 \times 10^9/L$. Postoperatively, reactive thrombocytosis led to a much greater increase in all treatment groups, and a dose-dependent effect was also not apparent in this phase.

Analysis of the laboratory variables creatinine, sGPT, sodium, potassium, prothrombin time, partial thromboplastin time, leukocytes, and differential blood count revealed no difference in the behavior of the rhEPO groups compared to the placebo group.

Adverse Events

One patient in the placebo group who had participated in the study without incident died of a myocardial infarction about 3 months after completing the treatment phase. Altogether, 11 patients (7% of the total study population) had an adverse event classified as serious (Table 6), of whom two patients were in the placebo group (6%), two in the 100 U group (6%), two in the 200 U group (7%), one in the 400 U group (3%), and four in the 800 U group (12%). Three of these serious adverse events occurred during the donation phase. In one of these cases, one patient in the 100 U group experienced anginal symptoms after the first autologous blood donation and was withdrawn from the study.

During the donation phase, the adverse events asthenia, headache, dizziness, and nausea were observed somewhat more frequently in the rhEPO group than in those on placebo (Table 7). Blood pressure increases were equally frequent in all groups. There were no other differences between the five treatment groups in terms of intra- and postoperative adverse events.

Table 6. Patients with serious adverse events

	Treatment group—U/kg (*n*)					
	Placebo	100	200	400	800	Total
No. of patients evaluable	31	31	28	30	34	154
No. of patients with serious adverse events	2	2	2	1	4	11
Adverse events:						
Angina pectoris	—	1[ab]	—	1	—	2
Syncope	—	—	—	—	1[a]	1
Hypertensive enzephalopathia	—	—	1	—	—	1
Heart failure	—	—	1	—	—	1
Myocardial infarction	1[c]	—	—	—	—	1
Apoplectic stroke	—	—	—	—	1	1
Thrombosis	—	—	—	1	—	1
Disturbed wound healing	—	—	1	—	—	1
Infection	1[ab]	—	—	—	—	1
Pneumonia	—	—	1	—	—	1
Lung embolism	—	—	—	—	1	1
Hemorrhage	—	—	—	—	1	1
Accidental injury	—	1	—	—	—	1

[a]Preoperative.
[b]Withdrew from study.
[c]Died.

Discussion

The stimulation of erythropoiesis is known to be influenced by anemia or hypoxia. Studies on erythropoietin levels in autologous blood donors have shown that when the hemoglobin concentration falls to levels between 11 and 12 g/dl, a moderate increase in the serum erythropoietin concentration to a maximum of double the baseline concentration occurs, which causes only a doubling of the erythropoietic rate. This can be interpreted as evidence of the low sensitivity of the erythropoietic system to the acute fall in hemoglobin during autologous blood donation, and invites the conclusion that exogenous supply of erythropoietin can additionally stimulate the erythropoietic rate [11]. The use of rhEPO in preoperative autologous blood donation has been demonstrated in both animal experiments and human studies. Goodnough et al. [7] observed an increase in donation volume of 41% in men and 29% in women with sixfold administration of 600 U/kg body weight twice weekly i.v. over a treatment period of 3 weeks. In our study, rhEPO was given eight times altogether. This schedule was chosen to suit

Table 7. Number of patients with adverse events during donation phase

	Treatment group—U/kg (*n*)					
	Placebo	100	200	400	800	Total
No. of patients evaluable	31	31	28	30	34	154
No. of patients with adverse events (%)	12 (38.7)	15 (48.4)	14 (50.0)	13 (43.3)	19 (59.9)	73 (47.4)
Adverse events:						
Angina pectoris	1	2	2	1	—	6
Arrythmia	1	—	—	—	1	2
Hypertension	3	1	3	2	4	13
Syncope	—	1	—	—	2	3
Headache	2	1	3	2	4	12
Edema	—	3	—	1	—	4
Asthenia	1	3	5	3	8	20
Dizziness	2	1	1	—	6	10
Sweating	—	—	1	1	1	3
Diarrhea	1	1	1	—	1	4
Nausea	1	2	—	2	3	8
Other	6	8	6	9	9	38

the 4-week period available for autologous blood donation with two donation visits per week. In order to establish the dose-response relationship in the therapeutically relevant dose range, we selected the dosages 100, 200, 400, and 800 U/kg body weight twice weekly i.v.

In our study, an increase in donation volume of 32% (400 U group) and 44.9% (800 U group) was found in the women in the two high-dose groups compared to placebo, slightly above the results obtained by Goodnough et al. (29%) [7]. In the men, the increase was only 20% (400 U group) and 18% (800 U group) above the result for the placebo group, which diverges from the findings of Goodnough (41%). In considering the results of these two studies, it should be remembered that numerous factors, such as total blood volume, baseline hematocrit value, and depletion of the $ERCR_B$ in autologous blood donation, have an impact on obtainable donation volume.

The two high-rhEPO-dose groups showed a much smaller decrease in hematocrit (approximately 3 vol %) in the donation phase than the placebo group and the two lower-rhEPO groups (5.5 to 7.5 vol %). This means that the red cell volume available in the patient at the beginning of the donation phase (endogenous red cell volume) was depleted less in the two high-dose groups in which, despite a larger donation volume, a better preoperative hematocrit value was achieved (median 38–39 vol % versus 36 vol %).

To take account of the varying degrees of hematocrit decrease in the donation phase, the net cumulative red cell volume was analyzed. This parameter describes the additional red cell volume obtained exclusively as a result of increased erythropoiesis in the donation phase. The occurrence of this net effect demonstrated the marked additional stimulation of erythropoiesis due to administration of rhEPO in the donation phase. A 79.6% higher net red cell volume was achieved in the 800 U rhEPO group compared to placebo and the administration of 400 U rhEPO led to a 61.4% higher red cell volume compared to placebo. As well as the rhEPO dose, the endogenous red cell reserve at the beginning of the donation phase (i.e., the product of baseline hematocrit minus 34 vol % multiplied by the patient's blood volume) was the decisive factor for the donated red cell volume.

Figures 5 and 6 demonstrate the relationship between $ERCR_B$ at the beginning of the donation phase, the rhEPO dose, and the preoperatively available red cell volume RCV_C (sum of RCV_D and $ERCR_F$) for men and women. Clearly, the need to use rhEPO increases with growing blood requirements and low baseline

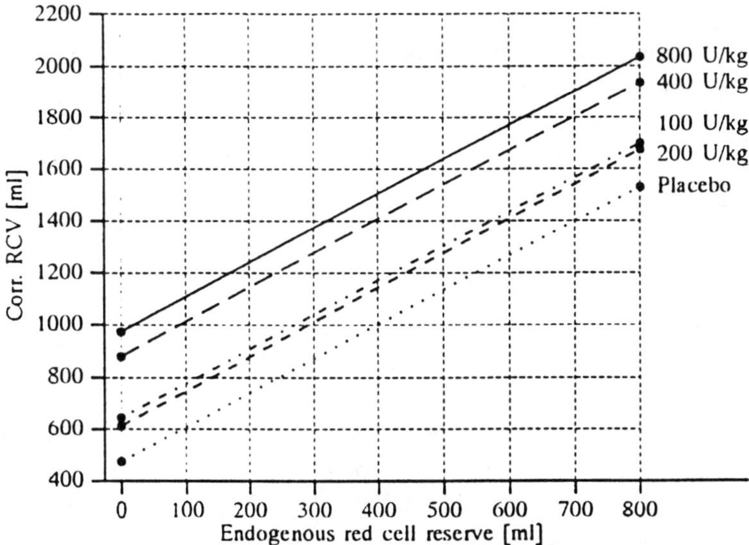

Fig. 5.   Relation between the endogenous red cell reserve at baseline ($ERCR_B$), the rhEPO dose, and the corrected red cell volume (RCV_C) in male patients (regression lines of analysis of covariance).

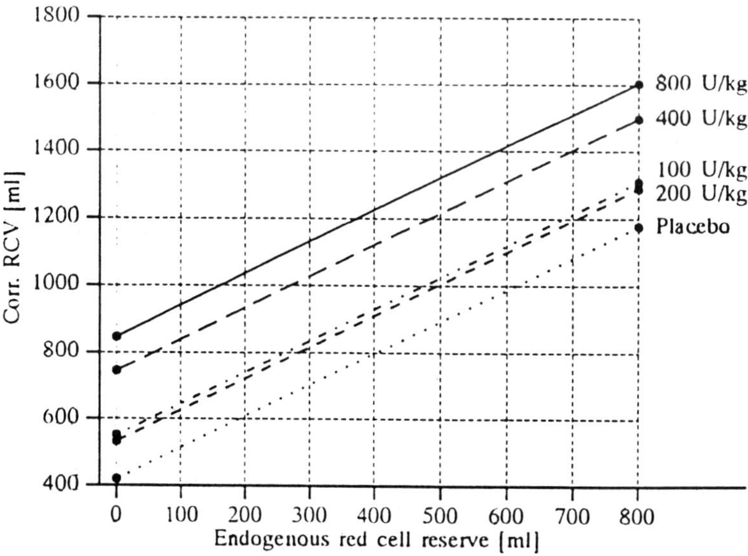

Fig. 6. Relation between the endogenous red cell reserve at baseline ($ERCR_B$), the rhEPO dose, and the corrected red cell volume (RCV_C) in female patients (regression lines of analysis of covariance).

reserve. Whereas patients with high baseline hematocrit levels and normal blood requirements are unlikely to have an indication for the use of rhEPO, patients with a low blood volume could profit from additional administration of rhEPO. Furthermore, rhEPO could be used prior to scheduled operations with a large anticipated blood loss. Patients who previously were excluded from autologous blood donation due to the risk of ischemia resulting from a pronounced fall in hematocrit could also be maintained within the safe range through the use of rhEPO. Further indications might be the use of rhEPO for operations in which only a short period is available for preoperative autologous blood donation, e.g., tumor surgery.

The study design, involving up to eight autologous blood donations in all treatment groups, was chosen with the aim of ascertaining the dose-responsive relationship and allowed the elective orthopedic operation to be carried out in 93% of patients without transfusion of homologous blood. Therefore, a difference in the frequency of homologous blood transfusions in the rhEPO groups compared to placebo could not be demonstrated. It should be noted in this connection that only patients with baseline hematocrit values within normal limits were enrolled, in accordance with the inclusion criteria.

Initial results [12,13] show that substantial savings of stored homologous blood are to be expected in patients with a lower baseline hematocrit.

The parameters of iron metabolism reflected the marked depletion of endogenous iron reserves due to autologous blood donation in all groups. Oral iron supplementation was not sufficient to compensate for the iron loss. Although blood donation obviously resulted in severe iron loss, the erythrocyte indices gave no evidence of microcytic or hypochromic changes in erythrocytes as a consequence of iron deficiency. Since a comparison of the treatment groups revealed a dose-dependent increase in donation volume despite successive depletion of iron stores, erythropoiesis does not appear to have been limited by iron deficiency during the investigational period.

Further studies will be necessary to establish the degree to which erythropoiesis can be further increased with the aid of adequate iron substitution. Platelet count increased within normal limits in all treatment groups, although the rise was rather more pronounced in the rhEPO groups. This increase was not dose-dependent and, with reference to the median, was slight in all treatment groups. The postoperative reactive thrombocytosis observed after the elective surgical procedure caused a much more marked but non-dose-dependent increase in platelet count in all treatment groups. Platelet values had largely normalized by the time of the follow-up examination, and an increased rate of thromboembolic complications was not detectable in the rhEPO groups. The distribution of the observed adverse events showed a higher incidence of asthenia, dizziness, headache, and nausea in the rhEPO groups. This is presumably related to the more frequent autologous blood donation in the rhEPO groups, since an increase in the rate of these adverse events is typically associated with blood donation. The frequency distributions of the adverse events in the intra- and postoperative phase yielded no evidence of an increased incidence of specific adverse events in patients on rhEPO compared to placebo.

Conclusions

1. The administration of rhEPO in the investigated dose range twice weekly i.v. causes dose-dependent stimulation of erythropoiesis in men and women. The lowest evaluated dosage of 100 U/kg body weight induces initial effects, and, from a dosage of 400 U/kg body weight upward, a clinically relevant increase of the preoperatively available red cell volume can be expected.

2. The necessity of using rhEPO increases when the patient has a lower baseline hematocrit and blood volume and is expected to suffer heavy blood loss

during surgery (e.g., in repeated operations). The indication for the use of rhEPO should be established with reference to these variables and the required donation volume.

3. According to the results of this study, no adverse events relevant to safety are likely to occur during the use of rhEPO in autologous blood donation programs. Relatively frequent autologous blood collection may presumably be expected to cause a higher incidence of asthenia, dizziness, headache, and nausea. Patients should be monitored for a possible rise in platelet count during the preoperative phase since the surgical procedure is likely to cause a further marked increase in platelet levels.

References

1 Osswald PM, Lorentz A, Jani L, Ehmer B, Scigalla P, Maßnahmen zur Einsparung homologer Transfusionen bei orthopädischen Eingriffen (Teil 1). Anaesthesiol Intensivmed 1991;32:168–173.
2 Osswald PM, Lorentz A, Jani L, Ehmer B, Scigalla P, Maßnahmen zur Einsparung homologer Transfusionen bei orthopädischen Eingriffen (Teil 2). Anaesthesiol Intensivmed 1991;32:204–209.
3 Wittig M: Stellenwert der Abnahmeintervalle der präoperativen Eigenblutspende auf die Effektivität der Spende zur Vermeidung von Fremdbluttransfusionen bei geplantem totalendoprothetischem Ersatz des Hüftgelenks. Dissertation. Fakultät für klinische Medizin Mannheim der Universität Heidelberg 1991.
4 Biesma D, Kraaijenhagen RJ, Poortman I, Marx IIM, Van de Wiel A: The effect of oral iron supplementation on erythropoiesis in autologous blood donors. Transfusion 1992;32:162–165.
5 Bommer J, Huber W, Tewes G, Ritz E, von Wedel S, Küppers S, Weinreich T, Bommer G: Treatment of polytransfused hemodialysis patients with recombinant human erythropoietin. In: Koch KM, Kühn K, Nonnast-Daniel B, Scigalla P, eds. Treatment of Renal Anemia with Recombinant Human Erythropoietin. Basel: Karger, 1988:131–138.
6 Eschbach J, Egrie J, Downing M, Browne J, Adamson J: Correction of the anemia of end-stage renal disease with recombinant human erythropoietin. N Engl J Med 1987;316:73–78.
7 Goodnough LT, Rudnick S, Price TH, Ballas SK, Collins ML, Crowley JP, Kosmin M, Kruskall MS, Lenes BA, Menitove JE, Silberstein LE, Smith KJ, Wallas CH, Abels R, von Tress M: Increased preoperative collection of autologous blood with recombinant human erythropoietin therapy. N Engl J Med 1989;321:1163–1168.
8 Levine EA, Rosen AL, Gould SA: Recombinant human erythropoietin and autologous blood donation. Surgery 1988;104:365–369.
9 Hothorn L, Lehmacher W: A simple testing procedure "control versus treatment" for one-sided ordered alternatives with application in toxicology. Biomet J 1991;33(2):179–189.

10 Nadler SB, Hidalgo MS, Bloch T: Prediction of blood volume in normal human adults. Surgery 1962;51(2):224–232.
11 Kickler TS, Spivak JL: Effect of repeated blood donations on serum immunoreactive erythropoietin levels in autologous donors. JAMA 1988;260:65–67.
12 Price TH, Goodnough LT, Vogler W, Sacher R: The impact of recombinant erythropoietin administration on the efficacy of autologous blood strategies in patients with low hematocrits. ASH 1992.
13 Mercuriali F, Bitti E: Potential role of erythropoietin in preoperative donation of autologous blood in anemic patients. Transfusion 1993;33:55–60.

P.M. Osswald, Institut für Anästhesiologie und Operative Intensivmedizin, Fakultät für Klinische Medizin Mannheim der Universität Heidelberg, Theodor-Kutzer-Ufer, 68167 Mannheim, Germany

Erythropoiesis in Autologous Blood Donors Treated with Recombinant Human Erythropoietin

Albert van de Wiel, Douwe H. Biesma

Department of Internal Medicine, Eemland Hospital, Amersfoort,
The Netherlands

Introduction

Blood transfusions are important therapeutic procedures in modern medicine and have contributed to the enormous expansion of the possibilities of surgical intervention. In many countries, blood banks guarantee the high quality of their blood products. Nonetheless, increasing attention is being paid to the limitations of blood loss and thus the need for blood transfusions. The reason for this is the increased insight into the disadvantages of homologous blood transfusions such as the induction of alloimmunization, the possible transfer of pathogenic micro-organisms, particularly viruses, and the possible suppression of the immune system. Autologous blood transfusions, whereby the patient serves as his or her own donor, form a logical alternative, which has already been widely adopted.

There are various forms of autologous blood transfusion, such as intra- and postoperative autotransfusion, preoperative hemodilution, and preoperative phlebotomies. In the last method, several units of blood are taken from the patient in the weeks preceding an elective procedure so that, if necessary, they can be transfused back during or after the operation. The more extensive orthopedic operations are particularly suitable for this form of autotransfusion. The number of units of blood needed is principally determined by the nature and extent of the operation. Limitations are placed on the technique by the length of time that erythrocyte concentrates can be stored (5–6 weeks) and the erythropoietic potential of the patient/donor. Important limiting factors in this erythropoietic potential are the available iron reserves and the endogenous erythropoietin production. The erythropoietic potential can be considerably increased by using exogenous recombinant human erythropoietin (rhEPO).

Endogenous Erythropoietin and Perioperative Anemia

Erythropoietin production appears to be regulated by the tissue oxygen tension at the side of the erythropoietin oxygen sensor in the kidney [1]. This tissue oxygen tension is the result of oxygen supply and oxygen consumption. The oxygen supply is determined by the red blood cell mass, the environmental oxygen tension, cardiopulmonary function, and hemoglobin oxygen affinity. If there are changes in one or more of these parameters leading to a fall in the oxygen tension in the kidney, an increase occurs in the production of erythropoietin. This hormone reaches the bone marrow via the bloodstream and stimulates the production of red blood cells.

Several studies have shown that the reduction of red blood cell mass that occurs after blood donation in the course of an autologous blood transfusion program provides only a very slight stimulus for increased erythropoietin production. Kickler and Spivak [2] studied the effect of repeated whole blood donations on erythropoietin levels in autologous donors. If the hematocrit remains above 0.34, a limit maintained by the American Association of Blood Banks, there is only a very slight increase in serum erythropoietin (s-EPO) levels even after the removal of 4 units of blood, each of 450 ml, within a 2-week period. The level of

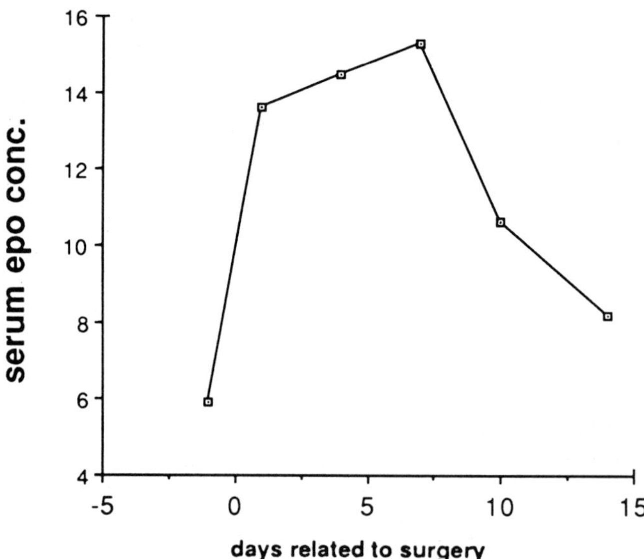

Fig. 1.   Serum erythropoietin concentrations in 53 patients undergoing total hip replacement.

s-EPO under these conditions rarely exceeds the upper limit of normal. Biesma et al. [3] found the same, whereby a hematocrit limit as low as 0.30 was accepted. No difference was found in this study in the erythropoietic response noted in patients with and without iron supplementation. Most likely, compensatory mechanisms such as an increase in the cardiac output can maintain the tissue oxygen tension at a reasonable level, thereby preventing an increase in s-EPO levels.

Postoperative anemia also rarely leads to a marked increase in erythropoietin production [4]. We followed the postoperative course of 54 patients who underwent a total hip replacement, recording not only the hemoglobin and hematocrit values but also the reticulocyte count and the s-EPO level. Despite the borderline values of hemoglobin and hematocrit, the increase in s-EPO is modest and within the normal range of the assay (Fig. 1). It can be concluded from this that a moderate anemia, induced by regular phlebotomies or operation, leads to a comparatively small s-EPO response. This implies delayed erythropoiesis and therefore a slow recovery from anemia. These observations also form the rationale for treatment with exogenous rhEPO if a more rapid correction of the red blood cell mass is required.

Application of rhEPO in Autologous Blood Transfusion

Levine et al. [5] studied the effectiveness of rhEPO in baboons that had been subjected to an aggressive autologous blood transfusion program. For a period of 5 weeks, 200 ml of blood were taken 3 times a week, provided that the hematocrit value remained above 0.30. The animals received 750 U/kg rhEPO intravenously or a placebo after each donation. The rhEPO-treated animals had an earlier onset of reticulocytosis and donated 35% more blood.

Goodnough et al. [6] conducted a randomized, controlled trial of rhEPO in 47 patients scheduled for elective orthopedic surgery. The patients received either rhEPO (600 U/kg body weight) or a placebo intravenously twice a week for 21 days during which time up to 6 units of blood were collected. The mean number of units collected per patient was 5.4 ± 0.2 for the rhEPO group and 4.1 ± 0.2 for the placebo group. Furthermore, the mean red cell volume donated by the patients who received rhEPO was 41% greater than that donated by the patients who received a placebo. In a study by Tasaki et al. [7], this rhEPO induced increase in red cell volume proved to be dose dependent. These studies clearly show that the addition of rhEPO to an autologous blood transfusion program allows an even larger number of units of blood to be drawn preoperatively. Furthermore, the red cell volume of the units of blood removed is higher, thus improving the yield of a transfusion. Finally, the hematocrit value during operation is higher in patients treated with rhEPO than in patients who have only supplied blood.

However, it is questionable if it is always necessary to remove a large number of units of blood, and the strategy of increasing this number to 6 has been criticized [8, 9]. The number of units necessary depends in the first place on the nature and extent of the procedure; moreover, local circumstances, such as the operative technique employed and the experience and skill of the surgeon, play a not unimportant role. However, there has been a noticeably more restrictive policy with regard to blood transfusion in the past few years. Some years ago, for example, it was the usual course of events in our hospital, a general regional hospital, to reserve 4 units of erythrocyte concentrate for a total hip operation. This has now been reduced to 2 units. The same applies to other orthopedic procedures such as total knee operation and laminectomy. A too aggressive donation program can lead to a high wastage rate of autologous blood units. There are other disadvantages to this approach. It is stressful for the patient and time consuming, and the blood bank has more to do with a higher chance of logistical errors. A large number of donations coupled with the use of rhEPO makes more demands on the iron reserves, which frequently requires adequate iron supplementation. In patients with minimal iron reserves, this could make intramuscular or even intravenous iron administration necessary, something not always without side effects. Finally, a significant drop in the hematocrit is seen in a number of patients. In older people, and orthopedic operations usually involve older people, this could lead to cardiovascular difficulties such as manifest or silent ischemia.

As a result of the more restrictive transfusion policy on the one hand, and the misgivings connected with an aggressive donation program on the other, we decided to implement another strategy. This approach comprises the preoperative removal and reserving of 2 units of blood in agreement with the blood ordering list and the administration of rhEPO so that the hemoglobin level can be completely restored by the time of the operation [10]. In 30 patients, 450 ml of blood were taken twice in the third week before operation. Half of these patients were given 500 U/kg body weight of rhEPO subcutaneously at the time of the donation and twice a week thereafter until the operation. Both the rhEPO group and the control group were prescribed ferrous sulfate (200 mg orally 3 × a day). Initial hemoglobin concentrations in the treatment group (14.2 ± 0.8 g/dl) were completely restored by the time of surgery (15.0 ± 1.6 g/dl) as compared to a decrease from 14.3 ± 0.8 to 12.6 ± 0.8 g/dl in the controls (Fig. 2). Reticulo-cyte counts showed a more than 5-fold increase in patients receiving rhEPO,

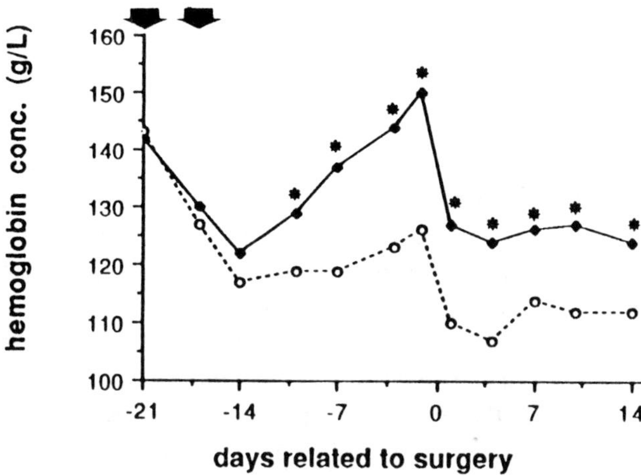

Fig. 2.   Hemoglobin concentrations in 14 patients treated with rhEPO ($\blacklozenge$---$\blacklozenge$) and in 14 controls (O---O). All patients were phlebotomized twice in the first week of the program (day -21 and -17).*p < 0.05.

whereas only a 2-fold increase was seen in the controls. Apart from flu-like symptoms in 4 patients in the rhEPO group, there were no serious side effects and no thromboembolic complications. No changes were seen in the rhEPO group with regard to systolic and diastolic blood pressures, platelet counts, and creatinine. It is concluded that such a regimen is safe and effective in compensating within a 3-week period for the loss of 2 units of blood. Blood donations took place 3 weeks preoperatively principally for logistical reasons, thus coordinating with the operation planning in the hospital. Furthermore, the blood could be kept should it be needed in the postoperative phase and could still be used even if the operation had to be delayed for one reason or another. The results of this study seem to indicate that a strategy in which rhEPO is combined with a limited number of blood donations satisfies the transfusion need.

Erythropoietic Response

RhEPO can be given both intravenously and subcutaneously. From a pharmocokinetic point of view, there appears to be a certain preference for the subcutaneous route, although peak values are lower and reached more slowly [1, 11]. Furthermore, the subcutaneous forms of administration are simpler, and it is possible to allow the patient to administer the substance himself.

The effect of the treatment can be measured from the recovery of the hemoglobin level and the hematocrit, the red cell volume of the units of blood taken, and the reticulocyte response. Both the intravenous and subcutaneous routes show a rapid and clear increase in the number of reticulocytes after the first injection. Although reticulocytes also increase in patients who have only donated blood, this increase is less impressive (Fig. 3). The difference between the two groups with regard to the reticulocytes increases up to the fourth injection using the regimen employed by us of 500 U/kg rhEPO given subcutaneously twice a week. It is noteworthy that there is no further increase in the reticulocyte count after the fourth injection. An upper limit seems to be reached. The curve even seems to indicate a certain decrease even though the patient is still receiving injections. Nowadays, the reticulocyte population can be further analyzed by flow cytometry using a Sysmex E-100 Reticulocyte-counter [12]. The presence of RNA permits the counter to distinguish three populations of reticulocytes whereby the youngest cells with the highest RNA content are referred to as highly fluorescent reticulocytes (HFR). If the HFR population is studied in the autologous donors treated with rhEPO, it can be seen that a significant fall in the number of HFR occurs after the fourth injection (Fig. 4). This implies that at that moment the maximum achievable effect on erythropoiesis has been reached. Although it cannot be excluded that a higher dose may produce extra stimulation, it would appear unlikely since the current dosage is high. Another possibility is a

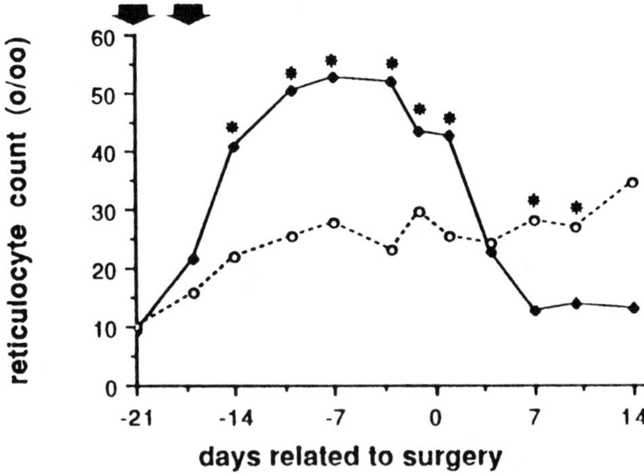

Fig. 3. Reticulocyte counts in 14 patients treated with rhEPO (◆---◆) and in 14 controls (○---○). All patients were phlebotomized twice in the first week of the program (day −21 and −17).*p < 0.05.

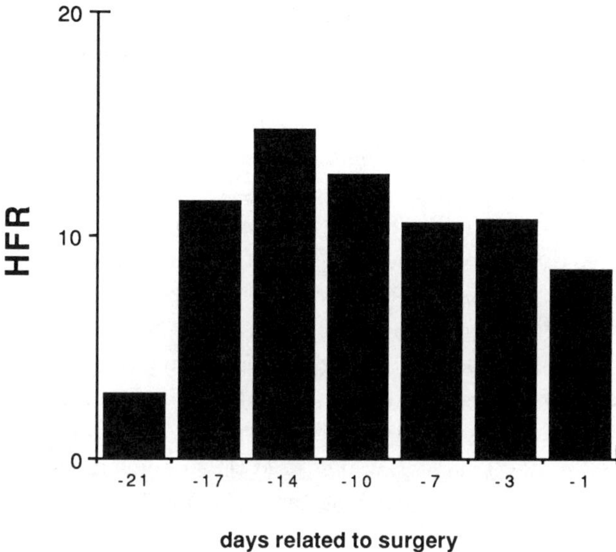

Fig. 4.   HFR fraction of reticulocytes measured in 23 patients who received rhEPO.

shortage of available iron, which is being studied currently. Furthermore, it might be possible that all the erythropoietin receptors on the erythroid progenitor cells in the bone marrow have been occupied. The decrease noted could even be a reflection of a down-regulation mechanism. Based on these observations, one might consider limiting the number of rhEPO injections in our regimen to 4.

Once the injections have been stopped, the s-EPO concentrations and thus the reticulocyte count fall rapidly. In the postoperative phase, we found very low s-EPO levels in the patients treated with rhEPO despite a still reduced hemoglobin level. This could indicate that the administration of exogenous rhEPO is accompanied by a suppression of endogenous rhEPO production [7, 13].

Impact of rhEPO on the Need for Homologous Transfusion

The aim of an autologous blood transfusion program with or without rhEPO is to avoid or greatly reduce the use of homologous blood. Several factors, partly of a general nature and partly of a local nature, play a part in the strategy to be chosen. The program should stress the patient as little as possible, and it must fit in with hospital and blood bank policies. Financial aspects should not be forgotten either. It is therefore useful to check the strategy chosen for effectiveness, safety, and costs. A study with this aim is presently being undertaken in our hospital. At the present time, 28 patients are evaluated in the program chosen by us, 14 with rhEPO treatment and 14 controls. Of the 14 treated with rhEPO, only 1 required homologous blood (4 units), while 10 patients required no blood transfusion at all. Of the 14 controls, 5 required homologous blood, while 3 patients needed no blood at all. After completion of the study, in which at least 90 patients will be evaluated, a more detailed picture can be given. These preliminary data already indicate that the need for homologous donation can be greatly reduced by a combined regimen of autologous blood donation and rhEPO. Autologous transfusion alone still requires the use of homologous blood in 36% of cases. However, there is greater wastage with the combined approach. The cost per patient of the 6 rhEPO injections in the dosage employed by us is $2000. It seems likely that this cost can be considerably reduced in the future. In a recently completed dose-finding study, it appears that a dosage of 250 U/kg rhEPO s.c. is just as effective as 500 U/kg [14]. As pointed out above, it is also possible that the number of injections can be reduced to 4.

Conclusion

In elective orthopedic surgery, autologous blood transfusion with a restrictive transfusion policy presents a good alternative to homologous blood. The number of autologous blood units yielded in the preoperative phase can be increased by using rhEPO. With the present operative techniques, it is sufficient to reserve 2 units of blood. If the donation of 2 units of blood is combined with rhEPO, then the hemoglobin level and the hematocrit can be completely restored within 3 weeks. There are strong indications that this type of less aggressive strategy can bring about a significant reduction in the use of homologous blood. Studies currently being undertaken will clarify the optimal dosage and frequency of injections, and will also provide a better picture of the costs attached to such a course of treatment. These will partly determine if this approach can be applied more widely. Furthermore, it is not yet clear whether we should treat all patients with rhEPO, or just a subgroup that is at risk for anemia, such as patients with a small build, a low initial hematocrit, or both [8, 15].

References

1 Goldberg MA: Biology of erythropoietin; in Garnick MB (ed): Erythropoietin in Clinical Applications. New York, Marcel Dekker, 1990, pp 59–104.
2 Kickler TS, Spivak JL: Effects of repeated whole blood donations on serum immunoreactive erythropoietin levels in autologous donors. JAMA 1988;260:65–67.

3 Biesma DH, Kraaijenhagen RJ, Poortman J, Marx JJM, van de Wiel A: The effect of oral iron supplementation on erythropoiesis in autologous blood donors. Transfusion 1992;32:162–165.

4 Levine EA, Rosen AL, Sehgal LR, Gould SA, Egrie JC, Moss GS: Erythropoietin deficiency after coronary artery bypass procedures. Ann Thorac Surg 1991;51:764–766.

5 Levine EA, Rosen AL, Gould SA, Sehgal LR, Egrie JC, Browne JK, Sehgal HL, Moss GS: Recombinant human erythropoietin and autologous blood donation. Surgery 1988;104:365–369.

6 Goodnough LT, Rudnick S, Price TH, Ballas SK, Collins ML, Crowley JP, Kosmin M, Kruskall MS, Lenes BA, Menitove JE, Silberstein LE, Smith KJ, Wallas CH, Abels R, von Tress M: Increased preoperative collection of autologous blood with recombinant human erythropoietin therapy. N Engl J Med 1989;321:1163–1168.

7 Tasaki T, Ohto H, Hashimoto C, Abe R, Saitoh A, Kikuchi S: Recombinant human erythropoietin for autologous blood donation: Effects on perioperative red-blood-cell and serum erythropoietin production. Lancet 1992;339:773–775.

8 Mintz PJ, Popovsky MA, Ness P: Erythropoietin and preoperative blood donation. N Engl J Med 1990;322:1157–1158.

9 Bell K, Gillon J: Erythropoietin and preoperative blood donation. N Engl J Med 1990;322:1158.

10 Biesma DH, van de Wiel A: Safety and effectiveness of recombinant human erythropoietin in correcting anemia of autologous blood donors. Actuar 1992;20:63–64.

11 Bommer J, Ritz E, Weinreich T, Bommer G, Ziegler T: Subcutaneous erythropoietin. Lancet 1988; ii:406.

12 Davies SV, Cavill I, Bently N, Fegan CD, Poynton CH, Whittaker JA: Evaluation of erythropoiesis after bone marrow transplantation: quantitative reticulocyte counting. Br J Haematol 1992;81:12–17.

13 Erslev AJ: Erythropoietin. N Engl J Med 1991;324:1339–1344.

14 Biesma DH, Kraaijenhagen RJ, Marx JJM, van de Wiel A: The correction of phlebotomy-induced anemia of autologous blood donors with recombinant human erythropoietin: A dose-finding study. (Submitted.)

15 Goodnough LT, Brittenham G: Limitations of the erythropoietic response to serial phlebotomy: Implications for autologous blood donor programs. J Lab Clin Med 1990;115:28–35.

Albert van de Wiel, Department of Internal Medicine, Eemland Hospital, Utrechtseweg 160, NL-3818 ES Amersfoort, The Netherlands

Discussion

to the Paper by A. van de Wiel and D.H. Biesma

Horina (Graz): You showed us a suppression of EPO levels in those patients receiving EPO at the time of surgery. My question is: Did the controls and did those patients on EPO get the same amount of packed cells during operation? If they did not, this might just be the effect of the packed cells you gave them and a down-regulation of endogenous EPO production.

Van de Wiel: I fully agree with you that when you evaluate EPO levels in the postoperative period, you should correct your figures for the blood they have been given during operation and for blood and hematocrit levels postoperatively. We did not do that, but in the major analysis we will do on 100 patients we are investigating at this moment we will do that, and then we will see what the difference is.

Wardrop (Cardiff): Could I suggest an additional tactic that might help you? If at the start of operation you venesected maybe one or two units and replace with colloids, then at the end of operation you can give "strong" blood replacing some of the most weak blood. This would help the economy of The Netherlands.

van de Wiel: Yes, I agree, and I would like to have the comment of Dr. Goodnough on that point. In our system it is also possible to do preoperative hemodilution, so you have a combination of preoperative phlebotomies and preoperative hemodilution, and I don't know whether you can do that in a more aggressive strategy—but maybe Dr. Goodnough can comment on that.

Goodnough (St. Louis): When I look at your 12 or 14 placebo patients and see that five received allogeneic blood, yet they were asked to store only two autologous units preoperatively, I am left with the conclusion that your surgeons are underestimating their blood-transfusion requirements.

Elective Surgery (Autologous Blood Donation; Transfusion Avoidance)

What are the recent incidence rates of infections (hepatitis, AIDS, etc.) induced by homologous blood transfusion? Are there any country-specific differences?

Adamson (New York): You heard from Dr. Kubanek some of the estimates of the incidence or frequency of certain infectious agents in tested units of blood and the possibility of transfusion-transmitted disease. I will answer the second part of this first. There are differences in the frequency of infectious-disease markers between countries, and even between regions within countries. However, there has been a dramatic reduction over time in the number of HIV-positive donors coming into centers such as ours. The current estimate of the likelihood of transfusion-transmitted HIV-1 is 1 in 220,000 units of product. Since this paper appeared in the *New England Journal of Medicine*, there has been another paper which has appeared in the literature, which has looked at the incidence post–HIV testing in individuals who have undergone coronary artery bypass grafting, and the results put the frequency of fully tested units of blood capable of transmitting HIV at around one in 60,000.

The problem with all of these studies, as any epidemiologist will recognize, is that these are low-frequency events, so that you have a fairly wide 95% confidence interval. Our disease-marker prevalences at the present time do not vary too much between large urban centers and suburban centers in the U.S. Even at the New York Blood Center, which I think everybody would agree was in the middle of a hotbed of HIV, we have only 1 in 10,000 donors who is HIV-positive by routine testing. But population prevalence is a bit more frightening. The one that we are still concerned about most is hepatitis C, and that is about 3 per 10,000 risks of transfusion-transmitted disease. This is what we have in the way of current estimates of frequency. This means in the U.S., if we assume one HIV-positive unit in 200,000, there would be five HIV transmissions per million, and there are 14 to 15 million transfusion events in the U.S. each year. Thus, there is some number of cases of HIV transmission which we can predict, and Dr. Kubanek said this very nicely in his presentation. But what is frequently left out of the equation is that patients who are being transfused very often die for the very reasons that they are being transfused, and the number of actual cases of AIDS which have appeared in the U.S. since testing is less than 20. In fact, in the U.S., one-half to two-thirds of individuals being transfused will be dead within 5 years due to their underlying or comorbid conditions and they never develop AIDS.

Kubanek (Ulm): A comment to the last remark you made. We did a look-back study in the frame of this study I was talking about and we found that about 50%—and this would confirm your figures—of the patients who got transfused died, so we transfuse a severely diseased population.

Blanchard (Shreveport): Would you address, rather than the relative risk of developing a disease, the actual incidence of posttransfusional hepatitis from a clinical standpoint and how that translates into long-term morbidity?

Adamson: The likelihood of posttransfusion hepatitis is probably on the order of 3 in 10,000. But hepatitis C carries with it the likelihood of about a 50% chronic active hepatitis phase, and many of those go on to other complications, including cirrhosis and carcinoma of the liver. But transfusion is a very, very small contributor to the spread of hepatitis C; in fact, the spread of hepatitis C is not well understood, but in the U.S., as you may have seen, 1 out of 200 individuals is hepatitis C–positive. That used to be 0.5% of blood donors. While hepatitis C is still being transmitted, we think the likelihood of transmission has been reduced in the U.S. by about over 90%.

Van de Wiel (Amersfoort): Data from The Netherlands indicate that the chance to become HIV-positive after a blood transfusion is 2 in 1 million; for hepatitis C it is 1 in 20,000. One in 1000 donors is a carrier for hepatitis C in The Netherlands. In Europe, there is quite a difference in this respect between the northern and southern parts, with a much higher prevalence of hepatitis C carriers in the southern countries.

Obladen (Berlin): How about cytomegalovirus? Have you figures on that?

Van de Wiel: Since Dr. Kubanek is a blood banker, he's more capable to answer this question.

Kubanek: About 50% of our donors—it depends on age—are CMV-positive. I think we only have to prevent CMV for some of our patients, as far as we know now, and this is easily done by testing and avoiding transfusing leukocytes. I think CMV is a problem, but it is not such a problem as the other viral infections.

Güse (Bremen): It seems to be very important to focus on additional justification to argue in favor of autologous predonation. This is the immune-modulating effect of homologous blood transfusions, which can be prevented by autologous predonation. And, of course, administration of EPO may extend the possibility to harvest more own blood from the patients. Many data have been collected and many well-controlled studies have been made that proved the connection between homologous transfusions and postoperative infections or recurrence of tumors. To my opinion, this subject becomes extremely more important for the future than the infectious side effects of homologous transfusions.

Can EPO be given pre- or postoperatively as an alternative to blood transfusions in nonelective surgery?

Adamson: The answer is yes, and although the data are unpublished, they have been presented at national and international meetings. There has been a large randomized and placebo-controlled clinical trial in the U.S. in which EPO was given 5 days before coronary artery bypass surgery, the day of surgery, and 2 days after surgery. The preliminary analysis of some 140 patients out of a total of 180 revealed a very striking reduction in the number of individuals exposed to homologous blood—in fact, a 50% reduction. That is a very important outcome. Hopefully, when the data have been fully analyzed, the results will provide a powerful indication that EPO can be used in the perisurgical setting as adjuvant therapy to reduce exposure to homologous blood. I believe there are similar clinical trials ongoing in orthopedic surgery patients in the U.S.

Van de Wiel: Certainly EPO can be given perioperatively even in nonelective surgery, but the question is when should we use it. In many cases anemia can be accepted to a certain extent. However, when a rapid correction is necessary, e.g., in cardiovascular, older, or obstetric patients, it might be an attractive alternative. In patients with symptomatic anemia, especially with angina pectoris, you cannot always avoid blood transfusions.

What could be the additional benefit of EPO treatment in comparison with the combined use of different means of autologous blood transfusions (autotransfusion, isovolemic hemodilution, retransfusion of drainage blood, and autologous blood donation)?

Van de Wiel: First of all, the combination of preoperative phlebotomies with isovolemic hemodilution or retransfusion of drainage blood is possible but not widely used. There are not too many reports on such a strategy. This probably has to do with the fact that some forms of autotransfusion are better suited for a particular type of surgery than others. Preoperative donation of blood is best suited for operations with a rather predictable and moderate blood loss, such as orthopedic surgery and some forms of plastic, cardiovascular, and cancer surgery. Retransfusion of drainage blood is especially applied in thoracic and transplantation surgery, in which the extent of blood loss is far more unpredictable. Application of EPO in preoperative phlebotomies permits more donations with a higher red blood cell volume. With a limited number of donations, initial hemoglobin levels can be restored at the time of surgery, thereby reducing the risk of manifest or silent ischemia. Finally, the quality of the blood products that are collected preoperatively is better than that of drainage blood.

Miller (*Baltimore*): Do they use drainage procedures and retransfusion of blood in oncology surgery? Or do they not use it because of the risk of tumor-cell contamination?

Van de Wiel: As far as I know from studies in Rotterdam, they don't use drainage systems in oncology surgery. They only use preoperatively donated blood and, in some cases, EPO.

How would you assess the combined use of EPO and autologous blood donation in cancer patients who must be operated?

Adamson: I think that's the general practice in New York City hospitals as well. I don't know that I would distinguish between the cancer patient and other patients if the decision was made that EPO was appropriate either to stimulate red cell production prior to surgery or to enable the patient to provide blood for autologous use. Again, I come back to a point that I have made before, which was that some judgment has to be given in terms of what the clinical status of the patient is and what the purpose of the surgery is. I take the point that was made a moment ago that we have not really talked about the opinions of people in the audience as to the noninfectious complications of the use of homologous blood in patients with malignancy. So, if the indications are there to collect autologous blood prior to surgery, then the same indications for the use of EPO would apply and the program should work.

Kubanek: I think the Dutch study I cited showed very clearly that an autologous program on colorectal carcinomas is feasible. And this was published too, very recently (*Vox Sang.* 62(2):102–107, 1992).

Goodnough (*St. Louis*): I think there are two circumstances in cancer patients undergoing resection for which autologous blood donation with or without EPO is very compelling—not on issues of blood safety but on issues of resection for cure—if you really want to avoid the immunosuppression associated with allogeneic blood transfusion. Those two circumstances would be colorectal carcinoma, a common cancer often requiring blood transfusion, and radical prostatectomy with lymphadenectomy, another increasingly common procedure that commonly requires blood transfusions. This may ultimately be addressed with filtration of blood components and leukodepletion techniques. But until that becomes widespread, I think that the compelling reason to do this for conservation in those circumstances is not so much because of our feelings about blood safety but going for cure at the primary resection.

Van de Wiel: As long as there is any doubt about immunomodulation and its clinical relevance, I think we should give these patients the benefit of the doubt and use autologous blood and, when necessary, EPO.

Miller: You must also consider in the cancer patients the data from our center and other places that have found that EPO levels may be suppressed even in cancer patients who are not receiving chemotherapy. So they may be more likely to be anemic going into their surgery and may not be able to manifest a normal EPO response if you use autologous blood collection without EPO.

Adamson: I quite agree and in fact, again, I would not separate out cancer from other patients with chronic anemia who may face elective surgery, such as patients with rheumatoid arthritis. Here, I think you have the same clinical requirements to raise the hematocrit, to allow autologous predonation and to prepare the patient for surgery. I think it will work.

Joven (Reus): We routinely include our patients with cancer who have to be operated into a predeposited autologous blood transfusion program. Our data suggest that these patients usually are not particularly anemic, and the problem is that frequently in these patients one has not so much time for the preoperative blood donation as one has for hip replacement or any other orthopedic surgery. Therefore, one has to conduct a much more aggressive autologous blood-donation program in order to be successful, with respect to elimination of homologous transfusion. Also, the response in the serum endogenous EPO level is the same as in other patients without cancer, and probably procedures should be the same as in other types of surgery.

Van de Wiel: What I know from the Rotterdam study is that only two units of blood are withdrawn from the patients with colorectal cancer. In some of the patients it was combined with EPO given postoperatively when hemoglobin levels were too low.

Joven: As far as I know, the group who has more experience is that from Houston, in the M.D. Anderson Center. They routinely perform autotransfusion and the level of homologous transfusion is very low.

What is the logistical procedure for autologous blood donation in your country—who is responsible for the diagnosis, blood collection, storage of the blood, monitoring and transport of the autologous blood, etc.?

Adamson: Dr. Goodnough, you wanted to reflect on two communities that you are close to. I can certainly say that the practice in New York is very hospital-specific. In the Hospital for Special Surgery, which is primarily an orthopedic hospital, over 70% of the blood used comes from predeposit programs. The New York Blood Center is responsible for collecting, testing, typing, storing, inventorying, and distribution. But that must vary from center to center and from country to country.

Goodnough: I can just briefly describe to you the way it works, and there may be a more ideal way. I think the way it usually works is the surgeon or the physician initiates the process. I was able to get it up to 75% utilization with a patient-education intervention by putting a letter in the pack of information materials they get when they are scheduled for surgery, introducing them to this as an option. You can extend that with your hospital transfusion committee developing policies and guidelines for whom it should be performed, so that it could be more automated. With respect to blood collection and storage, I published a survey of Ohio hospitals; only about a quarter of them had hospital-based autologous blood procurement facilities. So we very much depend on the regional blood center offering this as an alternative, as we should. I also have the bias, however, that a hospital-based procurement program for very large hospitals with big surgical programs is probably a good idea.

Van de Wiel: In the Netherlands, blood banks are autonomous and most of them operate outside the hospital. Some of the university hospitals have their own blood bank, but regional or local hospitals obtain their blood products from a regional blood bank. All hospitals keep a stock of the most current products. When an operation is indicated by the surgeon, he will order the various blood products (including autologous) which are needed in conformity with the blood-ordering list. Most of the patients will be screened preoperatively by an internist and, in case of autologous blood donation, by the physician of the blood bank. The blood bank is responsible for the donation, the storage, and distribution. A problem in this system is that blood banks are not used to work with older patients. For this reason we decided that donations as well as EPO injections take place within the hospital and then the blood is transported to the blood bank. This strategy needs a tight organization and a good cooperation between hospital and blood bank.

Blanchard: What is your rationale for dealing with unused autologous blood, both from an ethical and more legal standpoint, and how long do you have to hold it, and whether you transfuse it to other individuals?

Adamson: Our policy is not to cross over either autologous or directed units into the general inventory. The reason for that is relatively simple: We have determined that we do not consider these individuals "voluntary blood donors" by the standards which have been established by the American Association for Blood Banks, the American Red Cross, and the Council for Community Blood Centers. We are not unique, but it is also a position that is not shared by some blood centers which do cross over fully tested blood into the general inventory if it is clear that the blood is not going to be used for the patient for whom it was intended.

Van de Wiel: In our program we do cross, but that is possibly related to the distance between hospital and blood bank. We do not test on HIV.

Kubanek: We do not cross over and we do the autologous blood collection for the university hospital, but we do not have logistic problems in the regional hospital, the same situation as in Holland.

What are the indications for which you recommend the use of rhEPO in elective surgery?

Van de Wiel: I made a comment on that in my presentation. EPO should be used in elective surgery when you expect a considerable blood loss, e.g., in case the blood-ordering list indicates the reservation of at least 4 units of blood. When less than 4 units are required you should select patients with a low initial hemoglobin, a small blood volume, or those at increased risk to develop anemia.

Adamson: I happen to agree with you. I might just add one thing. We do not know yet if EPO given to targeted patients to enhance presurgical deposition of red cells followed by the use of EPO through the surgical procedure itself would further reduce the number of patients exposed to homologous blood. There may be some value there as well.

Unger (Vöcklabruck): I wonder whether freezing red blood cells would be a good alternative to EPO in this manner—when we have time enough for elective surgery but are limited, usually for bigger operations, by falling hematocrits. You would have the chance to freeze blood. I suppose this would be cheaper than using EPO in the short time of 42 days which is now the limit for liquid storage.

Adamson: You make a valid point, because currently we are freezing red cells for patients with rare antigens or antibodies, and Dr. Krantz has published a case report of giving EPO to a patient with multiple antibodies and then freezing away the blood prior to surgery. That patient, who would be impossible to cross-match in a blood-bank setting, now could be supported through surgery. We do the same thing in terms of freezing away blood for individuals who know that they have elective surgery scheduled well in advance. Right now the cost-effectiveness would favor EPO because freezing blood in the U.S. is not an inexpensive process. However, there are parallel technologies being developed at present which will very likely substantially reduce the cost of the freezing process. So, things will iron themselves out going forward, and your suggestion is a good one.

What is the current clinical knowledge about contraindications, dosage, route of administration and dose frequency, and iron supplementation during treatment with rhEPO in elective surgery?

Adamson: I think we have already covered most of these points. I cannot think of medical contraindications to the use of EPO. People might make decisions not to use EPO for a variety of reasons since clinical decision-making is more complex than just looking at contraindications. The dosage, I think we have seen, is probably going to be in the range of 100 to 200 units per kilogram three times weekly for most conditions. It is not yet precise. Certainly, the U.S. data of the perisurgical use of EPO had doses of 300 and 150 units per kilogram given daily, and one could not tell the difference between these two treatment arms. 150 units per kilogram are at least enough, and it may even be as low as 100 in that particular setting. The frequency depends on the application. If EPO is being given to stimulate a larger pool of red cells for autologous use, then probably two or three times a week is optimal. Subcutaneous dosing is certainly optimal; I think we have heard and agreed on that. Iron supplementation is a must, even if individuals have normal iron stores going on. If patients are in a predeposit program, it would appear as if aggressive parenteral iron administration would maximize the response to a given dose of EPO. We don't do that very much in the U.S. because there is concern about the safety of iron dextran preparations. The treatment duration, again, depends on the clinical setting. In the perisurgical setting, we have experience giving EPO a few days before surgery, the day of surgery, and a couple of days after surgery. Obviously, this schedule works, but fine-tuning will be necessary. Nevertheless, for the individual with reasonably responsive erythroid marrow, we are coming very close to the proper dose, to the proper route of administration, and to the timing of that dose. And EPO, I remind you, is an extraordinarily safe drug, particularly in the non-renal anemia patient.

Van de Wiel: In our group of orthopedic patients treated with EPO, no effect was observed on systolic or diastolic blood pressure. With regard to thrombocytosis, we did see a thrombocytosis. Since this can also be observed in the controls, who were not treated with EPO, we do relate this phenomenon to the surgical intervention and not to EPO treatment.

Cazzola (Pavia): Is anybody aware of studies evaluating the incidence of deep venous thrombosis after the use of EPO? Is there any difference in such incidence between patients who are treated with EPO and patients who are not?

Adamson: I will give the first short answer and then Dr. Goodnough may want to comment on this. In the U.S. multicenter trial of the perioperative use of EPO in patients undergoing coronary artery bypass surgery, that was looked for as an adverse event and there were no differences in the treatment groups.

Goodnough: It is well described that the prevalence of thromboembolic events after orthopedic surgery is about 2%. Of the 91 patients that I put on study in my institution we had two serious adverse events, both of them in the postoperative period. One was a myocardial infarction on postoperative day 3; another was a myocardial infarction and a stroke on postoperative day 17—in patients who had not been previously identified as having significant cardio-vascular disease. What amazed me was that they went through the entire preoperative collection interval (one placebo, one EPO), donating blood, and [they had] no complications preoperatively but did have those two events post-operatively. A third patient (EPO) had a pulmonary embolism 21 days after surgery.

The value of rhEPO in autologous blood transfusion in comparison with other measures is not to be measured in terms of the increased number of donations, but rather in the difference in the need for homologous transfusions.

Van de Wiel: I can fully agree with this statement.

Adamson: I agree, but there may be one other variable that has not been emphasized as a reason for giving EPO. I certainly agree that the value of giving EPO should not be measured in terms of increased numbers of donations. But, in addition to reduced exposure to homologous blood, the administration of EPO may enhance the rate of rehabilitation of individuals who are not quite so anemic after the surgical procedure as they otherwise might be.

Eschbach (Seattle): I would like to return to the last question. How effective is EPO after surgery? In the dialysis population, surgical inflammation interferes with the effectiveness of EPO. I am interested in whether studies have been done in a non-dialysis population to determine whether EPO is effective post-operatively.

Adamson: I have no idea. However, if you recall, we talked about the fact that experimental animal data suggest that even when hemoglobin synthesis may be limited by iron availability in the postsurgical period, the marrow may be primed in terms of the progenitor cell pool by continued administration of EPO. Unless our organizers know of trials which they are currently supporting which specifically look at the use of EPO after the surgical event, I know of no current studies in the U.S. that would directly address this question.

Scigalla (Mannheim): We also have no studies planned for this indication.

R. Huch (Zurich): Among postpartum treated women, we have analyzed the efficacy in patients after caesarean section, and this is to some extent postsurgical. There is no evidence that EPO is less effective, and there are other studies going on that show the same trend.

Index

Heart:
  anemia and, 93–105
    clinical and epidemiological
      aspects, 93–94
    compensatory cardiovascular
      mechanisms, 94–95
    discussion, 104–105
    hemodilution and myocardial
      ischemia, 101–102
    hemodynamic adaptions to anemia,
      95–97
    rheological considerations, oxygen
      transport, and myocardial
      perfusion, 97–100
  benefits of rhEPO therapy, 107–127
    chronic anemia and exercise
      capacity, 110–112
    discussion, 126–127
    hemodynamic effects of correcting
      anemia, 110
    hemodynamic effects of rhEPO
      therapy in patients with end-stage
      renal failure, 113–119
    hemodyanmic response to chronic
      anemia, 108–110
    rhEPO therapy and exercise
      capcity, 119–121
    subjective improvements of
      exercise capacity during rhEPO
      therapy, 121
Hematological deviations during
    pregnancy, 381–382
Hematological malignancies,
    311–323
  discussion, 321–323
  laboratory investigations useful for
      monitoring the erythroid marrow
      response to rhEPO, 312–313
  rhEPO in treatment of anemia
      associated with malignant
      lymphomas, 316–317
  rhEPO in treatment of anemia
      associated with multiple
      myeloma, 313–316
  rhEPO in treatment of
      myelodysplastic syndromes and
      idiopathic myelofibrosis, 313

Hematology, oncology and (See
    Oncology, hematology and)
Hematopoiesis, effect of EPO
    administration on, 178–180
Hemodialysis (See Dialysis)
Hemodilution, myocardial ischemia and,
    101–102
Hemodynamic adaptions to anemia,
    95–97
Hemodynamics of EPO-induced
    hypertension, 134
Hepatitis C virus (HCV), 393–394
Hepatic EPO mRNA accumulation in
    chronic renal failure, 73–75
Homologous blood transfusions:
  in elective orthopedic surgery, 402
  impact of rhEPO on need for, 449–450
  incidence rates of infections induced
    by, 453–455
  risks of, 389–399
Human fetus, EPO in, 365
Hypertension, 129–152
  discussion, 151–152
  effect of rhEPO on nonuremic
    patients, 132, 133
  hemodynamics of EPO-induced
    hypertension, 134
  incidence of rhEPO-induced
    hypertension, 129–132
  increase in hematocrit as cause of the
    hypertensinogenic effect of
    rhEPO, 137–138
  increase in total or effective blood
    volume as causative for rhEPO-
    induced hypertension, 134–135
  pathogenesis in uremics of, 132–134
  pathophysiology of rhEPO-induced
    hypertension, 135–137
  possible mediators of vasoconstrictor
    effects induced by rhEPO,
    138–141
  relation between hematocrit, viscosity,
    and vascular resistance, 137
  treatment, 141
Hypoferremia, 191–192
Hypoxia-inducible factor I, identification
    of, 26–27